Editors

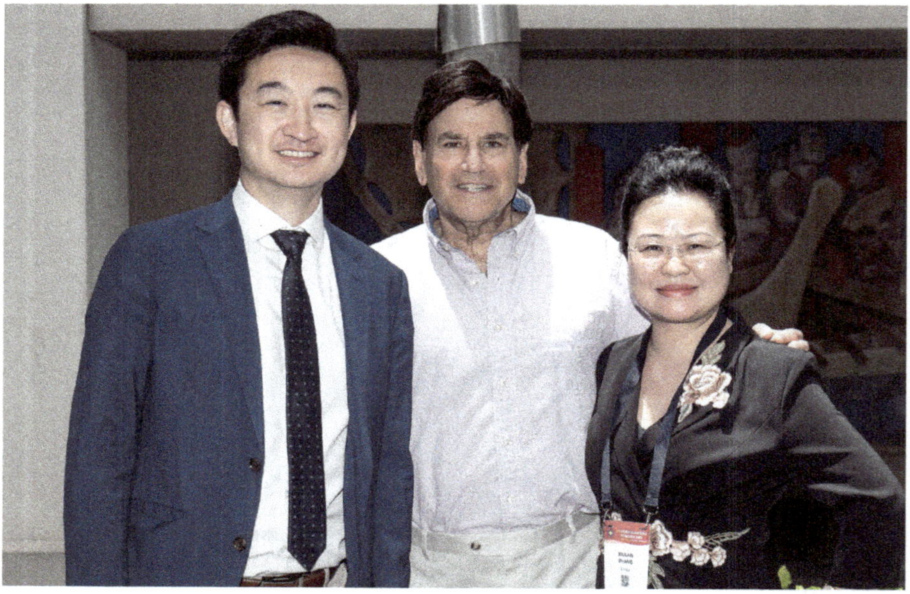

Benjamin Xu, Robert N. Weinreb and Xiulan Zhang

ANGLE CLOSURE AND ANGLE-CLOSURE GLAUCOMA

The 12th Consensus Report of the

World Glaucoma Association

Editors

Robert N. Weinreb
Benjamin Xu
Xiulan Zhang

Kugler Publications/Amsterdam/The Netherlands

ISBN 978-90-6299-339-0

Standard soft cover print-on-demand edition. See our website for premium editions of our books.

Kugler Publications
P.O. Box 20538
1001 NM Amsterdam, The Netherlands
www.kuglerpublications.com

This publication is the twelfth of a series of Consensus reports on Glaucoma under the auspices of the World Glaucoma Association

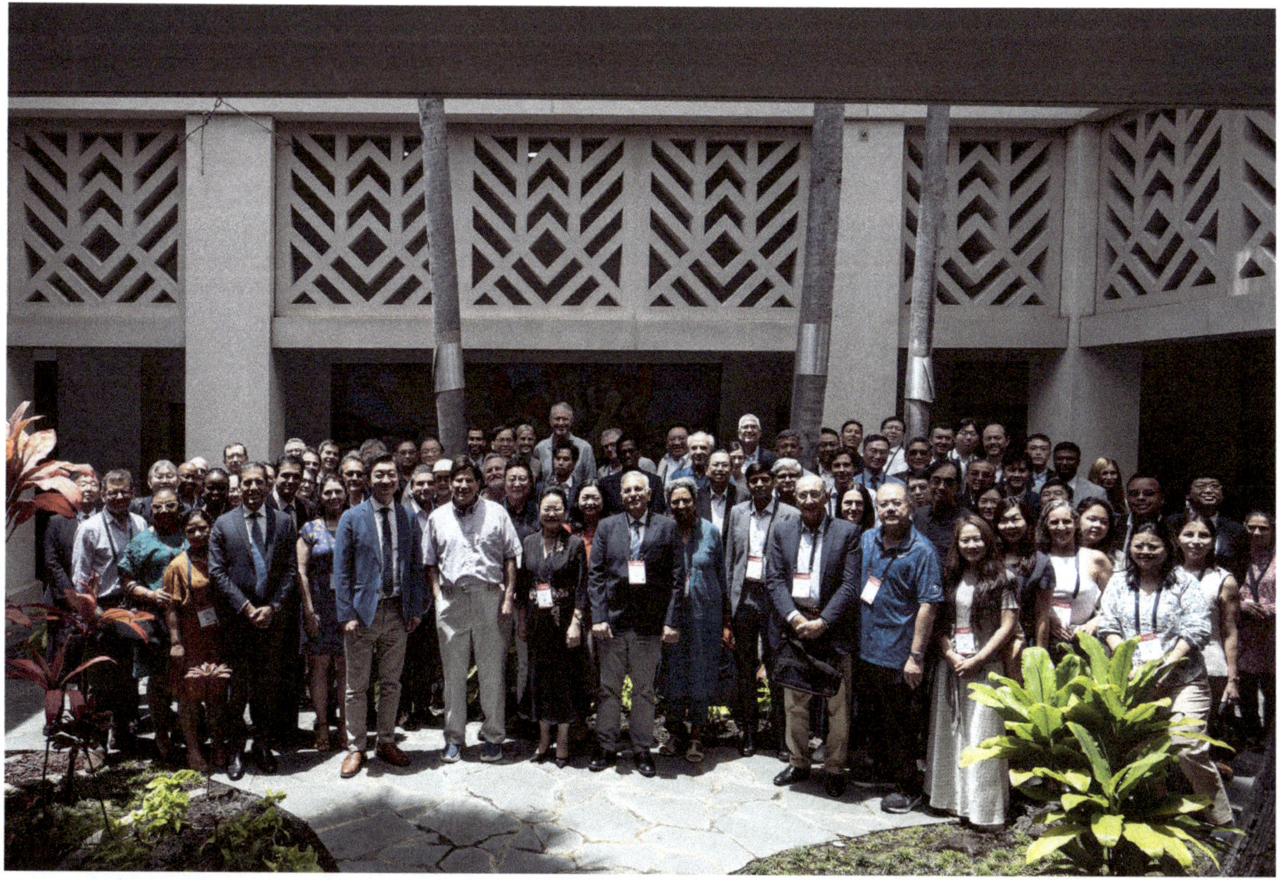

Consensus 12 participants

FACULTY

Consensus Initiative Chair
Robert N. Weinreb, USA

Co-Chairs
Tin Aung, Singapore
Paul Foster, UK
David S. Friedman, USA
Benjamin Xu, USA
Xiulan Zhang, PR China

Section Leaders
Mani Baskaran, India
Ching-Yu Cheng, Singapore
Tanuj Dada, India
Gus Gazzard, UK
Ronnie George, India
Mingguang He, Hong Kong, SAR
Christopher Leung, Hong Kong, SAR
Shan Lin, USA
Vijaya Lingam, India
Sasan Moghimi, USA
Monisha Nongpiur, Singapore
Lisandro Sakata, Brazil
Kyung Rim Sung, Korea
Do Tan, Vietnam
Clement C. Tham, Hong Kong SAR
Ningli Wang, PR China

Contributors
Iqbal Ike K. Ahmed, Canada
Bryan Ang, Singapore
Dewang Angmo, India
Dang Phuong Anh, Vietnam
Sanjay Asrani, USA
Augusto Azuara Blanco, UK
Eytan Blumenthal, Israel
Kyle Bolo, USA
Noel Chan, Hong Kong, SAR
Poemen Chan, Hong Kong, SAR
Sunee Chansangpetch, Thailand
Evan M. Chen, USA
Vikas Chopra, USA
Michael Coote, USA
Jazmine Denning, USA
Jiun Do, USA
Syril Dorairaj, USA
Seng Kheong Fang, Malaysia
Robert Feldman, USA
Theodoros Filippopoulos, Greece
Brock Flowers, Australia
Andrés Gerhard, Chile
Rodolfo Perez-Grossmann, Peru
Ying Han, USA
Marcelo Hatanaka, Brazil
Federico Hermes, Caribbean
Naoto Honda, Japan
Alex S. Huang, USA
Rahat Husain, Singapore
Parul Ichhpujani, India
Nazrul Islam, Bangladesh
Mona Khurana, India
Ko Eun Kim, Korea
Nkiru Kizor-Akaraiwe, Nigeria
Miriam Kolko, Denmark
George Kong, Australia
Yasuo Kurimoto, Japan
Guna Laganovska, Latvia
Eun Ji Lee, Korea
Fabian Lerner, Argentina
Fei Li, PR China

Shuning Li, PR China
Fengbin Lin, PR China
Jeff Liebmann,USA
Catherine Liu, Taiwan
Waldo Loaya-Gamboa, Peru
Austin Nakatsuka, USA
Akiko Narita, Japan
Winnie Nolan, UK
Van Nguyen, USA
Takashi Nishida, USA
Sara Okamoto, Japan
Olusola Olawoye, Nigeria
Mineo Ozaki, Japan
Vrundaben Patel, Zambia
Shamira Perera, Singapore
Claire Peterson, Singapore
Natalia Porporato, Singapore
Sayeh Pourjavan, Belgium
Maria Prazenicova, Slovakia
Chunyan Qiao, PR China
Harry Quigley, USA
Pradeep Ramulu, USA
Harsha Rao, India
Hitomi Saito, Japan
Ana Sanseau, Argentina
Rajesh Sasikumar, USA
Jovina See, Singapore
Arsham Sheybani, USA
Zi Da Soh, Singapore
Yunhe Song, PR China
Clemens Strohmaier, Austria
Xinghuai Sun, PR China
Remo Susanna Jr., Brazil
Masaki Tanito, Japan
Angelo P. Tanna, USA
Visanee Tantisevi, Thailand
Niklas Telinius, Denmark
Janey Wiggs, USA
John Thygesen, Denmark
Jolly Tsui, Hong Kong, SAR
Joseph Anthony Tumbocon, Philippines
Tin A. Tun, Singapore
Ana Maria Vasquez, Colombia
Roberto M. Vessani, Brazil
Eranga Vithana, Singapore
Sophia Wang, USA
Tina Wong, Singapore
Chungkwon Yoo, Korea
Ye Zhang, PR China

Participants
Luis Abegao Pinto, Portugal
Michael Chaglasian, USA
Henry Chan, Taiwan
Murray Fingeret, USA
Christopher Girkin, USA
Luis Alberto Guerra, Chile
Ahmad Khalil, Egypt
Daniel Laroche, USA
Kaweh Mansouri, Switzerland
Philip Phatudi, South Africa

Observers
Travis Brooks, USA
Chao Dai, PR China
Xuanchu Duan, PR China
Andrés Gerhard, Colombia
Eleonora Micheletti, Italy
Virna Dwi Oktariana, Indonesia
Emilio Suzuki, Brazil
Ping Zhao, PR China

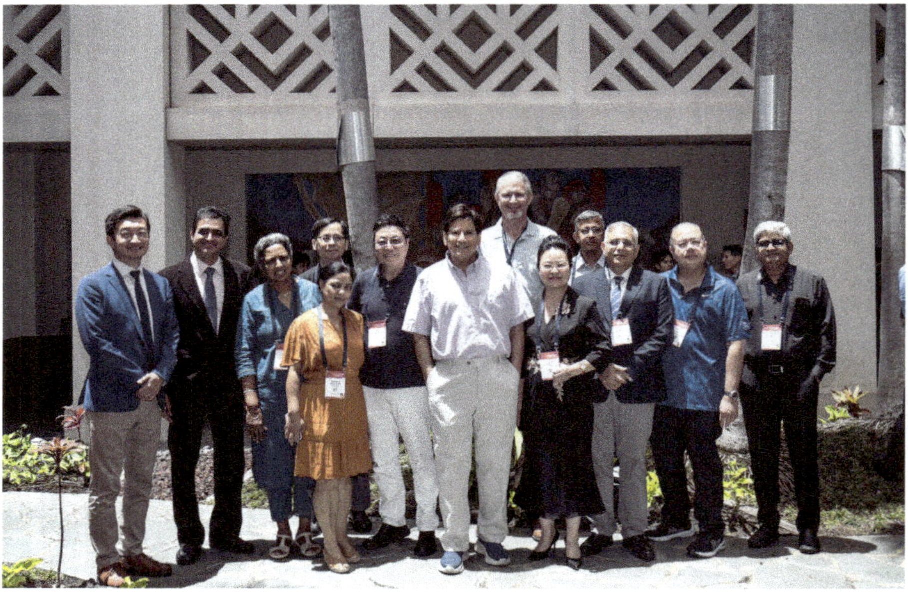

Consensus Co-Chairs and Section Leaders

TABLE OF CONTENTS

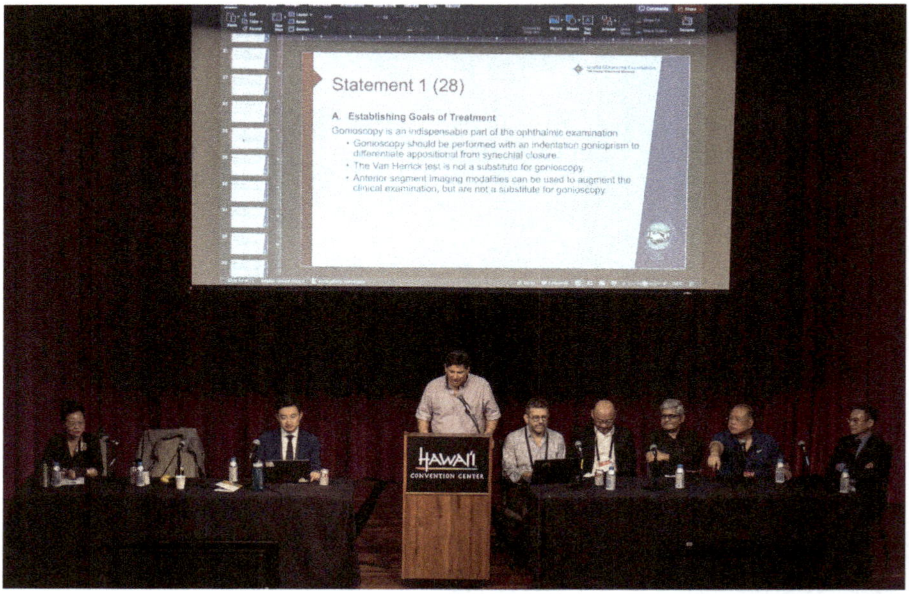
Statement 1 (28)
A. Establishing Goals of Treatment
Gonioscopy is an indispensable part of the ophthalmic examination
• Gonioscopy should be performed with an indentation gonioprism to differentiate appositional from synechial closure
• The Van Herrick test is not a substitute for gonioscopy
• Anterior segment imaging modalities can be used to augment the clinical examination, but are not a substitute for gonioscopy
HAWAI'I
CONVENTION CENTER

FOREWORD

The topic for World Glaucoma Association Consensus 12 was angle closure and angle-closure glaucoma. Global experts were invited and assembled by our international Co-Chairs, beginning in June 2024, to draft a literature review and participate in an online discussion on this topic. Consensus was reached for each of the six sections on key issues relating to definitions, diagnosis, and management. The results of these thoughtful discussions were then summarized with preliminary consensus statements for each section. The draft of the Consensus Report, including the preliminary consensus statements, was distributed to the Section Leaders prior to the Consensus Meeting, which took place in Honolulu on Tuesday June 25, 2025. During the meeting, the Co-Chairs, Section Leaders, and participants engaged in a lively and thought-provoking session to review and revise the consensus statements. With the foundational consensus statements, the Co-Chairs and Section Leaders oversaw the updating of their respective texts. The wisdom that emerged from the group surpassed the influence of any individual expert. The Consensus Report was then finalized by the Co-Chairs and editors.

Throughout the process, it was challenging to reach consensus on subject matters for which clinical opinions vary widely and practice patterns are highly diverse. In large part, this reflects the often limited evidence that guides current clinical practice. Hence, this Consensus is based not only on the published literature, but also on expert opinion. Although consensus does not replace, nor is it a surrogate for, scientific investigation, it does provide considerable value, especially when the desired evidence is lacking.

The goal of this Consensus is to provide a foundation for diagnosing and managing angle closure and angle closure glaucoma. It also seeks to identify those areas lacking in evidence where there is a need for additional research. In other words, this Consensus Report can serve as a benchmark of our understanding of what is known and what we would still like to know.

Robert N. Weinreb, Consensus Chair
Benjamin Xu, Consensus Co-Chair

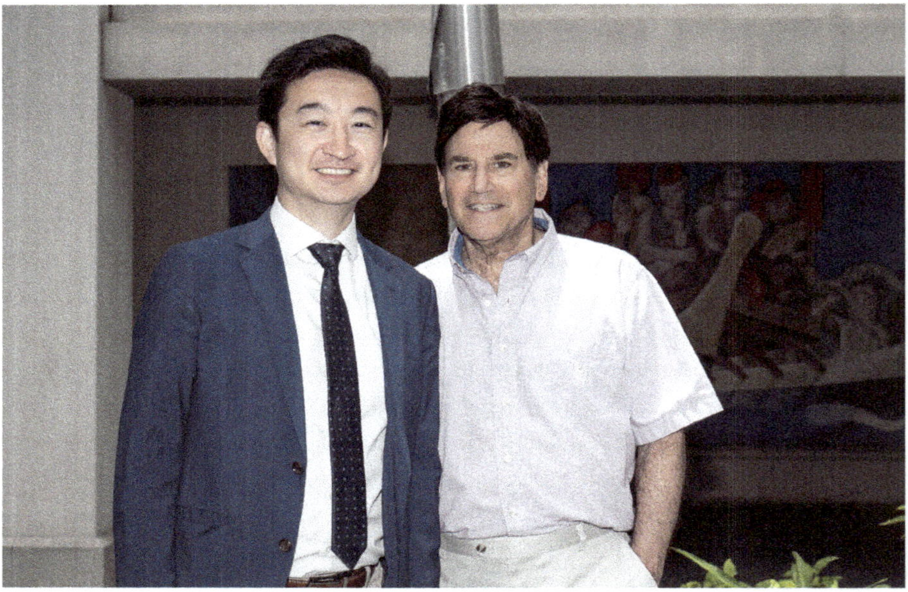

Robert N. Weinreb and Benjmin Xu

PREFACE

Primary angle-closure glaucoma (PACG) remains a leading cause of irreversible blindness worldwide. Even though primary open-angle glaucoma (POAG) is more prevalent, it has been estimated that nearly half of all global glaucoma-related blindness is attributable to PACG due to its greater severity and more aggressive course. As populations age, the number of individuals affected by PACG is expected to rise substantially, underscoring the need for clear, evidence-based strategies to address this growing global burden.

Since the last World Glaucoma Association (WGA) consensus on angle-closure glaucoma in 2006, numerous landmark studies have transformed our understanding of this potentially blinding disease. Population-based epidemiological studies have provided more accurate estimates of the prevalence, global distribution, and associated ocular morbidity of angle closure and PACG. Our understanding of disease pathogenesis, especially regarding racial anatomical differences and dynamic iris-related mechanisms, has also advanced. Anterior segment optical coherence tomography (AS-OCT) has emerged as a key modality for detecting and risk-stratifying individuals at risk for PACG, complementing gonioscopy, the long-standing clinical reference standard. The integration of artificial intelligence (AI) may further enhance the efficiency, accessibility, and scalability of OCT-based assessment. At the same time, landmark clinical trials such as EAGLE and ZAP have expanded the evidence base for managing angle closure, supporting more precise and individualized decision making across a growing range of treatment options, such as clear lens extraction. Goniosynechiolysis and minimally invasive glaucoma surgery (MIGS) show promise, but require further evaluation to define their precise role, benefits, and cost-effectiveness. Together, these developments underscore the need to synthesize recent clinical and scientific advances and identify the critical knowledge gaps that warrant future study.

Identifying best practices for angle closure and angle-closure glaucoma has become increasingly challenging as the literature expands at a rapid pace. As with prior WGA consensus statements, the current Angle Closure Consensus synthesizes both published evidence and expert clinical experience. Although consensus guidelines are not a substitute for rigorous scientific investigation, they serve an important function, particularly in areas where high-quality evidence remains limited. The aim of this consensus is to clarify what is currently established and highlight the key unanswered questions needed to advance our understanding of disease mechanisms and refine screening and treatment strategies for angle closure. This report is intended to serve as a reference point for the field, with the expectation that it will evolve as new data emerge and clinical practice continues to advance.

Consensus Co-Chairs
Benjamin Xu
Tin Aung
Paul Foster
David S. Friedman
Xiulan Zhang
Robert N. Weinreb

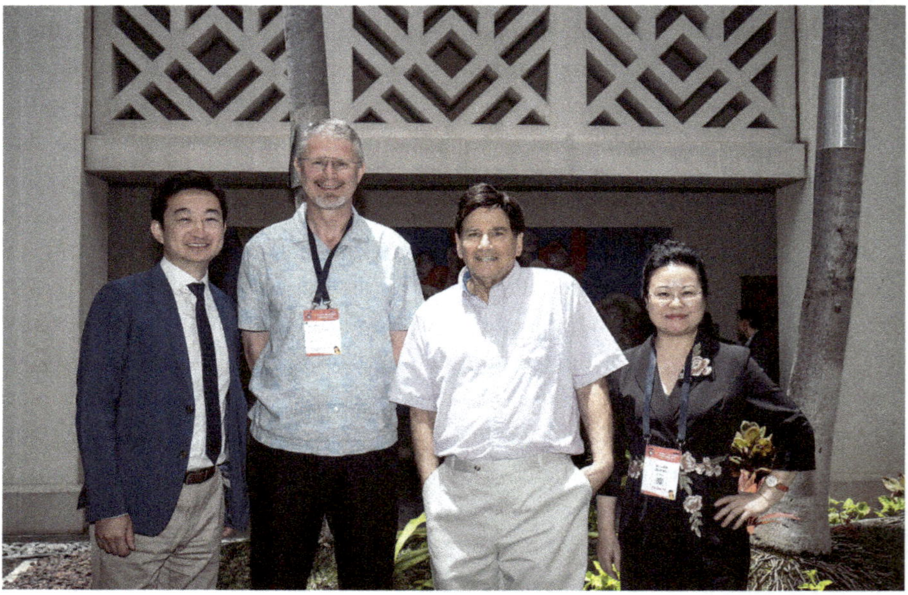

Co-Chairs Benjamin Xu, Paul Foster, Robert N. Weinreb, Xiulan Zhang (Tin Aund, and David S. Friedman, absent)

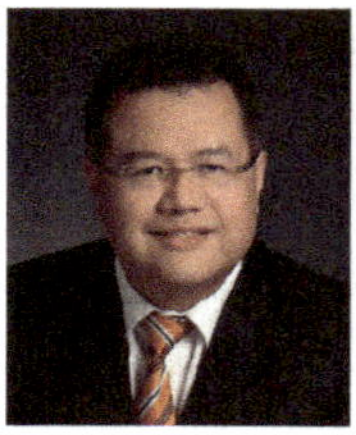

Tin Aung

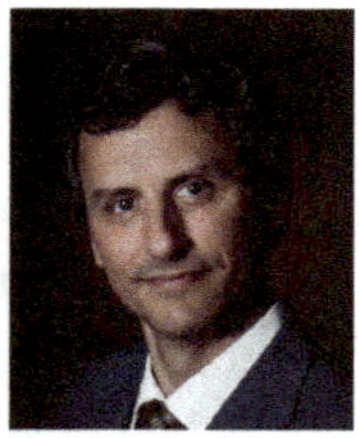

David S. Friedman

DEFINITIONS OF ANGLE CLOSURE

1. The definitions of the spectrum of primary angle closure (sPAC) are based on gonioscopy and clinical findings:
   - Angle closure on gonioscopy is defined as when the posterior, usually pigmented, trabecular meshwork is not visible, possibly indicating the presence of ITC.
   - Primary angle closure suspect (PACS): 2 or more quadrants of angle closure on gonioscopy.
   - Primary angle closure (PAC): PACS plus peripheral anterior synechiae (PAS) and/or elevated intraocular pressure (IOP), or an acute primary angle closure (APAC) attack.
   - Primary angle closure glaucoma (PACG): PACS or PAC plus glaucomatous optic neuropathy.
2. One way of characterizing the spectrum of PAC is:
   - The term primary angle closure disease (PACD) includes PAC and PACG.
   - The term sPAC includes PACS and PACD

Section Leaders

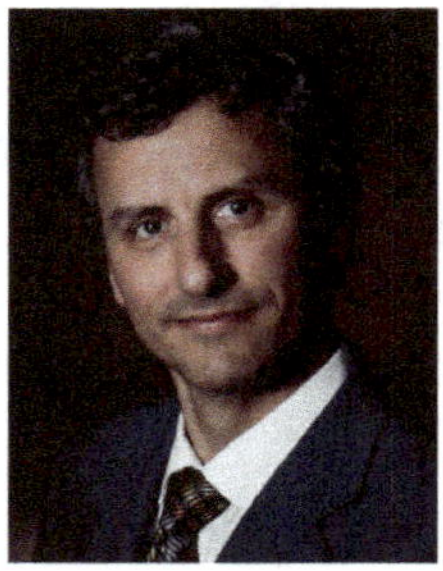

David Friedman

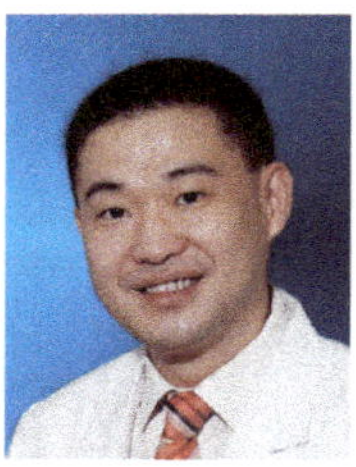

Mingguang He

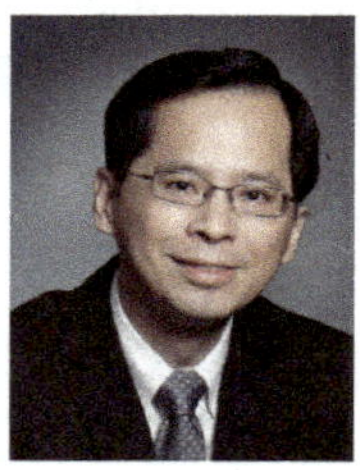

Ching-Yu Cheng

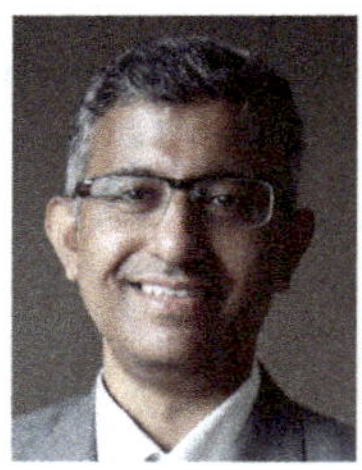

Ronnie George

1. EPIDEMIOLOGY

David Friedman, Mingguang He, Ching-Yu Cheng, Ronnie George

Abbreviations

ACA: anterior chamber angle
ACD: anterior chamber depth
AL: axial length
IOP: intraocular pressure
PAC: primary angle closure
PACD: primary angle-closure disease
PACG: primary angle-closure glaucoma
PACS: primary angle-closure suspect
PAS: peripheral anterior synechiae

Consensus statements

Angle closure

1. Angle closure prevalence appears to be increasing due to population aging.
2. Angle closure appears to be more common in many Asian populations than in European-derived or African-derived populations.
   - More epidemiologic data are needed, particularly in African-derived populations.
3. Women and the elderly are at higher risk of angle closure.
4. The risk of progression from PACS to PAC is low for most PACS eyes.
   - There is a higher risk of progression from PACS to PAC with older age.
   - The low rate of progression in clinical trials is not consistent with the prevalence of PACG in epidemiological studies.
5. PAC is a higher risk state for PACG.
   - Data on the clinical significance of PAS are limited.

Angle Closure and Angle-Closure Glaucoma, pp 1-19
Edited by Robert N. Weinreb, Benjamin Xu, Xiulan Zhang

PACG

6. The number of individuals with PACG is projected to rise.
   - Projections do not account for the increasing rates of cataract surgery and myopia prevalence, which are strongly protective against PACG.
7. PACG is most common among individuals of Asian ancestry.
   - Data in non-Asians are limited.
8. As blindness is associated with over 25% of PACG cases worldwide, a focus on detecting PACD (defined as PAC or PACG) at a treatable stage is needed to prevent vision loss from PACG.
9. PACG can occur in myopic eyes, although the proportion varies by race and ethnicity.
   - PACG is uncommon in high myopes.
   - The relationship between myopia and angle closure depends on the effects on anterior segment biometrics more than overall AL.

Future directions

- Data are sparse from individuals aged 70 years and older, which is a growing demographic group. Cross-sectional biometry in populations shows mean ACD declines with age, peaking between 30 to 50 years of age. This decline slows and potentially reverses at age 70 years, but more research is needed.
- Further research is required to investigate individuals who may be at higher risk of progression from PACS to PAC, such as those with connective tissue abnormalities.

Epidemiology summary

Zi Da Soh, Ching-Yu Cheng

The global prevalence of PACG in individuals 40 years of age and older is estimated at 0.5%, with 77% of cases located in Asia.[1] The aggregated prevalence of PACG was 1.09% in Asia, 0.85% in Latin America, 0.60% in Africa, 0.42% in Europe, 0.35% in Oceania, and 0.26% in North America.[1] Within Asia, the prevalence of PACG ranges between 0.24% and 2.05%, with a higher disease burden reported in East Asia (Table 1).[1,2] Prevalence figures range between 1.90% and 11.50% for PACS,[2-9] and between 0.32% and 3.70% for PAC.[2,4-8,10] An estimated 65% of PACG cases are undetected across different

Asian communities.[11] Globally, PACG affected 23 million adults in 2020.[1] This is projected to increase by 37% to 32 million adults by 2040, with steeper increases in Africa and West Asia.[1,12] Although the global prevalence of PACG is less than half that of primary open-angle glaucoma, but PACG is associated with a 2- to 3-fold increase in the risk of vision impairment (best-corrected visual acuity worse than 6/18 but better than 6/120) and blindness (best-corrected visual acuity worse than 6/120).[13]

The estimated annual incidence of angle-closure diseases in adults was 0.55% in the Singapore Epidemiology of Eye Disease Study, 0.67% in the Chennai Eye Disease in India, 1.06% in the Andhra Pradesh Eye Disease Study in India, and 2.05% in the Liwan Eye Study in China.[14-17] The incidence of PACS, PAC and PACG amongst these Asian populations (in Singapore, India and China) increased with longer follow-up time. [14-17] The incidence of acute angle-closure attacks in Asian populations ranged between 10.5 to 49.5 cases per 100,000 individuals annually,[18,19] compared to 2 to 4 cases per 100,000 individuals in European-derived populations.[20-22] Estimates of progression from prevalent PACS to more severe forms of angle closure vary widely, with recent prospective studies pointing to a lower progression rate than was found in prior clinic-based reports from a single observer (9% to 22% incidence of mostly PAS over 5 to 6 years).[17,23]

Epidemiological data on the prevalence and incidence of angle closure are limited outside of Asia and for PACS and PAC. However, the burden of angle closure among European-derived and Asian American populations may be greater than previously recognized.[24,25]

Risk factors summary

The risk of angle closure is higher with age, among Asians, females, and in eyes with shallower ACD and shorter AL. The prevalence of angle closure increases with age (Table 2), and the odds of PACG increase 2.2-fold for each decade of life.[12] This age-related increase in risk is likely due to the effect of lens enlargement, moving it forward relative to the iris-lens diaphragm.[26] Despite there being a higher prevalence of angle closure in older ages, the incidence of PACG among older populations over 40 years of age is similar to that in younger individuals. This paradox can likely be explained by cataract surgery leading to a reduction in incidence rates.[13-15]

The risk of angle closure is notably higher among Asian populations, particularly among Chinese individuals in East Asia and Inuits of Sino-Mongoloid ancestry.[1] The prevalence of PACG among Asians is 1.8 times greater than that in Africans and between 1.3 to 4.2 times higher than in European-derived populations.[1] Within Asia, the odds of PACG are 5.5 times greater in East Asia compared to Southeast Asia.[12] PACG is more prevalent in China and Mongolia than in South Korea and Japan in the East Asia region. This ethnic variation in angle-closure risk may be linked to differences in anterior chamber dimensions, but this remains inconclusive.[27,28]

Additionally, female adults have approximately 1.5 times the risk of PACG compared to males for angle closure in Asia (Table 3). This increased risk in females is often attributed to a smaller and more crowded anterior chamber.[27,29] Shallow ACD is recognized as a significant and consistent risk factor for angle closure, correlating with other demographic risk factors.[30] Although clinical trials have introduced other anatomical and physiological parameters for angle-closure assessment,[31-33] epidemiological studies have not fully integrated these findings. The observed ethnic and geographic disparities in angle-closure risk suggest potential familial associations or genetic predispositions that require further investigation.

Table 1. Prevalence of PACG in Asia

Study	Country	Year examined	Habitation	Response rate (%)	Age (years)	Sample size	Angle definition	PACG (%)
East Asia								
Liwan Eye Study[5]	China	2003	Urban	75.3	≥ 40	1405	≥ 270° PTM	1.53
Beijing Eye Study[34]	China	2001	Mixed	83.4	≥ 40	4315	≥ 270° PTM	1.02
Bin County Survey[4]	China	2000	Rural	80.0	≥ 40	4956	≥ 270° PTM	1.57
Handan Eye Study[35]	China	2007	Rural	90.4	≥ 40	5480	≥ 180° PTM	0.55
Yunnan Minority Eye Study[36]	China	2010	Rural	77.8	≥ 50	2133	≥ 270° PTM	0.94
Tajimi Study[10]	Japan	2000	Urban	78.1	≥ 40	3021	≥ 270° PTM	0.63
Kumejima Study[7]	Japan	2005	Rural	81.2	≥ 40	3762	≥ 270° PTM	2.00
Hisayama Study	Japan	2022	Urban	68.1	≥ 40	3405	≥ 270° PTM	0.70
Sangju Eye Study[37]	Korea	-	Rural	60.0	≥ 40	671	≥ 270° PTM	0.30
Namil Study[38]	Korea	2007	Rural	79.5	≥ 40	1426	≥ 270° PTM	0.70
Kailu Eye Study[8]	Mongolia	2009	Rural	87.4	≥ 40	5158	≥ 180° PTM	1.74
Hovsgol Eye Study[9]	Mongolia	1996	Mixed	94.2	≥ 40	942	≥ 270° PTM	1.49
Vientiane Eye Study	Laos	2021	Mixed	76.0	≥ 40	1264	≥ 180° PTM	0.55
West Asia								

Study	Country	Year examined	Habitation	Response rate (%)	Age (years)	Sample size	Angle definition	PACG (%)
Oman Eye Study[39]	Oman	2005	Mixed	79.5	≥ 30	3324	≥ 180° PTM	2.05
Qatar Eye Study[40]	Qatar	2009	Mixed	97.7	≥ 40	3149	≥ 270° PTM	0.44
South-East Asia								
Rom Klao Eye Study[41]	Thailand	1999	Urban	88.7	≥ 50	701	≥ 270° PTM	0.86
Meiktila Eye Study[42]	Myanmar	2005	Rural	83.7	≥ 40	2075	≥ 270° PTM	2.50
Singapore Malay Eye Study[43]	Singapore	2004	Urban	78.7	≥ 40	3280	≥ 180° PTM	0.12
Singapore Indian Eye Study[44]	Singapore	2007	Urban	75.6	≥ 40	3400	≥ 180° PTM	0.12
Singapore Chinese Eye Study[45]	Singapore	2011	Urban	72.8	≥ 40	3353	≥ 180° PTM	1.50
South Central Asia								
Aravind Comprehensive Eye Study[46]	India	1995	Rural	93	≥ 40	5150	≥ 90° PTM	0.50
West Bengal Glaucoma Study[47]	India	1998	Rural	83.1	≥ 50	1324	≥ 270° PTM	0.24
Chennai Glaucoma Study[3]	India	2001	Rural	80.2	≥ 40	3350	≥ 180° PTM	0.88
Andhra Pradesh Eye Disease Study[2]	India	1996	Mixed	87.3	≥ 40	3724	≥ 180° PTM	0.94
Central India Eye and Medical Study[48]	India	2006	Rural	87.3	≥ 30	4711	≥ 270° PTM	0.24
Bhaktapur Glaucoma Study[49]	Nepal	2007	Mixed	83.4	≥ 40	3991	≥ 270° PTM	0.39
Dhaka Eye Study[50]	Bangladesh	1997	Rural	65.9	35	2347	≥ 270° PTM	0.30
Yazd Eye Study[51]	Iran	2010	Mixed	90.4	≥ 40	1990	≥ 270° PTM	0.33

PACG: primary angle-closure glaucoma; PTM: pigmented trabecular meshwork

Table 2. Prevalence of PACD in population-based studies, stratified by disease stage and age group

Study	Country	Age (years)	Angle definition	40-49 years (%)	50–59 years (%)	60–69 years (%)	70–79 years (%)	≥ 80 years (%)
PACS								
Bin County Survey[4]	China	≥ 40	≥ 270° PTM	0.70	4.63	8.83	6.10*	-
Handan Eye Study[35]	China	≥ 40	≥ 180° PTM	5.60	14.30	21.90	20.10	17.20
Kailu Eye Study[8]	Mongolia	≥ 40	≥ 180° PTM	3.50	5.90	5.45	6.37*	-

Study	Country	Age (years)	Angle definition	40-49 years (%)	50–59 years (%)	60–69 years (%)	70–79 years (%)	≥ 80 years (%)
Andhra Pradesh Eye Disease Study[2]	India	≥ 40	≥ 180° PTM	1.19	1.90	2.50	3.10	-
PAC								
Bin County Survey[4]	China	≥ 40	≥ 270° PTM	0.28	1.42	2.47	1.43*	-
Liwan Eye Study[5]	China	≥ 50	≥ 270° PTM	-	1.10	2.90	2.90	3.70
Handan Eye Study[35]	China	≥ 40	≥ 180° PTM	0.50	1.70	3.20	3.70	-
Kailu Eye Study[8]	Mongolia	≥ 40	≥ 180° PTM	0.94	0.78	1.51	2.27*	-
Tajimi Study[10]	Japan	≥ 40	≥ 270° PTM	0.10	0.20	0.40	1.40	1.20
Andhra Pradesh Eye Disease Study[2]	India	≥ 40	≥ 180° PTM	0.14	0.57	0.33	0.28	-
PACG								
Bin County Survey[4]	China	≥ 40	≥ 270° PTM	0.06	0.99	2.29	4.54*	-
Liwan Eye Study[5]	China	≥ 50	≥ 270° PTM	-	0.00	1.20	3.30	1.90
Handan Eye Study[35]	China	≥ 40	≥ 180° PTM	0.10	0.50	1.70	2.60	-
Beijing Eye Study[34]	China	≥ 40	≥ 270° PTM	0.40	0.80	1.00	3.60*	-
Yunnan Minority Eye Study[52]	China	≥ 50	≥ 270° PTM	-	0.20	0.80	1.20	-
Kailu Eye Study[8]	Mongolia	≥ 40	≥ 180° PTM	0.63	1.99	2.18	2.97*	-
Tajimi Study[10]	Japan	≥ 40	≥ 270° PTM	0.00	0.20	0.90	1.40	3.00
Bhaktapur Glaucoma Study[50]	Nepal	≥ 40	≥ 270° PTM	0.00	0.00	0.84	1.67	2.06
Andhra Pradesh Eye Disease Study[2]	India	≥ 40	≥ 180° PTM	0.56	0.45	0.88	2.50*	-

PACD: primary angle-closure disease; PACS: primary angle-closure suspect; PAC: primary angle closure; PACG: primary angle-closure glaucoma; PTM: pigmented trabecular meshwork
*Represents prevalence in adults aged 70 years (not 70 to 79 years old).

Table 3. Prevalence of PACD in population-based studies, stratified by disease severity and gender

Study	Country	Age (years)	Angle definition	Male (%)	Female (%)
PACS					
Bin County Survey[4]	China	≥ 40	≥ 270° PTM	2.69	4.45
Handan Eye Study[35]	China	≥ 40	≥ 180° PTM	5.90	16.4
Kailu Eye Study[8]	Mongolia	≥ 40	≥ 180° PTM	4.05	5.98
Andhra Pradesh Eye Disease Study[2]	India	≥ 40	≥ 180° PTM	1.30	2.40
PAC					
Bin County Survey[4]	China	≥ 40	≥ 270° PTM	0.63	1.43
Liwan Eye Study[5]	China	≥ 50	≥ 270° PTM	1.10	3.30
Handan Eye Study[35]	China	≥ 40	≥ 180° PTM	0.90	2.30
Kailu Eye Study[8]	Mongolia	≥ 40	≥ 180° PTM	1.00	1.36
Tajimi Study[10]	Japan	≥ 40	≥ 270° PTM	0.10	0.90
Andhra Pradesh Eye Disease Study[2]	India	≥ 40	≥ 180° PTM	0.05	0.55
PACG					
Bin County Survey[4]	China	≥ 40	≥ 270° PTM	0.67	1.49
Liwan Eye Study[5]	China	≥ 50	≥ 270° PTM	1.30	1.60
Handan Eye Study[35]	China	≥ 40	≥ 180° PTM	0.50	1.00
Beijing Eye Study[34]	China	≥ 40	≥ 270° PTM	0.70	1.20
Kailu Eye Study[8]	Mongolia	≥ 40	≥ 180° PTM	1.09	2.27
Tajimi Study[10]	Japan	≥ 40	≥ 270° PTM	0.30	0.90
Bhaktapur Glaucoma Study[50]	Nepal	≥ 40	≥ 270° PTM	0.22	0.60
Andhra Pradesh Eye Disease Study[2]	India	≥ 40	≥ 180° PTM	0.79	1.06

PACD: primary angle-closure disease; PACS: primary angle-closure suspect; PAC: primary angle closure; PACG: primary angle-closure glaucoma; PTM: pigmented trabecular meshwork

References

1. Tham Y-C, Li X, Wong TY, Quigley HA, Aung T, Cheng C-Y. Global prevalence of glaucoma and projections of glaucoma burden through 2040: a systematic review and meta-analysis. Ophthalmology. 2014;121(11):2081-2090. https://doi.org/10.1016/j.ophtha.2014.05.013
2. Senthil S, Garudadri C, Khanna RC, Sannapaneni K. Angle closure in the Andhra Pradesh eye disease study. Ophthalmology. 2010;117(9):1729-1735. https://doi.org/10.1016/j.ophtha.2010.01.021
3. Vijaya L, George R, Arvind H, et al. Prevalence of primary angle-closure disease in an urban south Indian population and comparison with a rural population: the Chennai Glaucoma Study. Ophthalmology. 2008;115(4):655-660. https://doi.org/10.1016/j.ophtha.2007.05.034
4. Qu W, Li Y, Song W, et al. Prevalence and risk factors for angle-closure disease in a rural Northeast China population: a population-based survey in Bin County, Harbin. Acta Ophthalmologica. 2011;89(6):e515-e520. https://doi.org/10.1111/j.1755-3768.2011.02146.x
5. He M, Foster PJ, Ge J, et al. Prevalence and clinical characteristics of glaucoma in adult Chinese: a population-based study in Liwan District, Guangzhou. Invest Ophthalmol Vis Sci. 2006;47(7):2782-2788. https://doi.org/10.1167/iovs.06-0051
6. Liang Y, Friedman DS, Zhou Q, et al. Prevalence and characteristics of primary angle-closure diseases in a rural adult Chinese population: the Handan Eye Study. Invest Ophthalmol Vis Sci. 2011;52(12):8672-8679. https://doi.org/10.1167/iovs.11-7480
7. Sawaguchi S, Sakai H, Iwase A, et al. Prevalence of primary angle closure and primary angle-closure glaucoma in a southwestern rural population of Japan: the Kumejima Study. Ophthalmology. 2012;119(6):1134-1142. https://doi.org/10.1016/j.ophtha.2011.12.038
8. Song W, Shan L, Cheng F, et al. Prevalence of glaucoma in a rural northern China adult population: a population-based survey in Kailu county, inner Mongolia. Ophthalmology. 2011;118(10):1982-1988. https://doi.org/10.1016/j.ophtha.2011.02.050
9. Foster PJ, Baasanhu J, Alsbirk PH, Munkhbayar D, Uranchimeg D, Johnson GJ. Glaucoma in Mongolia: a population-based survey in Hövsgöl Province, northern Mongolia. Arch Ophthalmol. 1996;114(10):1235-1241. https://doi.org/10.1001/archopht.1996.01100140435011
10. Yamamoto T, Iwase A, Araie M, et al. The Tajimi Study report 2: prevalence of primary angle closure and secondary glaucoma in a Japanese population. Ophthalmology. 2005;112(10):1661-1669. https://doi.org/10.1016/j.ophtha.2005.05.012
11. Soh ZD, Yu M, Betzler BK, et al. The global extent of undetected glaucoma in adults: a systematic review and meta-analysis. Ophthalmology. 2021;128(10):1393-1404. https://doi.org/10.1016/j.ophtha.2021.04.009
12. Chan EWe, Li X, Tham Y-C, et al. Glaucoma in Asia: regional prevalence variations and future projections. Br J Ophthalmol. 2016;100(1):78-85. https://doi.org/10.1136/bjophthalmol-2014-306102

13. Friedman DS, Foster PJ, Aung T, He M. Angle closure and angle-closure glaucoma: what we are doing now and what we will be doing in the future. Clin Exp Ophthalmol. 2012;40(4):381-387. https://doi.org/10.1111/j.1442-9071.2012.02774.x
14. Choudhari NS, Khanna RC, Marmamula S, et al. Fifteen-year incidence rate of primary angle closure disease in the Andhra Pradesh Eye Disease Study. Am J Ophthalmol. 2021;229:34-44. https://doi.org/10.1016/j.ajo.2021.02.030
15. Vijaya L, Asokan R, Panday M, et al.-. Am J Ophthalmol. 2013;156(6):1308-1315. https://doi.org/10.1016/j.ajo.2013.07.027
16. Wang L, Huang W, Huang S, et al. Ten-year incidence of primary angle closure in elderly Chinese: the Liwan Eye Study. Br J Ophthalmol. 2019;103(3):355-360. https://doi.org/10.1136/bjophthalmol-2017-311808
17. Teo ZL, Da Soh Z, Tham Y-C, et al. Six-year incidence and risk factors for primary angle-closure disease: the Singapore Epidemiology of Eye Diseases Study. Ophthalmology. 2022;129(7):792-802. https://doi.org/10.1016/j.ophtha.2022.03.009
18. Lai JS, Liu DT, Tham CC, Li RT, Lam DS. Epidemiology of acute primary angle-closure glaucoma in the Hong Kong Chinese population: prospective study. Hong Kong Medical Journal = Xianggang Yi Xue Za Zhi/Hong Kong Academy of Medicine. 2001.
19. Chiu S-L, Chu C-L, Muo C-H, Chen C-L, Lan S-J. The prevalence and the incidence of diagnosed open-angle glaucoma and diagnosed angle-closure glaucoma: changes from 2001 to 2010. J Glaucoma. 2016;25(5):e514-e519. https://doi.org/10.1097/IJG.0000000000000381
20. Chua PY, Day AC, Lai KL, et al. The incidence of acute angle closure in Scotland: a prospective surveillance study. Br J Ophthalmol. 2018;102(4):539-543. https://doi.org/10.1136/bjophthalmol-2017-310725
21. Keenan TDL, Salmon JF, Yeates D, Goldacre M. Trends in rates of primary angle closure glaucoma and cataract surgery in England from 1968 to 2004. J Glaucoma. 2009;18(3):201-205. https://doi.org/10.1097/IJG.0b013e318181540a
22. Bojiæ L, Mandiæ Z, Ivaniševiæ M, et al. Incidence of acute angle-closure glaucoma in Dalmatia, southern Croatia. Ophthalmology. 2004;45(3):279-282.
23. Thomas R, George R, Parikh R, Muliyil J, Jacob A. Five year risk of progression of primary angle closure suspects to primary angle closure: a population based study. Br J Ophthalmol. 2003;87(4):450-454. https://doi.org/10.1136/bjo.87.4.450
24. Day AC, Baio G, Gazzard G, et al. The prevalence of primary angle closure glaucoma in European-derived populations: a systematic review. Br J Ophthalmol. 2012;96(9):1162-1167. https://doi.org/10.1136/bjophthalmol-2011-301189
25. Xu B, Burkemper B, Grisafe D, et al. Prevalence and Characteristics of Primary Angle Closure Disease in an Adult Chinese American Population: The Chinese American Eye Study. Invest Ophthalmol Vis Sci. 2018;59(9):2725-2725.
26. Stamper RL, Lieberman MF, Drake MV. Chapter 15: Primary angle-closure glaucoma. In:

Becker-Shaffer's diagnosis and therapy of the glaucomas E-Book. Elsevier Health Sciences; 2009. https://doi.org/10.1016/B978-0-323-02394-8.00015-2
27. Congdon NG, Youlin Q, Quigley H, et al. Biometry and primary angle-closure glaucoma among Chinese, white, and black populations. Ophthalmology. 1997;104(9):1489-1495. https://doi.org/10.1016/S0161-6420(97)30112-2
28. Devereux JG, Foster PJ, Baasanhu J, et al. Anterior chamber depth measurement as a screening tool for primary angle-closure glaucoma in an East Asian population. Arch Ophthalmol. 2000;118(2):257-263. https://doi.org/10.1001/archopht.118.2.257
29. Foster PJ, Broadway DC, Hayat S, et al. Refractive error, axial length and anterior chamber depth of the eye in British adults: the EPIC-Norfolk Eye Study. Br J Ophthalmol. 2010;94(7):827-830. https://doi.org/10.1136/bjo.2009.163899
30. Foster PJ. The epidemiology of primary angle closure and associated glaucomatous optic neuropathy. Semin Ophthalmol. 2002 Jun;17(2):50-8. https://doi.org/10.1076/soph.17.2.50.14718
31. Nongpiur ME, He M, Amerasinghe N, et al. Lens vault, thickness, and position in Chinese subjects with angle closure. Ophthalmology. 2011;118(3):474-479. https://doi.org/10.1016/j.ophtha.2010.07.025
32. Seager FE, Jefferys JL, Quigley HA. Comparison of dynamic changes in anterior ocular structures examined with anterior segment optical coherence tomography in a cohort of various origins. Invest Ophthalmol Vis Sci. 2014;55(3):1672-1683. https://doi.org/10.1167/iovs.13-13641
33. Koh V, Chua J, Shi Y, et al. Association of iris crypts with acute primary angle closure. Br J Ophthalmol. 2017;101(10):1318-1322. https://doi.org/10.1136/bjophthalmol-2016-309842
34. Wang YX, Xu L, Yang H, Jonas JB. Prevalence of glaucoma in North China: the Beijing eye study. Am J Ophthalmol. 2010;150(6):917-924. https://doi.org/10.1016/j.ajo.2010.06.037
35. Liang Y, Friedman DS, Zhou Q, et al. Prevalence and characteristics of primary angle-closure diseases in a rural adult Chinese population: the Handan Eye Study. Invest Ophthalmol Vis Sci. 2011;52(12):8672-8679. https://doi.org/10.1167/iovs.11-7480
36. Zhong H, Li J, Li C, et al. The prevalence of glaucoma in adult rural Chinese populations of the Bai nationality in Dali: the Yunnan Minority Eye Study. Invest Ophthalmol Vis Sci. 2012;53(6):3221-3225. https://doi.org/10.1167/iovs.11-9306
37. Kim JH, Kang SY, Kim NR, et al. Prevalence and characteristics of glaucoma among Korean adults. Korean J Ophthalmol. 2011;25(2):110-115. https://doi.org/10.3341/kjo.2011.25.2.110
38. Kim YY, Lee JH, Ahn MD, Kim CY, Group NS. Angle closure in the Namil study in central South Korea. Arch Ophthalmol. 2012;130(9):1177-1183. https://doi.org/10.1001/archophthalmol.2012.1470
39. Khandekar R, Jaffer M, Al Raisi A, et al. Oman Eye Study 2005: prevalence and determinants of glaucoma. EMHJ-Eastern Mediterranean Health Journal. 2008;14(6):1349-1359.
40. Al-Mansouri FA, Kanaan A, Gamra H, et al. Prevalence and determinants of glaucoma in

citizens of Qatar aged 40 years or older: a community-based survey. Middle East Afr J Ophthalmol. 2011;18(2):141. https://doi.org/10.4103/0974-9233.80703

41. Bourne R, Sukudom P, Foster P, et al. Prevalence of glaucoma in Thailand: a population-based survey in Rom Klao District, Bangkok. Br J Ophthalmol. 2003;87(9):1069-1074. https://doi.org/10.1136/bjo.87.9.1069
42. Casson R, Newland H, Muecke J, et al. Prevalence of glaucoma in rural Myanmar: the Meiktila Eye Study. Br J Ophthalmol. 2007;91(6):710-714. https://doi.org/10.1136/bjo.2006.107573
43. Shen SY, Wong TY, Foster PJ, et al. The prevalence and types of glaucoma in Malay people: the Singapore Malay eye study. Invest Ophthalmol Vis Sci. 2008;49(9):3846-3851. https://doi.org/10.1167/iovs.08-1759
44. Narayanaswamy A, Baskaran M, Zheng Y, et al. The prevalence and types of glaucoma in an urban Indian population: the Singapore Indian Eye Study. Invest Ophthalmol Vis Sci. 2013;54(7):4621-4627. https://doi.org/10.1167/iovs.13-11950
45. Baskaran M, Foo RC, Cheng C-Y, et al. The prevalence and types of glaucoma in an urban Chinese population: the Singapore Chinese eye study. JAMA Ophthalmol. 2015;133(8):874-880. https://doi.org/10.1001/jamaophthalmol.2015.1110
46. Ramakrishnan R, Nirmalan PK, Krishnadas R, et al. Glaucoma in a rural population of southern India: the Aravind comprehensive eye survey. Ophthalmology. 2003;110(8):1484-1490. https://doi.org/10.1016/S0161-6420(03)00564-5
47. Raychaudhuri A, Lahiri S, Bandyopadhyay M, Foster P, Reeves B, Johnson G. A population-based survey of the prevalence and types of glaucoma in rural West Bengal: the West Bengal Glaucoma Study. Br J Ophthalmol. 2005;89(12):1559-1564 https://doi.org/10.1136/bjo.2005.074948
48. Nangia V, Jonas JB, Matin A, et al. Prevalence and associated factors of glaucoma in rural central India. The Central India Eye and Medical Study. PloS One. 2013;8(9):e76434. https://doi.org/10.1371/journal.pone.0076434
49. Thapa SS, Paudyal I, Khanal S, et al. A population-based survey of the prevalence and types of glaucoma in Nepal: the Bhaktapur Glaucoma Study. Ophthalmology. 2012;119(4):759-764. https://doi.org/10.1016/j.ophtha.2011.10.021
50. Rahman M, Rahman N, Foster P, et al. The prevalence of glaucoma in Bangladesh: a population-based survey in Dhaka division. Br J Ophthalmol. 2004;88(12):1493-1497. https://doi.org/10.1136/bjo.2004.043612
51. Pakravan M, Yazdani S, Javadi M-A, et al. A population-based survey of the prevalence and types of glaucoma in central Iran: the Yazd eye study. Ophthalmology. 2013;120(10):1977-1984. https://doi.org/10.1016/j.ophtha.2013.02.029
52. Pan CW, Zhao CH, Yu MB, et al. Prevalence, types and awareness of glaucoma in a multi-ethnic population in rural China: the Yunnan Minority Eye Study. Ophthalmic Physiol Opt. 2016;36(6):664-670. https://doi.org/10.1111/opo.12319

Racial differences in prevalence

As noted above, angle closure is more common in Asian populations than in those of European and African descent. PACG is estimated to occur in approximately 0.5% of Whites and Blacks and possibly at lower rates in Hispanics over the age of 40.[1-4] Unpublished data from the Baltimore Eye Survey in the United States indicate that 0.4% of Whites and 0.6% of Blacks over the age of 40 have PACG (James Tielsch, personal communication). Similar rates were reported in the Egna-Neumarkt study of angle closure. Data on these populations are limited, especially among Hispanics and African-derived peoples, and prevalence rates likely vary across the Americas and in African populations.

References

1. Salmon JF, Mermoud A, Ivey A, Swanevelder SA, Hoffman M. The prevalence of primary angle-closure glaucoma and open angle glaucoma in Mamre, Western Cape, South Africa. Arch Ophthalmol. 1993;111:1263-9.
2. Quigley HA, West SK, Rodriguez J, Munoz B, Klein R, Snyder R. The prevalence of glaucoma in a population-based study of Hispanic subjects: Proyecto VER. Arch Ophthalmol. 2001 Dec;119(12):1819-26. https://doi.org/10.1001/archopht.119.12.1819
3. Bonomi L, Marchini G, Marrafa M, et al. Epidemiology of angle-closure glaucoma. Prevalence, clinical types, and association with peripheral anterior chamber depth in the Egna-Neumarkt glaucoma study. Ophthalmology. 2000;107:998-1003.
4. Day AC, Baio G, Gazzard G, et al. The prevalence of primary angle closure glaucoma in European-derived populations: a systematic review. Br J Ophthalmol. 2012 Sep;96(9):1162-7. https://doi.org/10.1136/bjophthalmol-2011-301189

Risk factors for primary angle-closure glaucoma

Major demographic risk factors for angle closure have been discussed above and include older age, female gender, and Asian ancestry. Ocular risk factors predisposing to angle closure relate to a smaller, more crowded anterior segment. Limbal and axial ACD strongly correlate with angle closure and angle-closure glaucoma.

Ocular risk factors include:

- Shallower axial and limbal ACD.
- Thicker lens and greater anterior lens vault.
- Shorter AL.
- Smaller corneal diameter.
- Hypermetropic refraction (largely owing to shorter AL).
- Many iris factors, including iris thickness, curvature, and area, are measured using optical coherence tomography.

Dynamic factors have also been associated with angle closure. These include less iris area reduction in response to illumination, leaving the angle crowded. There is also less angle opening in response to pilocarpine in angle-closure eyes. Family history is also a strong risk factor, with an estimated 8-fold risk in first-degree relatives. The genetics of angle closure are reviewed elsewhere.

Socioeconomic disadvantage, lower educational achievement and racial minority status are risk factors for acute angle closure and blindness from PACG. Those with lower body mass index are also at higher risk of acute angle closure.

Natural history of primary angle-closure disease

The natural history of angle closure can be ascertained from population-based studies with longitudinal follow-up or from randomized controlled trials on laser peripheral iridotomy for PACS that have followed up PACS eyes with and without intervention. There are few reports on the natural history of PACD progressing through all stages of the disease. The challenges of studying the natural history of PACD include the slow rates of progression, inter-observer variability in gonioscopic angle assessment (with some studies reporting a 15% reclassification rate on follow-up), and that very few studies have had the same observers for both baseline and follow-up assessments.[1] Variability in cataract surgery rates in the different study populations also makes assessment of true progression rates and comparisons between studies challenging.

Most population-based studies on the progression of PACD have been conducted in Asia, given the higher prevalence of the disease on the continent. There are only a few clinic-based studies from the West and 1 population-based study from Italy that have reported progression rates. PACS is not uncommon in susceptible populations, making it possible to get an adequate sample size for assessing progression to PAC in population-based studies. This is supported by the consensus that most such eyes can be safely observed without treatment.

However, the number of individuals with PAC in the population is relatively small, and therefore, fewer researchers study this condition. Most studies that examine PAC progression have small sample sizes, resulting in limited information on how untreated PAC progresses to PACG. This difficulty in studying the natural history of PAC is further compounded by the accepted clinical protocol, which requires a laser iridotomy or other interventions in all eyes with PAC, making longitudinal data on untreated PAC scarce. The significance of PAS also remains unclear, as they often do not result in IOP elevation. While the Ocular Hypertension Treatment Study demonstrated limited benefit to early treatment of ocular hypertension in open angles, results from this study cannot be extrapolated to those with angle closure, and many treat patients with PAC who have elevated IOP.

The progression rates of PACS to PAC in population-based and clinic-based studies have ranged from 6% to 22% (Table 1).[2,3] These studies have used different definitions for progression and different definitions for angle-closure disease, ranging from 180° to 270° of closure. The follow-up has also varied from 1 year to 14 years.[4,5] The estimated annual incidence varied from 0.67% to 4.4%.[3,6] Many of the studies had small sample sizes and few participants at final follow-up because of dropouts and cataract surgery.

In randomized trials studying the impact of laser peripheral iridotomy on PACS progression, the estimated annual incidence of PAC or PACG in the control arms ranged from 0.86% to 3.75%.[4,7] While the Zhongshan Angle-Closure Prevention study had exclusion criteria for eyes potentially at high risk for progression, only 1 subject was excluded for a large increase in IOP after dark-prone testing. Definitions of PAS were stringent (1 or more clock hours), which could have resulted in underestimates of PAS-based progression. In the Zhongshan Angle-Closure Prevention study, the estimated annual incidence was 0.87% at 6 years follow-up and 1.75% at the 14-year follow-up based on phakic eyes who completed the 6- and 14-year follow-up.[5] This increase in estimated annual incidence over a longer follow-up is similar to the higher annual incidence rates for incident PAC/PACG reported by the population-based studies with longer durations of follow-up, such as 0.11% in the Liwan Eye Study at 10 years[8] and 0.10% in the Andhra Pradesh Eye Disease Study at 15 years[9] compared with 0.05% in the Chennai Eye Diseases Incidence Study [10] and 0.04% in the Singapore Epidemiology of Eye Diseases Study,[1] both with 6 years of follow-up. This indicates a nonlinear increase in risk of progression/incidence of disease, which could be secondary to progressive lens thickening resulting in narrowing of the angle and progression. It is also possible that initial screening for PACS led to a population enriched for stable PACS (*i.e.*, tolerance of iridotrabecular contact) with a lower risk of progression to PAC/PACG, and that the low risk of progression reflects selection for eyes unlikely to progress.

Progression from PAC to PACG has been reported less frequently, with progression rates ranging from 8% to 28.5%,[11,12] again with varying follow-up rates and small numbers in each cohort. The only population-based study is from India and reported 28.5% progression in a small study of eyes with untreated PAC over 5 years. When the duration of follow-up is accounted for, the estimated annual incidence in individuals with previously open angles ranges from 2% to 5.7%.[11,12]

Incident angle-closure disease rates have been reported by 5 studies, 2 from India and 1 each from China, Italy, and Singapore (Table 2). The Liwan Eye Study, which reported the highest rates, also had the highest baseline age of 50 years compared with all other studies, which included participants 40 years or older. The estimated annual incidence of PACD was between 0.5% and 2%.[1,8] The annual incidence of PACG ranged from 0.04% to 0.11%.[8,13] A very low incidence of PACG of 0.25% and 0.3% was reported from Singapore and Chennai, respectively, at 6 years of follow-up, comprising less than 10% of the reported incidence for any form of PACD in these studies.[1,10] The age-adjusted incidence of PACD in individuals with previously open angles in 3 different Asian ethnicities in the Singapore Epidemiology of Eye Diseases study cohort was 3.22% for Indians, 3.33% for Chinese, and 3.20% for Malays.[1] The age-adjusted incidence of PACG was 0.43% in Indian adults, 0.03% in Chinese adults, and 0.16 in Malay adults from the same study. While this was statistically significant, the small number of converting participants makes it difficult to assess whether these are true differences.

The rates of incident PACD are variable across different studies but represent approximately one-third the rate of progression of established disease. Few cases of incident PACG are reported to occur within a 5–6-year follow-up. These could be related to a misdiagnosis at baseline or a small subset of rapidly progressing eyes. Disease progression rates were higher in studies with longer follow-up; these findings could have implications for follow-up protocols in individuals with long-standing PACS.

Table 1. Progression of PACS or PAC

Author (country)	Year	Number at baseline	Follow-up (years)	Age range	Change in disease stage	Rate of progression to PAC(G) %	Estimated annual incidence rate of PAC(G) %
Hospital-based studies							
Wishart (UK)[11]	1992	25	4	36.9–84.3	PAC to PACG	8	2
Wilensky (USA)[14]	1993	129	5	NA	PACS/PAC to PACG	19.38	3.88
Population-based studies							
Alsbirk (Greenland)[6]	1994	75	10	40–70+	PACS to PACG	6.67	0.67
Thomas (India)[3]	2003	50	5	36–65	PACS to PAC	22	4.4
Thomas (India)[12]	2003	28	5	36–65	PAC to PACG	28.57	5.71
Teo (Singapore)[1]	2021	222	6	≥ 40	PACS to PAC/(G)	9.38	1.56
Zhang (China)[2]	2022	526	5	≥ 30	PACS to PAC/(G)	6.08	1.21
From control arms of RCTs on PACS progression							
He (China)[7]	2019	(889) 664*	6	50-70	PACS to PAC/(G)	5.2	0.87
Mou (China)[4]	2021	(184) 80*	1	60 (mean age)	PACS to PAC/(G)	3.75	3.75
Baskaran (Singapore)[15]	2022	(480) 435*	5	50+	PACS to PAC/(G)	10.3	2.06
Yuan (China)[5]	2023	(889) 427*	14	50–70	PACS to PAC/(G)	24.5	1.75

PAC: primary angle closure; PACG: primary angle-closure glaucoma; PACS: primary angle-closure suspect; RCT: randomized controlled trial
*Numbers in parenthesis indicate the numbers enrolled at baseline; all rates are calculated based on the numbers seen at the final examination visit.

Table 2. Incidence of PACD

Study (country)	Year	Number at baseline	Follow-up (years)	Baseline age (years)	PACD incidence	PACG incidence	Estimated annual incidence			
							PACD	PACS	PAC	PACG
Ponza Eye Study (Italy)[13]	2012	411	12	≥ 40	NR	0.49	NR	NR	NR	0.04
CEDIS (India)[10]	2013	3350	6	≥ 40	4	0.3	0.67	0.43	0.18	0.05
Liwan Eye Study (China)[8]	2019	1405	10	≥ 50	20.48	1.13	2.05	1.69	0.21	0.11
APEDS (India)[9]	2021	1470	15	≥ 40	15.87	1.56	1.06	0.56	0.4	0.1
SEED (Singapore)[1]	2022	5065	6	≥ 40	3.26	0.25	0.54	0.4	0.08	0.03

APEDS: Andhra Pradesh Eye Diseases Incidence Study; CEDIS: Chennai Eye Diseases Incidence Study; PAC: primary angle closure; PACD: primary angle-closure disease; PACG: primary angle-closure glaucoma; PACS: primary angle-closure suspect; SEED: Singapore Epidemiology of Eye Diseases Study

References

1. Teo ZL, Soh ZD, Tham YC, et al. Six-Year Incidence and Risk Factors for Primary Angle-Closure Disease. Ophthalmology. 2022 Jul;129(7):792-802. https://doi.org/10.1016/j.ophtha.2022.03.009
2. Zhang Y, Thomas R, Zhang Q, Li SZ, Wang NL. Progression of Primary Angle Closure Suspect to Primary Angle Closure and Associated Risk Factors: The Handan Eye Study. Invest Opthalmol Vis Sci. 2021 Jun 1;62(7):2. https://doi.org/10.1167/iovs.62.7.2
3. Thomas R. Five-year risk of progression of primary angle closure suspects to primary angle closure: a population-based study. Br J Ophthalmol. 2003 Apr 1;87(4):450-4. https://doi.org/10.1136/bjo.87.4.450
4. Mou DP, Liang YB, Fan SJ, Peng Y, Wang NL, Thomas R. Progression rate to primary angle closure following laser peripheral iridotomy in primary angle-closure suspects: a randomised study. Int J Ophthalmol. 2021 Aug 18;14(8):1179-1184. https://doi.org/10.18240/ijo.2021.08.07
5. Yuan Y, Wang W, Xiong R, et al. Fourteen-Year Outcome of Angle-Closure Prevention with Laser Iridotomy in the Zhongshan Angle-Closure Prevention Study. Ophthalmology. 2023 Aug;130(8):786-94. https://doi.org/10.1016/j.ophtha.2023.03.024
6. Alsbirk PH. Anatomical risk factors in primary angle-closure glaucoma. A ten-year follow-up survey based on limbal and axial anterior chamber depths in a high-risk population. Int Ophthalmol. 1992 Sep;16(4-5):265-72. https://doi.org/10.1007/BF00917973
7. He M, Jiang Y, Huang S, et al. Laser peripheral iridotomy for the prevention of angle closure: a single-centre, randomised controlled trial. The Lancet. 2019 Apr;393(10181):1609-18. https://doi.org/10.1016/S0140-6736(18)32607-2
8. Wang L, Huang W, Huang S, et al. Ten-year incidence of primary angle closure in elderly Chinese: the Liwan Eye Study. Br J Ophthalmol. 2019 Mar;103(3):355-60. https://doi.org/10.1136/bjophthalmol-2017-311808
9. Choudhari NS, Khanna RC, Marmamula S, et al. Fifteen-Year Incidence Rate of Primary Angle Closure Disease in the Andhra Pradesh Eye Disease Study. Am J Ophthalmol. 2021 Sep;229:34-44. https://doi.org/10.1016/j.ajo.2021.02.030
10. Vijaya L, Asokan R, Panday M, et al. Six-Year Incidence of Angle-Closure Disease in a South Indian Population: The Chennai Eye Disease Incidence Study. Am J Ophthalmol. 2013 Dec;156(6):1308-1315.e2. https://doi.org/10.1016/j.ajo.2013.07.027
11. Wishart PK, Batterbury M. Ocular hypertension: correlation of anterior chamber angle width and risk of progression to glaucoma. Eye (Lond). 1992;6 (Pt 3):248-56. https://doi.org/10.1038/eye.1992.48
12. Thomas R, Parikh R, Muliyil J, Kumar RS. Five-year risk of progression of primary angle closure to primary angle closure glaucoma: a population-based study. Acta Ophthalmol Scand. 2003 Oct;81(5):480-5. https://doi.org/10.1034/j.1600-0420.2003.00135.x
13. Cedrone C, Mancino R, Ricci F, Cerulli A, Culasso F, Nucci C. The 12-year Incidence of

Glaucoma and Glaucoma-related Visual Field Loss in Italy: The Ponza Eye Study. J Glaucoma. 2012 Jan;21(1):1-6. https://doi.org/10.1097/IJG.0b013e3182027796

14. Wilensky JT, Kaufman PL, Frohlichstein D, et al. Follow-up of Angle-closure Glaucoma Suspects. Am J Ophthalmol. 1993 Mar;115(3):338-46. https://doi.org/10.1016/S0002-9394(14)73585-8
15. Baskaran M, Kumar RS, Friedman DS, et al. The Singapore Asymptomatic Narrow Angles Laser Iridotomy Study. Ophthalmology. 2022 Feb;129(2):147-58. https://doi.org/10.1016/j.ophtha.2021.08.017

Projected rise in primary angle-closure glaucoma prevalence

Ronnie George

The pooled prevalence of PACG among adults aged 40–80 years is estimated to be 0.50%, with approximately 34 million people with PACG in 2040 (Table 1).[1] Demographic changes globally with increasing longevity will result in an increase in these numbers, and meta-analysis has reported projections for the number of persons with PACG in 2040 and 2050. These reports have applied prevalence rates from studies that have used the International Society for Geographical and Epidemiological Ophthalmology definitions for glaucoma to generate these estimates. Most of the prevalence papers were published in the late 1990s. While estimates vary, predictions range from 26.3 million persons with PACG by 2050 to 32 million a decade earlier in 2040.[1,2]

Meta-analysis suggests that 70%–80% of the PACG caseload is in Asia. Estimates from other regions are less precise, as noted above.[3] Most studies from Africa and among Hispanic populations have reported low rates of angle closure. That said, population-based data from these regions are sparse, making it difficult to accurately determine the number of individuals with PACG in the Americas and Africa.

Several factors could result in current projections being overestimates. The COVID pandemic was associated with significant mortality in older age groups, so estimates of population growth among older populations may be too high. This could result in a dip in PACD numbers in the post-pandemic years, but its impact on long-term disease projections is uncertain. Another major factor is the increasing availability of cataract surgery in Asia, which should result in lower rates of PACG than projected, since earlier cataract surgery would alter the course of the disease by opening a closed angle.

Furthermore, the large increase in myopia prevalence, especially in Asia (see next section *Effects of myopia on the prevalence of PACG* for more detail), is yet another important factor that could reduce the prevalence of PACG. Myopia is associated with an increase in AL, which may potentially reduce the incidence of PACG in the future. However, the presence of myopia does not rule out PACG. In a simulation study using random sampling to generate cohorts with varying prevalences of myopia (from 10% to 60%), the projected prevalence of occludable angles in the cohorts with myopia prevalence of 10% to 60% was between 11.1% and 9.6% (95% CI, 8.9%–10.3%) suggesting a not very significant decline in PACG rates attributable to longer AL with myopia.[4] Spherical equivalent has been used to define myopia in most population-based studies, and nuclear cataract can induce index myopia. Since many studies from Asia had substantial numbers of people with unoperated cataracts (including nuclear cataract) this could confound both estimates of myopia and overestimate the occurrence of angle-closure disease in myopic eyes.

Many parts of Asia are also undergoing rapid economic growth, and improvements in healthcare and nutrition could translate into increased height. Since AL and height are weakly correlated,[5] this increase in AL could result in reduced angle-closure numbers over time.

Given that untreated PAC and high-risk PACS carry a higher risk of developing PACG, low eye examination rates in some Asian populations could potentially result in higher numbers of individuals developing PACG than projected.

These projections are for PACG alone. Going by population estimates from China and India,[6,7] the number of people with any form of PACD could be 8 to 10 times the number with PACG or close to 300 million individuals, most of them in Asia. This high prevalence could stress the eyecare infrastructure in the region.

Table 1. Projected prevalence of PACG by region

Study	Year	Projection year	Region	Prevalence (%)	Global number (million)	Regional number (million)
Tham et al.[1]	2014	2040	Global	0.50	32.04	24.5
Zhang et al.[2]	2021	2050	Global	0.6	26.26	18.47
Chan et al.8	2015	2040	Asia	0.73		17.51
Song et al.[9]	2017	2050	China	1.41		14.49
Day et al.[3]	2012	2050	Europe, USA	0.4		3.24

PACG: primary angle-closure glaucoma

References

1. Tham YC, Li X, Wong TY, Quigley HA, Aung T, Cheng CY. Global Prevalence of Glaucoma and Projections of Glaucoma Burden through 2040. Ophthalmology. 2014 Nov;121(11):2081-90. https://doi.org/10.1016/j.ophtha.2014.05.013
2. Zhang N, Wang J, Chen B, Li Y, Jiang B. Prevalence of Primary Angle Closure Glaucoma in the Last 20 Years: A Meta-Analysis and Systematic Review. Front Med. 2021 Jan 18;7:624179. https://doi.org/10.3389/fmed.2020.624179
3. Day AC, Baio G, Gazzard G, et al. The prevalence of primary angle closure glaucoma in European derived populations: a systematic review. Br J Ophthalmol. 2012 Sep;96(9):1162-7. https://doi.org/10.1136/bjophthalmol-2011-301189
4. Jin G, Ding X, Guo X, Chang BHW, Odouard C, He M. Does Myopia Affect Angle Closure Prevalence. Investig Opthalmology Vis Sci. 2015 Aug 27;56(9):5714. https://doi.org/10.1167/iovs.15-16914
5. Jiang Y, He M, Friedman DS, et al. Associations between Narrow Angle and Adult Anthropometry: The Liwan Eye Study. Ophthalmic Epidemiol. 2014 Jun;21(3):184-9. https://doi.org/10.3109/09286586.2014.903500
6. Foster PJ. Glaucoma in China: how big is the problem? Br J Ophthalmol. 2001 Nov 1;85(11):1277-82. https://doi.org/10.1136/bjo.85.11.1277
7. George R, Ve RS, Vijaya L. Glaucoma in India: Estimated Burden of Disease. J Glaucoma. 2010 Aug;19(6):391-7. https://doi.org/10.1097/IJG.0b013e3181c4ac5b
8. Chan EW, Li X, Tham YC, et al. Glaucoma in Asia: regional prevalence variations and future projections. Br J Ophthalmol. 2016 Jan;100(1):78-85. https://doi.org/10.1136/bjophthalmol-2014-306102
9. Song P, Wang J, Bucan K, Theodoratou E, Rudan I, Chan KY. National and subnational prevalence and burden of glaucoma in China: A systematic analysis. J Glob Health. 2017 Dec;7(2):020705. https://doi.org/10.7189/jogh.07.020705

Effects of myopia on the prevalence of PACG

Mingguang He

Over the past 3 decades, the rapid rise in myopia prevalence has led to a “myopia epidemic.” Currently, 10%–30% of adults in many countries are affected by myopia, with prevalence in East and Southeast Asia exceeding 80% among young adults in urban regions.[1] By 2050, myopia is projected to affect 4.76 billion (49.8%) individuals globally, with nearly 1 billion (9.8%) cases of high myopia anticipated.[2] The rise in myopia prevalence is largely attributed to modern lifestyle factors, such as increased near-work activities and reduced time spent outdoors, both of which are associated with higher levels of educational attainment.

Myopia is considered "protective" against PACG. Myopia is characterized by features such as longer AL, deeper ACD, larger anterior chamber volume, and a wider ACA. These characteristics are considered the opposite of established risk factors for PACG (*e.g.*, hyperopia, short AL, shallow ACD, and thicker lenses).

The observed increase in myopia prevalence in Asia, especially axial myopia, may potentially decrease the future risk of PACG. For instance, eyes with longer AL tend to have a lower prevalence of iris-trabecular meshwork contact, a factor associated with PACG risk.[3] As myopia prevalence increases and populations shift towards longer AL, assessing its influence on PACG prevalence is essential. The impact of increasing myopia on glaucoma prevalence (both primary open-angle glaucoma and PACG) is a research priority.

Could the myopia epidemic shift the risk of PACG?

The Liwan Eye Study on elderly Chinese populations previously demonstrated an inverse relationship between ACD and spherical equivalent, with per diopter spherical equivalent increase corresponding to a mean 0.03 mm decrease in ACD.[4] Similar studies on multiethnic populations demonstrated a protective effect of myopia on PACG, with each 1-diopter decrease in spherical equivalent associated with a 22% reduction in PACG prevalence.[5,6] More recently, in a large population consisting of over 10,000 individuals aged 30 and older, Jonas *et al.* found that myopia and longer AL were associated with lower PACG prevalence.[7]

Notably, studies on populations in China and Alaskan Eskimos, 2 groups with increasing myopia prevalence, have documented shallower ACA depth in older age groups.[8,9] This difference may be due to higher myopia prevalence among younger individuals, resulting in greater axial elongation and deeper ACA than older cohorts. There is a hypothesis that if these trends persist, the future burden of PACG in younger, myopic populations may decrease.

Does the myopia epidemic lower the prevalence of PACG?

Based on the evidence that myopia lowers PACG risk, one might expect a lower PACG prevalence with the myopia epidemic, especially in Asia. However, there remains some uncertainty around this. One simulation study modeled myopia prevalence levels from 10% to 60% to assess the impact on occludable angle prevalence—a surrogate marker for PACG.[10] Although increased ACD with higher myopia prevalence was observed in this simulation, this resulted in a reduction of PACG prevalence remained by only 1.5%, which is unlikely to impact disease numbers significantly.

Furthermore, despite the high myopia prevalence, Chinese populations continue to experience significant PACG.[11] Comparatively, PACG patients in Asia show a higher prevalence of myopia than those in Western populations, with 22%–37% of PACG patients in Asia having myopia, contrasting with a 0.05%–1.9% prevalence in the United States.[11-13] High myopia, however, remains uncommon among PACG patients, comprising only 1.1%–2.5% of cases in Asian populations.[13,14]

Possible mechanisms of angle closure in PACG patients with axial myopia

Not all myopic eyes have deep ACDs despite their longer AL and vitreous length, especially when considering relative dimensions within the eye. Some myopic eyes may present anterior segment characteristics similar to those of hyperopic or emmetropic eyes, such as shallow ACD and narrow ACA, as they have small anterior segment dimensions.[13,15,16] Studies suggest that when myopia primarily results from vitreous cavity elongation, the effect on PACG prevalence may be less, reinforcing that ACD—not AL or refractive status—is the primary risk factor for angle closure.[17] Additional anterior segment features, including ciliary body thickness, iris parameters, and anterior chamber width and volume, may also contribute to angle-closure risk among myopic eyes with shallow ACD.[10]

Lens position is another factor to consider; myopic eyes often have a more anterior lens position despite longer AL, while hyperopic eyes tend to have thicker lenses positioned slightly posteriorly.[11,15] In some myopic PACG cases, the lens is excessively thick and anteriorly positioned, crowding the anterior segment and contributing to a shallow ACD.[14] Zonular laxity may also contribute to PACG risk in myopic eyes, underscoring the need to comprehensively evaluate lens and anterior segment characteristics in myopic PACG patients.[18]

Conclusions for myopia and PACG

The role of myopia in PACG prevalence remains complex and controversial, as evidence from existing studies indicates differing associations (Table 1). Although longer AL in myopic eyes is associated with reduced PACG risk, some epidemiological studies show a relatively high proportion of myopia among PACG patients, suggesting that the myopia epidemic may have minimal impact on overall PACG prevalence. Anterior segment characteristics—such as ACD and lens position—appear to exert a stronger influence on PACG risk than AL or refractive status. Thus, even in myopic patients, it is essential to carefully assess anterior segment and lens characteristics to evaluate PACG risk accurately.

Table 1. Literature comparison on myopia's effect on PACG prevalence

No	Study	Population	Sample size	Age (years)	Findings	Conclusion
Evidence suggesting myopia decreases PACG risk						
1	Wojcie-chowski et al., 2003	Alaskan Eskimos	133	40+	A pronounced age-related decline in ACA depth was observed in Eskimos and Chinese, populations with high myopia prevalence.	Deeper ACA in younger populations may be linked to higher myopia prevalence compared to older individuals.
2	Yip et al., 2011	Mongolian	1,892	50+	Lower educational levels were significantly associated with increased PACG risk.	Low education may independently increase PACG risk in East Asia, possibly by influencing ocular biometric traits such as AL.
3	Shen et al., 2016	Multiethnic cohort in the USA	34,040 cases and 403,398 controls	35+	Each 1-diopter decrease in spherical equivalent was linked to a 22% reduction in PACG prevalence.	Hyperopia substantially increases PACG risk.
4	Zhou et al., 2023	Chinese Americans	3970	50+	Hyperopic eyes had over 5 times the PACG risk of myopic eyes, with ACD as a stronger PACG predictor than refractive error.	Myopia is linked to lower PACG risk, with ACD being a key factor in angle-closure risk.
5	Jonas et al., 2024	Multiethnic cohort from Russia, China, and India	15,049	30+	Longer AL, representing myopia, correlated with a lower prevalence of ACG.	Myopia appears protective against ACG.

No	Study	Population	Sample size	Age (years)	Findings	Conclusion
Evidence suggesting myopia does not affect PACG prevalence						
6	Yong et al., 2014	Asian	427	41–93	Approximately 22% of angle-closure patients were myopic: 29.8% had moderate and 11.7% had high myopia. Myopic angle-closure patients had longer AL and VL but similar ACD, lens thickness, and lens vault as non-myopic counterparts.	A substantial proportion of angle-closure patients have myopia. Despite longer AL, the shallow ACD in myopic patients may still lead to angle closure.
7	Jin et al., 2015	Chinese	1160	50+	As myopia prevalence rose, mean ACD increased slightly, but OA prevalence reduction was minimal (from 11.1% to 9.6%).	Increasing myopia prevalence minimally affects OA prevalence.
8	Mohamed-Noor et al., 2017	Malaysian	137	21–88	Myopia (37.2%) and hyperopia (35.8%) were similarly distributed among PACD patients. Myopic PACD patients had shallower ACD than non-myopic patients.	Myopia is common in PACG patients, and shallow ACD in myopic PACG patients underscores the need to monitor anterior chamber characteristics in this group.
9	Li et al., 2018	Chinese	138	36–94	PAC patients with longer AL (10.9%) were with unique traits like flatter corneas, larger ACW, and more anterior lens positions. Despite larger absolute anterior segments, they had smaller relative dimensions.	In eyes with longer AL, specific anterior segment characteristics, such as relative lens positioning, can contribute to angle closure.

No	Study	Population	Sample size	Age (years)	Findings	Conclusion
10	Loh et al., 2020	Malaysian	171	30+	Among PACD eyes, 51% were hyperopic, 31% were emmetropic, and 18% were myopic. Myopic PACD eyes had longer AL and VL but similar ACD across groups. Anterior lens position contributes to angle closure in myopic eyes.	Anterior lens positioning may predispose myopic eyes to angle closure.
11	Liang et al., 2022	Chinese	6791	30+	Myopia prevalence was 13.7% among PACD cases, with higher rates in PACG (62.5%) versus PAC (21.6%) and PACS (11.6%).	Myopia presence in PACD cases with shallow ACD and thick lenses indicates significant risk factors, especially in myopic patients.
12	Chen et al., 2023	Chinese	742	65.98 (average)	Among PACG eyes, 33.9% were myopic, and 12% had long AL ($\geq$ 23.5 mm). PACG eyes with long AL had lower keratometry values, larger ACD, and a more anterior lens position (both absolute and relative).	An anteriorly positioned lens could predispose myopic eyes with long AL to angle closure.

ACA: anterior chamber angle; ACD: anterior chamber depth; ACG: angle-closure glaucoma; AL: axial length; OA: occludable angle; PAC: primary angle closure; PACD: primary angle-closure disease; PACG: primary angle-closure glaucoma; PACS: primary angle-closure suspect; VA: visual acuity; VL: vitreous length; RLP: relative lens position

References

1. Baird PN, Saw SM, Lanca C, et al. Myopia. Nat Rev Dis Primers. 2020; 6(1):99. https://doi.org/10.1038/s41572-020-00231-4
2. Holden BA, Fricke TR, Wilson DA, et al. Global Prevalence of Myopia and High Myopia and Temporal Trends from 2000 through 2050. Ophthalmology. 2016;123(5):1036-42. https://doi.org/10.1016/j.ophtha.2016.01.006
3. Liu X, Ye H, Zhang Q, et al. Association between Myopia, Biometry and Occludable Angle: The Jiangning Eye Study. PLoS One. 2016;11(10):e0165281.https://doi.org/10.1371/journal.pone.016528
4. He M, Huang W, Zheng Y, Alsbirk PH, Foster PJ. Anterior chamber depth in elderly Chinese: the Liwan eye study. Ophthalmology. 2008; 115(8):1286-90, 90.e1-2. https://doi.org/10.1016/j.ophtha.2007.12.003
5. Shen L, Melles RB, Metlapally R, et al. The Association of Refractive Error with Glaucoma in a Multiethnic Population. Ophthalmology. 2016; 123(1):92-101. https://doi.org/10.1016/j.ophtha.2015.07.002
6. Zhou S, Pardeshi AA, Burkemper B, et al. Refractive Error and Anterior Chamber Depth as Risk Factors in Primary Angle Closure Disease: The Chinese American Eye Study. J Glaucoma. 2023;32(4):257-64. https://doi.org/10.1097/IJG.0000000000002154
7. Jonas JB, Bikbov MM, Kazakbaeva GM, et al. Positive and Negative Associations of Myopia with Ocular Diseases in Population-Based Studies. Ophthalmology. 2024 Dec;131(12):1427-1435. https://doi.org/10.1016/j.ophtha.2024.07.003
8. Zhao LL, Lu XZ, Tang GD, et al. Anterior chamber and angle characteristics in Chinese children (6-11 years old) with different refractive status using swept-source optical coherence tomography. BMC Ophthalmol. 2024;24(1):259. https://doi.org/10.1186/s12886-024-03520-8
9. Wojciechowski R, Congdon N, Anninger W, Teo Broman A. Age, gender, biometry, refractive error, and the anterior chamber angle among Alaskan Eskimos. Ophthalmology. 2003;110(2):365-75. https://doi.org/10.1016/S0161-6420(02)01748-7
10. Jin G, Ding X, Guo X, Chang BH, Odouard C, He M. Does Myopia Affect Angle Closure Prevalence. Invest Ophthalmol Vis Sci. 2015;56(9):5714-9. https://doi.org/10.1167/iovs.15-16914
11. Loh CC, Kamaruddin H, Bastion MC, Husain R, Mohd Isa H, Md Din N. Evaluation of Refractive Status and Ocular Biometric Parameters in Primary Angle Closure Disease. Ophthalmic Res. 2021;64(2):246-52. https://doi.org/10.1159/000510925
12. Li S, Shao M, Wan Y, Tang B, Sun X, Cao W. Relationship between ocular biometry and severity of primary angle-closure glaucoma: relevance for predictive, preventive, and personalized medicine. EPMA J. 2019;10(3):261-71. https://doi.org/10.1007/s13167-019-00174-1
13. Mohamed-Noor J, Abd-Salam D. Refractive errors and biometry of primary angle-closure disease in a mixed Malaysian population. Int J Ophthalmol. 2017;10(8):1246-50.
14. Chen J, Zhang Y, Huang Y, Ng TK, Huang C. Relatively anterior lens position in primary

angle-closure glaucoma eyes with long axial length. Indian J Ophthalmol. 2023;71(5):1941-7. https://doi.org/10.4103/ijo.IJO_1890_22

15. Li M, Chen Y, Jiang Z, Chen X, Chen J, Sun X. What Are the Characteristics of Primary Angle Closure With Longer Axial Length? Invest Ophthalmol Vis Sci. 2018;59(3):1354-9. https://doi.org/10.1167/iovs.17-23711
16. Yong KL, Gong T, Nongpiur ME, et al. Myopia in asian subjects with primary angle closure: implications for glaucoma trends in East Asia. Ophthalmology. 2014;121(8):1566-71. https://doi.org/10.1016/j.ophtha.2014.02.006
17. Shon K, Sung KR, Yoon JY. Implications of the Relationship Between Refractive Error and Biometry in the Pathogenesis of Primary Angle Closure. Invest Ophthalmol Vis Sci. 2021;62(10):38. https://doi.org/10.1167/iovs.62.10.38
18. Dagi LR, Walton DS. Anterior axial lens subluxation, progressive myopia, and angle-closure glaucoma: recognition and treatment of atypical presentation of ectopia lentis. J AAPOS. 2006;10(4):345-50. https://doi.org/10.1016/j.jaapos.2006.01.218

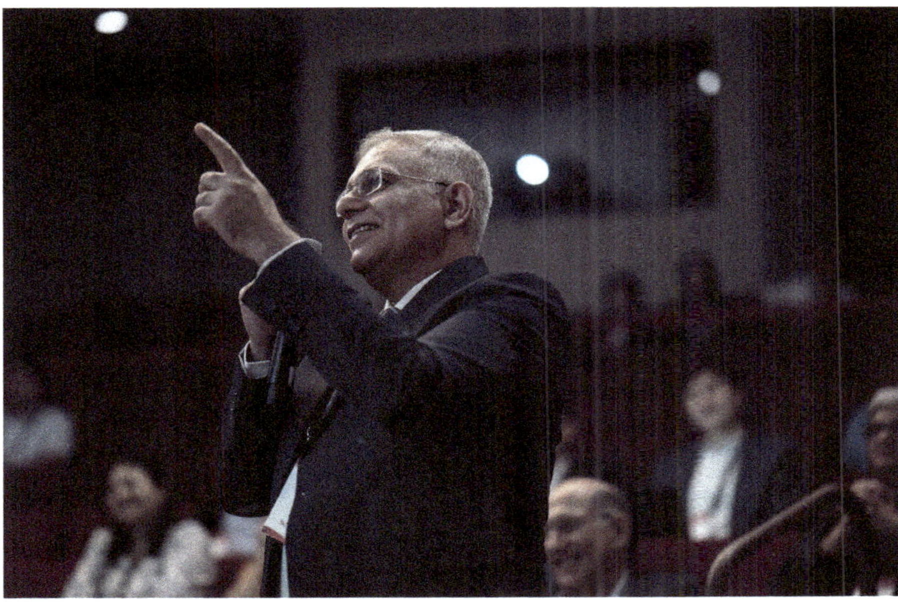

Tanuj Dada

Section Leaders

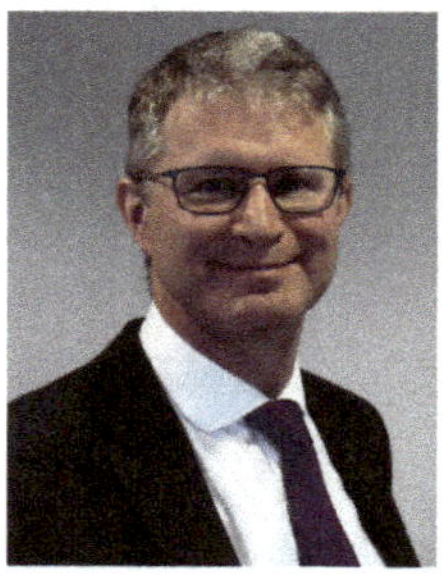

Paul Foster

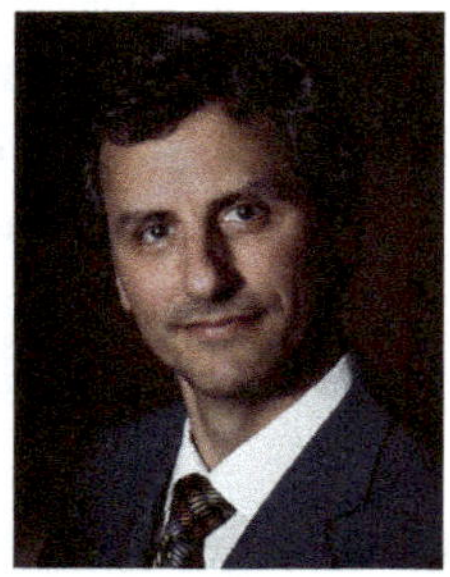

David Friedman

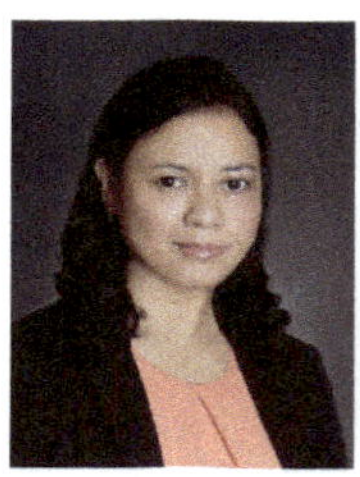

Monisha Nongpiur

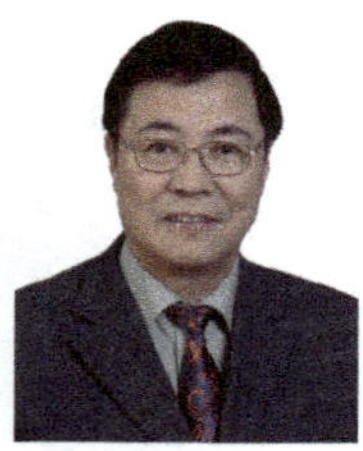

Ningli Wang

2. GENETICS AND PATHOPHYSIOLOGY

David Friedman, Paul Foster, Monisha Nongpiur, Ningli Wang

Abbreviations
AAC: acute angle closure
ACD: anterior chamber depth
ACW: anterior chamber width
AL: axial length
AS-OCT: anterior segment optical coherence tomography
ECM: extracellular matrix
GWAS: genome-wide association studies
IOP: intraocular pressure
LV: lens vault
PAC: primary angle closure
PACD: primary angle-closure disease
PACG: primary angle-closure glaucoma
PACS: primary angle-closure suspect
SNP: single nucleotide polymorphism
sPAC: spectrum of primary angle closure

Consensus statements

1. First-degree relatives of individuals with sPAC, defined as PACS, PAC, or PACG, are at significantly higher risk of angle closure supporting its genetic basis.
    - Large-scale GWAS have identified genetic loci associated with PACG.
    - Known genetic variants associated with PACG have small effect sizes.
2. Evidence to recommend genetic testing for PACD, defined as PAC or PACG, is limited.

Angle Closure and Angle-Closure Glaucoma, pp 1-19
Edited by Robert N. Weinreb, Benjamin Xu, David Friedman, Xiulan Zhang

3. Risk conferred by hyperopic refractive error is secondary to its association with ocular biometrics, specifically shorter AL and shallower ACD.
    - ACD alone does not explain racial and ethnic differences in angle-closure prevalence.
4. Pupillary block is the major mechanism, accounting for 75% of all PAC.
5. Association studies suggest that dynamic changes in iris and choroidal volume are involved in the pathogenesis of PACD.
    - Choroidal effusion can be found in PAC and PACG eyes.
    - PACS, PAC, and PACG are associated with greater choroidal thickness.
    - Supraciliary effusion can result in anterior rotation of the ciliary body and angle closure.
    - Accumulation of aqueous in the vitreous cavity and greater resistance to fluid exchange across the anterior hyaloid can precipitate angle closure from aqueous misdirection (also sometimes termed vitreous block).
    - Malignant glaucoma is an ambiguous term that is not adequately descriptive of the disease process.
6. Vitreous block, collagen abnormalities, autonomic dysfunction, and zonulopathy likely contribute to angle-closure pathogenesis but are not directly measurable using available tools.

Future directions

- More research is needed on iris thickness, which has emerged as an important anatomical risk factor for PACD.
- Serial studies, including follow-up on the Zhongshan Angle Closure Prevention study cohort, are needed to establish the precise nature of the relationship between PACG with dynamic changes in iris volume and choroidal volume.

Genetics

Monisha Nongpiur, Tin Aung, Janey Wiggs, Eranga Vithana, Ching-Yu Cheng

Genetic basis of angle-closure glaucoma

PACG is, in part, genetically determined with higher risk among first-degree relatives[1-4] and significant heritability of ocular risk factors related to angle closure.[5-8]

Heritability of PACG-related ocular parameters

Heritability measures the proportion of phenotypic variation due to genetic factors. The heritability for ACD and AL ranges from 50%–90%, depending on the population.[5,7,8,12] The Beaver Dam Eye Study estimated heritability at 0.67 for AL and 0.78 for ACD.[7] Other studies, including those on twins from Australia and China, confirmed high heritability estimates, with Chinese populations showing heritability for ACD as high as 90.1%.[5] ACW demonstrated a high heritability of 98%,[12] while heritability estimates for iris parameters ranged from 44% to 80%.[12,13] Biometric features of the eye have been demonstrated to have much stronger heritability than AS-OCT parameters, though inter-sibling agreement in several AS-OCT parameters (iris curvature, ACD, anterior chamber area, anterior chamber volume, LV) strongly predicts concordance of angle-closure phenotype across siblings.[8]

Familial predisposition

Family history is an important risk factor of PACD.[2,4] Certain ocular traits, such as shallower anterior chambers and thicker lenses, are more common in these relatives.[1,2, 9-11] Studies from Singapore highlight the high heritability (approximately 60%) of narrow angles, with a sibling recurrence risk of nearly 50% and a sibling relative risk of 7.57.[3] A study from South India found that siblings of a proband with PAC/PACG have a 14 fold greater odds of having angle closure (as opposed to open angle control).[12] Further investigation found that siblings of those with PAC or PACG, but not those with PACS, also had a higher risk of PAC/(G), suggesting that heritability of iridotrabecular contact and its sequelae (*e.g.*, IOP elevation and glaucomatous optic neuropathy) may be under differential genetic control.

Genes associated with PACG

Candidate gene approach and GWAS have been used to identify genes associated with PACG.

Candidate gene approach

Over 50 candidate genes have been studied for their association with PACG, typically using small case-control studies with fewer than 500 samples. These genes were selected based on their potential involvement in mechanisms relevant to PACG, such as ECM remodeling, or those that influence AL, IOP, and optic nerve changes in glaucoma.[14,15]

A missense variant (rs17576, Gln279Arg) in Matrix metalloproteinase-9 (*MMP9*), a gene involved in ECM remodeling, has shown varying associations with PACG across populations.[16-19] A meta-analysis identified *MMP9* and 4 other genes/loci (*HGF*, *HSP70*, *MFRP*, *NOS3*) as linked to PACG, with pathways involving *MMP9* being particularly significant.[20] A more recent meta-analysis identified 11 SNPs in 10 genes/loci (*ABCC5*, *ATOH7*, *CALCRL*, *FBN1*, *HGF*, *IL6*, *LOXL1*, *MMP19*, *PLEKHA7*, and *VAV3*) associated with PACG.[21] *MMP9* is a zinc-dependent proteolytic enzyme that plays a key role in ECM degradation and tissue remodeling,[20] thereby playing an important role in the pathogenesis of PACG. Altered *MMP9* levels have been implicated in abnormal ECM degradation and dysfunction of the trabecular meshwork.[21] Smaller eye dimensions, often associated with nanophthalmos and microphthalmia, also increase the risk of angle closure. Genetic factors influencing eye size, such as the *MFRP* gene, have been implicated in PACG, with SNP rs3814762 (missense change) in *MFRP* showing an association in a meta-analysis.[20] Other genes of interest include *HGF*, which plays a role in anterior segment morphology and has been linked to PACG in populations with smaller eyes.[22] Studies have also explored the roles of *CHX10*, *TMEM98*, and loci associated with nanophthalmos.[23-26]

GWAS

GWAS are useful for identifying genes related to complex diseases by comparing allele frequencies between cases and controls.

A 2-stage PACG GWAS by Vithana *et al.*[27] analyzed 1,854 PACG cases and 9,608 controls across 5 Asian countries, with replication in 1,917 cases and 8,943 controls from additional countries. They found significant associations with 3 novel genetic loci: *PLEKHA7* (rs11024102), *COL11A1* (rs3753841), and a region between *PCMTD1* and *ST18* on chromosome 8q (rs1015213).[27] A subsequent GWAS, combining data from 10,404 PACG cases and 29,343 controls across 23 countries, identified 5 new significant loci: *EPDR1* (rs3816415), *CHAT* (rs1258267), *GLIS3* (rs736893), *FERMT2* (rs7494379), and a locus between *DPM2* and *FAM102A* on chromosome 9 (rs3739821).[28] These loci showed consistent associations with PACG across multiple study populations and low heterogeneity.[28] It is important to note that these loci are named for the nearest gene, which may not always be the "causal" gene.

Selected genes from these loci are expressed in ocular tissues involved in PACG, such as the iris and trabecular meshwork, and play roles in key processes like cell adhesion, ECM remodeling, and fluid dynamics. Following is a brief overview of the function of selected genes from these loci (usually the gene closest to the

SNP with the best evidence for association and may not be the causal for PACG at this locus):

- *PLEKHA7* encodes a protein involved in the maintenance and stability of adherens junctions,[29] playing a key role in regulating paracellular permeability, the blood-aqueous barrier (BAB), and fluid dynamics. The reduced expression of *PLEKHA7* in ocular tissues of PACG patients suggests that a compromised BAB may contribute to impaired aqueous humor outflow.[30,31] This finding aligns with earlier research linking BAB dysfunction, characterized by the leakage of inflammatory factors, to increased IOP in PACG.[32,33] It is plausible that the resulting inflammatory response may also promote the formation of peripheral anterior synechiae. Importantly, *PLEKHA7* has also been identified associated with IOP and POAG,[34 35] suggesting that it may influence disease risk by contributing to elevated IOP.
- *COL11A1* encodes the alpha-1 chain of type XI collagen, a key interstitial ECM component.[36] Dominant negative mutations of *COL11A1* are linked to Marshall syndrome, type 2 Stickler syndrome, and Stickler-like syndrome,[37] where abnormal collagen in the sclera is likely responsible for axial myopia, a common characteristic of these conditions. A common variant in the coding region of *COL11A1* has been associated with PACG in GWAS.[27] In PACG, eyes typically exhibit hyperopia and a shorter AL, suggesting that the common *COL11A1* variant may produce a different phenotypic effect, which remains to be fully understood.
- *PCMTD1-ST18* locus, includes *PCMTD1*, which has an unknown function, and *ST18*, which is involved in apoptosis and inflammation.[38, 39] This locus is associated with early stages of angle-closure disease, suggesting a role in narrow angle configuration.[40]
- *EPDR1* encodes ependymin-related 1, a cell adhesion molecule,[41] ubiquitously expressed in ocular tissues.[28] Although its specific role in PACG is not fully elucidated, it may be involved in cell adhesion processes within the eye. *EPDR1* is associated with severe PACG and has also been linked to PACS, albeit with lower significance and effect size.[42] This suggests that *EPDR1* may have a dual function in PACD, potentially contributing to both the predisposition for narrow drainage angles and the development of severe glaucomatous optic neuropathy, with a more pronounced role in the development of severe disease.[42]
- For the *DPM2-FAM102A* locus, *DPM2* is involved in glycosylation,[43] while *FAM102A* has an unclear function. The study that identified the association between *PCMTD1-ST18* and PACS status also highlighted *DPM2-FAM102A*,

indicating that both loci may play a similar role in angle-closure disease.[40]

- *CHAT* encodes the enzyme choline acetyltransferase, which is crucial for synthesizing the neurotransmitter acetylcholine. Acetylcholine plays a vital role in the autonomic nervous system and is involved in parasympathetic pupillary reflexes as well as various other ocular functions.[44, 45]
- *GLIS3* encodes a transcription factor involved in regulating apoptosis and autophagy.[46,47] *GLIS3* is highly expressed in the brain and plays a dynamic role during embryonic neurulation.[46] *GLIS3* mutations are linked to various disorders, including congenital hypothyroidism, osteoarthritis, Alzheimer's disease types 1 and 2, and neonatal diabetes.[48-51] Although *GLIS3* has been repeatedly associated with IOP,[34,35,52,53] the precise mechanism by which it contributes to PACG remains unclear.
- *FERMT2* encodes for a protein called pleckstrin homology domain-containing family C member 1 (*PLEKHC1*), involved in cell adhesion and ECM remodeling.[54] *PLEKHC1*, similar to *PLEKHA7*, is crucial in maintaining the vascular barrier by stabilizing adherens junctions.[55] In a knockdown mouse model, disruption of *PLEKHC1* led to impaired wound healing and increased neovascular permeability.[56]

While the 2 PACG GWAS primarily included Asian populations, emerging evidence suggests that the genetic profile of PACG differs in Caucasians. Luben *et al.* (ARVO meeting abstract)[57] conducted the first PACG GWAS in Europeans, analyzing 440,611 discovery and 8,536 replication participants, including 1,783 and 694 PACG cases, respectively. They identified novel loci at *HERC2* and *SEMA3A*, genes associated with iris morphology and pigmentation,[58,59] indicating that these loci may influence PACG risk through alterations in iris anatomy.

Quantitative trait locus analysis

Another approach to uncovering genetic factors in complex diseases involves studying heritable quantitative traits or endophenotypes associated with the disease. GWAS for quantitative traits generally use linear regression to analyze trait data.

Using GWAS, an ACD quantitative trait locus was identified in a region on chromosome 3 that includes the ATP-binding Cassette Subfamily C Member 5 (*ABCC5*) gene.[60] SNP rs1401999, the lead variant in this locus, is linked to an increased risk for PACG in a separate case-control study. *ABCC5*, or multidrug resistance protein 5,[61,62] plays a role in cellular processes, such as drug efflux, and is expressed in ocular structures relevant to PACG, such as the iris, ciliary body, and lens. Its involvement in eye development and its association with shallower

ACD suggest it may influence eye growth, particularly in the anterior segment.[63] However, the exact role of *ABCC5* in PACG is still unclear. Further research with a larger GWAS dataset revealed only a nominal association between *ABCC5* and PACG.[60]

Deep sequencing to identify large effect mutations in PACG patients

Given the technological advances and reducing costs of next-generation sequencing methods, it should be considered a future method of molecular diagnosis and early treatment for PACG. Utility of this method requires the genetic analysis of patients with PACG to determine the contribution of rare variants and alleles associated with glaucoma. Through exome sequencing of 10,000 PACG patients and matched controls, Loo *et al.* identified novel variants in the gene *UBOX5* (U-box domain containing 5) that are associated with PACG.[64] Proving causality of discovered rare variants would necessitate segregation analyses and functional studies.

Clinical implications of PACG genetics

Despite the identification of susceptibility genes and loci for PACG, their precise role in disease pathogenesis and progression remains elusive. The initial GWAS for PACG identified 3 susceptibility loci and highlighted 3 candidate genes for causality, *COL11A1*, *PLEKHA7*, and *PCMTD-ST18*.[27] However, subsequent studies have not consistently demonstrated a correlation between these genes or variants located within these loci and variations in ocular biometric factors[65,66] or as markers of disease severity and progression.[67] This inconsistency may be due to limited study power or the possibility that these genes influence the disease through mechanisms not yet understood.

Two of the 8 PACG loci, specifically *PCMTD1-ST18* and *DPM2-FAM102A*, are significantly associated with PACS status, the earliest stage of the spectrum of PAC.[40] This association implies that these loci may contribute to susceptibility to a narrow-angle configuration. A subsequent study examining the relationship between PACG loci and disease severity found that the *EPDR1* locus was significantly associated with severe PACG, indicating that it may increase susceptibility to more aggressive disease progression.[42] Additionally, individuals with PACG who had a higher genetic risk score were more likely to experience severe PACG compared to those with early to moderate forms of the disease.[42] Another study comparing the diagnostic value of these 8 susceptibility genes with that of ACD alone found only a marginal improvement (0.5%) in PACG detection when including these susceptibility loci.[68]

Currently, genetic risk scoring offers limited clinical utility because the combined influence of the 8 GWAS genes explains only 1.8% of the genetic risk for PACG.[28] Recent reports highlighting the effectiveness of polygenic risk scores for POAG demonstrate that at least 50–100 genetic loci are necessary to create a useful clinical tool.[69-71] Notably, the confirmation of overlap between POAG and PACG in IOP-related genes suggests shared pathways, altering our understanding of these 2 types of glaucoma.[35] Leveraging this expanding genetic knowledge could lead to more personalized management strategies and improved clinical applications for PACG.

References

1. Lowe RF. Primary angle-closure glaucoma. Inheritance and environment. Br J Ophthalmol. 1972;56:13-20. https://doi.org/10.1136/bjo.56.1.13
2. Alsbirk PH. Primary angle-closure glaucoma. Oculometry, epidemiology, and genetics in a high-risk population. Acta Ophthalmol. 1976;Suppl:5-31.
3. Amerasinghe N, Zhang J, Thalamuthu A, et al. The heritability and sibling risk of angle closure in Asians. Ophthalmology. 2011;118:480-5. https://doi.org/10.1016/j.ophtha.2010.06.043
4. Kavitha S, Zebardast N, Palaniswamy K, et al. Family history is a strong risk factor for prevalent angle closure in a South Indian population. Ophthalmology 2014;121:2091-7. https://doi.org/10.1016/j.ophtha.2014.05.001
5. He M, Wang D, Zheng Y, et al. Heritability of anterior chamber depth as an intermediate phenotype of angle-closure in Chinese: the Guangzhou Twin Eye Study. Invest Ophthalmol Vis Sci. 2008;49:81-6. https://doi.org/10.1167/iovs.07-1052
6. He M, Ge J, Wang D, et al. Heritability of the iridotrabecular angle width measured by optical coherence tomography in Chinese children: the Guangzhou twin eye study. Invest Ophthalmol Vis Sci. 2008;49:1356-61. https://doi.org/10.1167/iovs.07-1397
7. Klein AP, Suktitipat B, Duggal P, et al. Heritability analysis of spherical equivalent, axial length, corneal curvature, and anterior chamber depth in the Beaver Dam Eye Study. Arch Ophthalmol. 2009;127:649-55. https://doi.org/10.1001/archophthalmol.2009.61
8. Dirani M, Chamberlain M, Shekar SN, et al. Heritability of refractive error and ocular biometrics: the Genes in Myopia (GEM) twin study. Invest Ophthalmol Vis Sci. 2006;47:4756-61. https://doi.org/10.1167/iovs.06-0270
9. Lowe RF. Primary Angle-Closure Glaucoma. Family Histories and Anterior Chamber Depths. Br J Ophthalmol. 1964;48:191-5. https://doi.org/10.1136/bjo.48.4.191
10. Tomlinson A, Leighton DA. Ocular dimensions in the heredity of angle-closure glaucoma. Br J Ophthalmol. 1973;57:475-86. https://doi.org/10.1136/bjo.57.7.475
11. Leighton DA. Survey of the first-degree relatives of glaucoma patients. Trans Ophthalmol Soc U K (1962). 1976;96:28-32.

12. Ciociola EC, Kavitha S, Sengupta S, et al. The Heritability of Primary Angle Closure Anatomic Traits and Predictors of Angle Closure in South Indian Siblings. Am J Ophthalmol. 2021;230:188-199. https://doi.org/10.1016/j.ajo.2021.04.038
13. He M, Wang D, Console JW, Zhang J, Zheng Y, Huang W. Distribution and heritability of iris thickness and pupil size in Chinese: the Guangzhou Twin Eye Study. Invest Ophthalmol Vis Sci. 2009;50:1593-7. https://doi.org/10.1167/iovs.08-2735
14. Vranka JA, Kelley MJ, Acott TS, Keller KE. Extracellular matrix in the trabecular meshwork: intraocular pressure regulation and dysregulation in glaucoma. Exp Eye Res. 2015;133:112-25. https://doi.org/10.1016/j.exer.2014.07.014
15. Wallace DM, O'Brien CJ. The role of lamina cribrosa cells in optic nerve head fibrosis in glaucoma. Exp Eye Res. 2016;142:102-9. https://doi.org/10.1016/j.exer.2014.12.006
16. Wang IJ, Chiang TH, Shih YF, et al. The association of single nucleotide polymorphisms in the MMP-9 genes with susceptibility to acute primary angle closure glaucoma in Taiwanese patients. Mol Vis. 2006;12:1223-32.
17. Aung T, Yong VH, Lim MC, et al. Lack of association between the rs2664538 polymorphism in the MMP-9 gene and primary angle closure glaucoma in Singaporean subjects. J Glaucoma. 2008;17:257-8. https://doi.org/10.1097/IJG.0b013e31815c3aa5
18. Cong Y, Guo X, Liu X, et al. Association of the single nucleotide polymorphisms in the extracellular matrix metalloprotease-9 gene with PACG in southern China. Mol Vis. 2009;15:1412-7.
19. Awadalla MS, Burdon KP, Kuot A, Hewitt AW, Craig JE. Matrix metalloproteinase-9 genetic variation and primary angle closure glaucoma in a Caucasian population. Mol Vis. 2011;17:1420-4.
20. Rong SS, Tang FY, Chu WK, et al. Genetic Associations of Primary Angle-Closure Disease: A Systematic Review and Meta-analysis. Ophthalmology. 2016;123:1211-21. https://doi.org/10.1016/j.ophtha.2015.12.027
21. Liang YJ, Wang YY, Rong SS, et al. Genetic Associations of Primary Angle-Closure Disease: A Systematic Review and Meta-Analysis. JAMA Ophthalmol. 2024;142:437-444. https://doi.org/10.1001/jamaophthalmol.2024.0363
22. Hu DN, Ritch R. Hepatocyte growth factor is increased in the aqueous humor of glaucomatous eyes. J Glaucoma. 2001;10:152-7. https://doi.org/10.1097/00061198-200106000-00002
23. Aung T, Lim MC, Wong TT, et al. Molecular analysis of CHX10 and MFRP in Chinese subjects with primary angle closure glaucoma and short axial length eyes. Mol Vis. 2008;14:1313-8.
24. Awadalla MS, Burdon KP, Souzeau E, et al. Mutation in TMEM98 in a large white kindred with autosomal dominant nanophthalmos linked to 17p12-q12. JAMA Ophthalmol. 2014;132:970-7. https://doi.org/10.1001/jamaophthalmol.2014.946
25. Khorram D, Choi M, Roos BR, et al. Novel TMEM98 mutations in pedigrees with autosomal dominant nanophthalmos. Mol Vis. 2015;21:1017-23.

26. Hu Z, Yu C, Li J, et al. A novel locus for congenital simple microphthalmia family mapping to 17p12-q12. Invest Ophthalmol Vis Sci. 2011;52:3425-9. https://doi.org/10.1167/iovs.10-6747
27. Vithana EN, Khor CC, Qiao C, et al. Genome-wide association analyses identify three new susceptibility loci for primary angle closure glaucoma. Nat Genet. 2012;44:1142-1146. https://doi.org/10.1038/ng.2390
28. Khor CC, Do T, Jia H, et al. Genome-wide association study identifies five new susceptibility loci for primary angle closure glaucoma. Nature genetics 2016;48:556-62. https://doi.org/10.1038/ng.3540
29. Pulimeno P, Bauer C, Stutz J, Citi S. PLEKHA7 is an adherens junction protein with a tissue distribution and subcellular localization distinct from ZO-1 and E-cadherin. PloS One. 2010;5:e12207. https://doi.org/10.1371/journal.pone.0012207
30. Lee MC, Chan AS, Goh SR, et al. Expression of the primary angle closure glaucoma (PACG) susceptibility gene PLEKHA7 in endothelial and epithelial cell junctions in the eye. Invest Ophthalmol Vis Sci. 2014;55:3833-41. https://doi.org/10.1167/iovs.14-14145
31. Lee MC, Shei W, Chan AS, et al. Primary angle closure glaucoma (PACG) susceptibility gene PLEKHA7 encodes a novel Rac1/Cdc42 GAP that modulates cell migration and blood-aqueous barrier function. Hum Mol Genet. 2017;26:4011-4027. https://doi.org/10.1093/hmg/ddx292
32. Kong X, Liu X, Huang X, Mao Z, Zhong Y, Chi W. Damage to the blood-aqueous barrier in eyes with primary angle closure glaucoma. Mol Vis. 2010;16:2026-32.
33. Chua J, Vania M, Cheung CM, et al. Expression profile of inflammatory cytokines in aqueous from glaucomatous eyes. Mol Vis. 2012;18:431-8.
34. Khawaja AP, Cooke Bailey JN, Wareham NJ, et al. Genome-wide analyses identify 68 new loci associated with intraocular pressure and improve risk prediction for primary open-angle glaucoma. Nat Genet. 2018;50:778-782. https://doi.org/10.1038/s41588-018-0126-8
35. MacGregor S, Ong JS, An J, et al. Genome-wide association study of intraocular pressure uncovers new pathways to glaucoma. Nat Genet. 2018;50:1067-1071. https://doi.org/10.1038/s41588-018-0176-y
36. Birk DE, Bruckner P. Collagens, suprastructures, and collagen fibril assembly. In: Mecham RP, editor. The Extracellular Matrix: an Overview. New York: Springer-Verlag, 2011:77-155. https://doi.org/10.1007/978-3-642-16555-9_3
37. Richards AJ, Yates JR, Williams R, et al. A family with Stickler syndrome type 2 has a mutation in the COL11A1 gene resulting in the substitution of glycine 97 by valine in alpha 1 (XI) collagen. Hum Mol Genet. 1996;5:1339-43. https://doi.org/10.1093/hmg/5.9.1339
38. Jandrig B, Seitz S, Hinzmann B, et al. ST18 is a breast cancer tumor suppressor gene at human chromosome 8q11.2. Oncogene. 2004;23:9295-302. https://doi.org/10.1038/sj.onc.1208131
39. Yang J, Siqueira MF, Behl Y, Alikhani M, Graves DT. The transcription factor ST18 regulates proapoptotic and proinflammatory gene expression in fibroblasts. FASEB J. 2008;22:3956-67. https://doi.org/10.1096/fj.08-111013

40. Nongpiur ME, Cheng CY, Duvesh R, et al. Evaluation of Primary Angle-Closure Glaucoma Susceptibility Loci in Patients with Early Stages of Angle-Closure Disease. Ophthalmology 2018;125:664-670. https://doi.org/10.1016/j.ophtha.2017.11.016
41. Gregorio-King CC, McLeod JL, Collier FM, et al. MERP1: a mammalian ependymin-related protein gene differentially expressed in hematopoietic cells. Gene. 2002;286:249-57. https://doi.org/10.1016/S0378-1119(02)00434-1
42. Liu C, Nongpiur ME, Cheng CY, et al. Evaluation of Primary Angle-Closure Glaucoma Susceptibility Loci for Estimating Angle Closure Disease Severity. Ophthalmology. 2021;128:403-409. https://doi.org/10.1016/j.ophtha.2020.07.027
43. Barone R, Aiello C, Race V, et al. DPM2-CDG: a muscular dystrophy-dystroglycanopathy syndrome with severe epilepsy. Ann Neurol. 2012;72:550-8. https://doi.org/10.1002/ana.23632
44. Dobransky T, Rylett RJ. Functional regulation of choline acetyltransferase by phosphorylation. Neurochem Res. 2003;28:537-42. https://doi.org/10.1023/A:1022873323561
45. McDougal DH, Gamlin PD. Autonomic control of the eye. Compr Physiol. 2015;5:439-73. https://doi.org/10.1002/j.2040-4603.2015.tb00603.x
46. Kim YS, Nakanishi G, Lewandoski M, Jetten AM. GLIS3, a novel member of the GLIS subfamily of Kruppel-like zinc finger proteins with repressor and activation functions. Nucleic Acids Res. 2003;31:5513-25. https://doi.org/10.1093/nar/gkg776
47. Senee V, Chelala C, Duchatelet S, et al. Mutations in GLIS3 are responsible for a rare syndrome with neonatal diabetes mellitus and congenital hypothyroidism. Nat Genet. 2006;38:682-7. https://doi.org/10.1038/ng1802
48. Kang HS, Kumar D, Liao G, et al. GLIS3 is indispensable for TSH/TSHR-dependent thyroid hormone biosynthesis and follicular cell proliferation. J Clin Invest 2017;127:4326-4337. https://doi.org/10.1172/JCI94417
49. Casalone E, Tachmazidou I, Zengini E, et al. A novel variant in GLIS3 is associated with osteoarthritis. Ann Rheum Dis. 2018;77:620-623. https://doi.org/10.1136/annrheumdis-2017-211848
50. Cruchaga C, Kauwe JS, Harari O, et al. GWAS of cerebrospinal fluid tau levels identifies risk variants for Alzheimer's disease. Neuron. 2013;78:256-68. https://doi.org/10.1016/j.neuron.2013.02.026
51. Duarte GCK, Assmann TS, Dieter C, de Souza BM, Crispim D. GLIS3 rs7020673 and rs10758593 polymorphisms interact in the susceptibility for type 1 diabetes mellitus. Acta Diabetol. 2017;54:813-821. https://doi.org/10.1007/s00592-017-1009-7
52. Choquet H, Thai KK, Yin J, et al. A large multi-ethnic genome-wide association study identifies novel genetic loci for intraocular pressure. Nat Commun. 2017;8:2108. https://doi.org/10.1038/s41467-017-01913-6
53. Huang L, Chen Y, Lin Y, et al. Genome-wide analysis identified 17 new loci influencing intraocular pressure in Chinese population. Sci China Life Sci. 2019;62:153-164. https://doi.org/10.1007/s11427-018-9430-2

54. Artym VV, Swatkoski S, Matsumoto K, et al. Dense fibrillar collagen is a potent inducer of invadopodia via a specific signaling network. J Cell Biol. 2015;208:331-50. https://doi.org/10.1083/jcb.201405099
55. Pluskota E, Bledzka KM, Bialkowska K, et al. Kindlin-2 interacts with endothelial adherens junctions to support vascular barrier integrity. J Physiol. 2017;595:6443-6462. https://doi.org/10.1113/JP274380
56. Ying J, Luan W, Lu L, Zhang S, Qi F. Knockdown of the KINDLIN-2 Gene and Reduced Expression of Kindlin-2 Affects Vascular Permeability in Angiogenesis in a Mouse Model of Wound Healing. Med Sci Monit. 2018;24:5376-5383. https://doi.org/10.12659/MSM.910059
57. Luben RB, Stuart K, Wagner S, et al. Genome-wide association study for primary angle closure glaucoma in Europeans identifies novel loci related to iris colour and morphology. ARVO Meeting Abstract 2023.
58. Simcoe M, Valdes A, Liu F, et al. Genome-wide association study in almost 195,000 individuals identifies 50 previously unidentified genetic loci for eye color. Sci Adv. 2021;7. https://doi.org/10.1126/sciadv.abd1239
59. Kayser M, Liu F, Janssens AC, et al. Three genome-wide association studies and a linkage analysis identify HERC2 as a human iris color gene. Am J Hum Genet. 2008;82:411-23. https://doi.org/10.1016/j.ajhg.2007.10.003
60. Nongpiur ME, Khor CC, Jia H, et al. ABCC5, a gene that influences the anterior chamber depth, is associated with primary angle closure glaucoma. PLoS Genet. 2014;10:e1004089. https://doi.org/10.1371/journal.pgen.1004352
61. Jedlitschky G, Burchell B, Keppler D. The multidrug resistance protein 5 functions as an ATP-dependent export pump for cyclic nucleotides. J Biol Chem. 2000;275:30069-74. https://doi.org/10.1074/jbc.M005463200
62. Wijnholds J, Mol CA, van Deemter L, et al. Multidrug-resistance protein 5 is a multispecific organic anion transporter able to transport nucleotide analogs. Proc Natl Acad Sci U S A. 2000;97:7476-81. https://doi.org/10.1073/pnas.120159197
63. Long Y, Li Q, Li J, Cui Z. Molecular analysis, developmental function and heavy metal-induced expression of ABCC5 in zebrafish. Comp Biochem Physiol B Biochem Mol Biol. 2011;158:46-55. https://doi.org/10.1016/j.cbpb.2010.09.005
64. Loo YC, Chng WL, Liu Z, Aung T, Khor CC, Wang Z. Identification of a new genetic loci associated with Primary Angle Closure Glaucoma. ARVO Annual Meeting Abstract 2024.
65. Nongpiur ME, Wei X, Xu L, et al. Lack of association between primary angle-closure glaucoma susceptibility loci and the ocular biometric parameters anterior chamber depth and axial length. Invest Ophthalmol Vis Sci. 2013;54:5824-8. https://doi.org/10.1167/iovs.13-11901
66. Day AC, Luben R, Khawaja AP, et al. Genotype-phenotype analysis of SNPs associated with primary angle closure glaucoma (rs1015213, rs3753841 and rs11024102) and ocular biometry in the EPIC-Norfolk Eye Study. Br J Ophthalmol. 2013;97:704-7. https://doi.org/10.1136/bjop-

hthalmol-2012-302969

67. Wei X, Nongpiur ME, de Leon MS, et al. Genotype-phenotype correlation analysis for three primary angle closure glaucoma-associated genetic polymorphisms. Invest Ophthalmol Vis Sci. 2014;55:1143-8. https://doi.org/10.1167/iovs.13-13552
68. Nongpiur ME, Khor CC, Cheng CY, et al. Integration of Genetic and Biometric Risk Factors for Detection of Primary Angle Closure Glaucoma. Am J Ophthalmol. 2019;208:160-165. https://doi.org/10.1016/j.ajo.2019.07.022
69. Craig JE, Han X, Qassim A, et al. Multitrait analysis of glaucoma identifies new risk loci and enables polygenic prediction of disease susceptibility and progression. Nat Genet. 2020;52:160-166. https://doi.org/10.1038/s41588-019-0556-y
70. Siggs OM, Qassim A, Han X, et al. Association of High Polygenic Risk With Visual Field Worsening Despite Treatment in Early Primary Open-Angle Glaucoma. JAMA Ophthalmol. 2022;141:73-7. https://doi.org/10.1001/jamaophthalmol.2022.4688
71. Tran JH, Kang J, Han E, et al. Use of Diagnostic Codes for Primary Open-Angle Glaucoma Polygenic Risk Score Construction in Electronic Health Record-Linked Biobanks. Am J Ophthalmol. 2024;267:204-212. https://doi.org/10.1016/j.ajo.2024.06.007

Static risk factors for angle-closure disease and angle-closure glaucoma

Paul Foster

"Static" risk factors for angle-closure disease include demographic factors such as older age and female sex.[1] Asians are at greater risk than Europeans, both in terms of prevalence and incidence of disease.[2–4] Chinese individuals are at higher risk than Southeast Asians and South Asians (*e.g.*, India, Pakistan, Bangladesh).[3,5] The highest-risk populations anywhere on Earth are the Inuit people of Alaska, northern Canada, and Greenland.[1,6,7] Hypermetropic refractive error is also a risk factor, but cases also occur in people who are myopic.[8] This includes cases of common "simple" axial myopia and cases related to microspherophakia.[9]

Socioeconomic disadvantage, lower educational achievement, and racial minority status are risk factors for AAC and blindness from PACG.[10–12] Those with lower body mass index are at higher risk of AAC.[10,13] The seminal studies of Alsbirk and Lowe have shown that all these factors are related to the biometric characteristics of the eye and ACD in particular.[1] All the sociodemographic risk factors associated with angle closure are also associated with a shallow anterior chamber, a surrogate for an occluded iridocorneal angle. A shallow anterior chamber is the most well-characterized risk factor for angle closure. It is a heritable phenomenon believed to be under genetic control, probably via a polygenic mechanism.[1,14] In turn, ACD is determined by the size as well as the relative and absolute position of the lens within the eye. The concept of "relative lens position" (RLP) was developed by Lowe and is defined as the ACD plus half of the lens thickness (LT) divided by the AL of the eye.[15]

RLP = (ACD + 0.5*LT) / AL (no units).

The relationship between a hypermetropic refraction and higher risk of angle closure is a consequence of hypermetropic eyes having a shorter AL. This is a determinant of the absolute lens position within the eye (the geometric center of the lens + ACD, measured in mm). A lens will, on average, be closer to the corneal endothelium of a smaller hypermetropic eye than in a larger myopic eye. The concept of absolute lens position is less well documented in studies of the risk of angle closure. However, a similar characteristic that helps capture the relationship between the lens size and position and its impact on the angle configuration is the LV. This is defined as the distance between the anterior lens pole and a line drawn between the scleral spurs on an axial, cross-sectional image of the anterior chamber. The greater the LV, the narrower the iridocorneal angle and the greater the risk of angle-closure disease.[16] Zonulopathy is a prevalent finding (7%) in people with angle-closure disease.[17]

The distribution of ACD has been carefully documented in many populations. ACD is less in women than in men. ACD increases from birth to approximately 20 years of age and then declines. This decline occurs in 2 phases, the steepest being between the ages of 20 and 40 and then a slower decline from 40 to 60 and 70 years.[1] It has been observed from 70 years onwards that there may be a gradual increase in ACD, but whether this is a phenomenon that occurs within individuals or is a consequence of differential mortality currently remains unclear.[18] Populations with high rates of angle closure have shallower mean ACD than populations with low rates of the disease.[18] Studies conducted between the 1970s and 2000s found a clear pattern of Asian people having shallower anterior chambers than Europeans.[18] However, the increase in myopic refraction that is currently underway, particularly in East Asian countries, will likely alter this relationship.

A thicker iris takes up more space in the anterior chamber and brings the surface of the iris closer to the trabecular meshwork, increasing the risk of closure.[19] Pupil block mechanism and disc margin hemorrhages confer a higher risk of progression to PACG than does plateau iris.[20,21] Risk factors for progression of PACG after lens extraction include higher IOP and thinner retinal nerve fiber layer.[22]

References

1. Alsbirk PH. Primary angle-closure glaucoma. Oculometry, epidemiology, and genetics in a high risk population. Acta Ophthalmol Suppl. 1976;(127):5-31.
2. Chua PY, Day AC, Lai KL, et al. The incidence of acute angle closure in Scotland: a prospective surveillance study. Br J Ophthalmol. 2018;102(4):539-543. https://doi.org/10.1136/bjophthalmol-2017-310725
3. Seah SK, Foster PJ, Chew PT, et al. Incidence of acute primary angle-closure glaucoma in Singapore. An island-wide survey. Arch Ophthalmol. 1997;115(11):1436-1440. https://doi.org/10.1001/archopht.1997.01100160606014
4. Quigley HA, Broman AT. The number of people with glaucoma worldwide in 2010 and 2020. Br J Ophthalmol. 2006;90(3):262-267. https://doi.org/10.1136/bjo.2005.081224
5. Wong TY, Foster PJ, Seah SK, Chew PT. Rates of hospital admissions for primary angle closure glaucoma among Chinese, Malays, and Indians in Singapore. Br J Ophthalmol. 2000;84(9):990-992. https://doi.org/10.1136/bjo.84.9.990
6. Arkell SM, Lightman DA, Sommer A, Taylor HR, Korshin OM, Tielsch JM. The prevalence of glaucoma among Eskimos of northwest Alaska. Arch Ophthalmol. 1987;105(4):482-485. https://doi.org/10.1001/archopht.1987.01060040052031
7. Drance SM. Angle closure glaucoma among Canadian Eskimos. J Can Ophtalmol. 1973;8(2):252-254.
8. Zhou S, Pardeshi AA, Burkemper B, et al. Refractive Error and Anterior Chamber Depth as Risk Factors in Primary Angle Closure Disease: The Chinese American Eye Study. J Glaucoma. 2023;32(4):257-264. https://doi.org/10.1097/IJG.0000000000002154
9. Senthil S, Rao HL, Hoang NTQ, et al. Glaucoma in microspherophakia: presenting features and treatment outcomes. J Glaucoma. 2014;23(4):262-267. https://doi.org/10.1097/IJG.0b013e3182707437
10. Nessim M, Denniston AK, Nolan W, Holder R, Shah P. Research into Glaucoma and Ethnicity (ReGAE) 8: is there a relationship between social deprivation and acute primary angle closure? Br J Ophthalmol. 2010;94(10):1304-1306. https://doi.org/10.1136/bjo.2009.160721
11. Shah SN, Zhou S, Sanvicente C, et al. Prevalence and Risk Factors of Blindness Among Primary Angle Closure Glaucoma Patients in the United States: An IRIS Registry Analysis. Am J Ophthalmol. 2024;259:131-140. https://doi.org/10.1016/j.ajo.2023.11.007
12. Saxby E, Cheng K, O'Connell N, Sanders R, Agarwal PK. Is there an association of socioeconomic deprivation with acute primary angle closure? Eye Lond Engl. 2022;36(6):1246-1252. https://doi.org/10.1038/s41433-021-01615-w

13. Wang Y, Dong XX, Hou XW, Pan CW. Risk Factors for Primary Angle-closure Glaucoma: A Systematic Review and Meta-analysis of 45 Studies. Optom Vis Sci Off Publ Am Acad Optom. 2023;100(9):606-613. https://doi.org/10.1097/OPX.0000000000002050
14. Alsbirk PH. Anterior chamber depth and primary angle-closure glaucoma. II. A genetic study. Acta Ophthalmol (Copenh). 1975;53(3):436-449. https://doi.org/10.1111/j.1755-3768.1975.tb01175.x
15. Lowe RF. Aetiology of the anatomical basis for primary angle-closure glaucoma. Biometrical comparisons between normal eyes and eyes with primary angle-closure glaucoma. Br J Ophthalmol. 1970;54(3):161-169. https://doi.org/10.1136/bjo.54.3.161
16. Nongpiur ME, He M, Amerasinghe N, et al. Lens vault, thickness, and position in Chinese subjects with angle closure. Ophthalmology. 2011;118(3):474-479. https://doi.org/10.1016/j.ophtha.2010.07.025
17. Salimi A, Fanous A, Watt H, Abu-Nada M, Wang A, Harasymowycz P. Prevalence of zonulop athy in primary angle closure disease. Clin Experiment Ophthalmol. 2021;49(9):1018-1026. https://doi.org/10.1111/ceo.13983
18. Foster PJ, Alsbirk PH, Baasanhu J, Munkhbayar D, Uranchimeg D, Johnson GJ. Anterior chamber depth in Mongolians: variation with age, sex, and method of measurement. Am J Ophthalmol. 1997;124(1):53-60. https://doi.org/10.1016/S0002-9394(14)71644-7
19. Wang BS, Narayanaswamy A, Amerasinghe N, et al. Increased iris thickness and association with primary angle closure glaucoma. Br J Ophthalmol. 2011;95(1):46-50. https://doi.org/10.1136/bjo.2009.178129
20. Wan-Ezatul-Arisha WM, Diana-Toh SJ, Huwaina AS, et al. Visual field progression in Malay patients with primary glaucoma: survival analysis and prognostic factors. Graefes Arch Clin Exp Ophthalmol. 2022;260(6):2003-2012. https://doi.org/10.1007/s00417-021-05466-9
21. Song MK, Sung KR, Shin JW. Glaucoma Progression After Lens Extraction in Primary Angle-closure Glaucoma According to Angle-closure Mechanism. J Glaucoma. 2022;31(4):261-267. https://doi.org/10.1097/IJG.0000000000001992
22. Song MK, Shin JW, Sung KR. Factors Associated with Deterioration of Primary Angle Closure after Lens Extraction. J Clin Med. 2022;11(9):2557. https://doi.org/10.3390/jcm11092557

Dynamic factors participating in angle-closure disease

Harry Quigley, David Friedman

While many known features of static ocular structure are associated with angle-closure disease, most eyes that have these anatomic risk factors do not develop disease.[1,2] Risk factors for angle-closure disease include lower

LV, shallower ACD, shorter AL, thicker choroid, narrow angle viewed by gonioscopy, and associated angle parameters measured by AS-OCT. However, these features have been generally treated as if they were immutable. In fact, all these parameters are affected by the size of the pupil—principally determined by lighting conditions. It has been known and taught for decades that gonioscopy must be performed taking into account the illumination of the pupil.[3] Yet, many reports of findings using AS-OCT do not account for pupil size in their findings, and significant differences in AS-OCT parameters are found between lighted and dark conditions.[4] In addition, many parameters measured by AS-OCT are dependent on identification of the position of the scleral spur. Very small changes in the marked position of the scleral spur can produce dramatic changes in angle opening distances and single location thicknesses of the iris.[5] By contrast, the iris area measurement is affected minimally by variation in scleral spur marking. Dynamic mechanisms leading to angle-closure disease as described in the section below, have been proposed for over 2 decades.[6]

Clinical examinations and research studies show that dynamic changes in the iris and choroid contribute to angle-closure disease

Pupillary block

Physiological or pharmacological events leading to pupil dilation cause angle-closure disease and can be measured as changes by gonioscopy, AS-OCT, and ultrasound biomicroscopy. Resistance through the iris-lens channel increases with dynamic change in its length and width, producing higher IOP behind the iris than in the anterior chamber.[7] Both forward lens movement (greater LV) and the mid-pupil position increase this pressure differential. The flattening of iris curvature in the majority of angle-closure disease eyes that undergo laser iridotomy confirms this physiological mechanism.

Iris area/volume loss

An important physiological feature of the iris is its exchange of interstitial fluid with the aqueous humor, leading to loss of iris area (volume) on pupil dilation.[8,9] In adult eyes, nearly half of the iris volume is exchanged almost immediately as the pupil dilates, a finding confirmed in multiple racial (derivation) groups. Research now documents that lower iris volume decrease with pupil dilation is a contributing risk factor in angle-closure disease.[10] AAC attack eyes with angle closure-disease and their fellow eyes show less iris area loss than controls in both European[11] and Chinese[12] individuals. While early calculations of iris volume change suggested that its volume could actually increase in the most susceptible eyes to AAC attack, this finding derived from how iris volume was calculated from iris area images using the centroid of iris mass. In fact, the most susceptible eyes to acute attack not only lose less iris area/volume, but they redistribute iris mass more into the iris periphery, intensifying angle closure.[13] Less iris area/volume loss has been confirmed in angle-closure disease eyes in all derivation groups, including Indian,[14] Chinese,[15-17] European, and African-derived individuals.[13] Low iris permeability and increased iris stiffness have been suggested by finite element models as contributing to angle-closure disease.[18] The major, prospective Zhongshan Angle Closure Prevention study confirmed that loss of iris area is a significant risk factor for conversion from PACS to PAC and that this dynamic factor is additive to static measurements.[19]

Choroidal expansion

With the advent of enhanced depth imaging-OCT imaging of the choroid, the thickness (and hence the volume) of the choroid became a measurement of interest in ocular disease. Most of the reports in the retinal literature did not account for the dynamic changes in choroidal thickness that occur with change in IOP and perfusion pressure,[20] pharmacological exposure, or other ocular conditions. Temporary choroidal expansion in Valsalva,[21] breath-holding playing wind instruments,[22] and head stand posture[23] have been documented, but are transient effects from increased vortex venous pressure. The fact that choroidal expansion causes secondary angle closure is well known, such as with choroidal hemorrhage, metastatic tumors, uveal inflammation, scleral buckling surgery, central retinal vein occlusion, carotid-cavernous fistula, and oral therapy with topiramate and sulfa-derived medications. There is residual reluctance to equate choroidal expansion with higher IOP due to the common association of choroidal detachment with low IOP.

The potential contribution of dynamic change in choroidal volume to angle-closure disease was proposed in 2009.[24] In ocular development, choroidal thickness is managed actively to respond to retinal image blur, dynamically altering scleral growth to maximize emmetropia.[25] Thus, there are active mechanisms for maintaining and altering choroidal volume, including the regulation of permeability to large proteins at the choriocapillaris. Such mechanisms are subject to individual variability and to abnormal function. Cross-sectional studies demonstrated that angle-closure disease eyes often have expanded choroidal volume,[26] more often in those with acute angle closure, but even in asymptomatic PACG.[27,28] Again, this was found in different derivation groups, so it is not unique to individuals from one continent. More importantly, eyes with angle-closure disease had more exaggerated choroidal thickening after provocation by water-drinking,[29] demonstrating that there was dynamic hyperresponsiveness to their choroid. By raising the IOP in the posterior chamber, choroidal expansion likely contributes to the pupillary block mechanism and angle-closure disease.

Malignant glaucoma is related to choroidal expansion and abnormal vitreous physiology

Choroidal expansion has now been documented in eyes with malignant glaucoma (also called vitreous block). While initial reports did not assume that the choroidal expansion had occurred prior to the onset of high IOP,[30,31] there are now multiple published series in which the expansion of the choroid is recognized as a contributing event leading to malignant glaucoma.[32-34] The sequence of events by which choroidal expansion leads to malignant glaucoma are similar to its role in pupillary block intensification, but include abnormal fluid conductivity in the vitreous humor in eyes predisposed to vitreous block. It has been experimentally demonstrated that water movement through the vitreous is hindered when a pressure differential is placed across it, setting up a vicious cycle.[35] Epstein and others performed experimental studies that confirmed vitreous compaction and anterior chamber flattening with posterior to anterior IOP differential in normal eyes.[36,37] Epstein concluded: "In malignant glaucoma,...there must be factors other than, or in addition to, diversion of aqueous humor through the vitreous body to explain this condition. It seems in malignant glaucoma that the permeability of the vitreous humor or of the anterior hyaloid membrane must be less than normal." There being no evidence that aqueous humor diverted from the ciliary body could explain malignant glaucoma, the term "aqueous misdirection" has been incorrectly applied. That mechanism would require a one-way valve for which there is no evidence. Instead, it is now clear that hyperreactive choroidal expansion, as seen in angle-closure disease eyes, could produce a high IOP. With consequent exit of aqueous from the anterior chamber, a pressure differential would be produced from behind to in front of the vitreous. If vitreous fluid conductivity is normal, water exits the vitreous and then through the outflow channels, and no malignant glaucoma occurs. If vitreous fluid conductivity is abnormally low, the vicious cycle continues, the vitreous compacts forward, carrying the lens and iris into the anterior chamber until the angle and chamber are flat. The mechanism is compatible with the curative effect of vitrectomy,[38] particularly by iridozonulohyaloidectomy,[39] in malignant glaucoma.

References

1. Baskaran M, Kumar RS, Friedman DS, et al. The Singapore Asymptomatic Narrow Angles Laser Iridotomy Study: Five-Year Results of a Randomized Controlled Trial. Ophthalmology. 2022 Feb;129(2):147-158. https://doi.org/10.1016/j.ophtha.2021.08.017
2. Yuan Y, Wang W, Xiong R, et al. Fourteen-Year Outcome of Angle-Closure Prevention with Laser Iridotomy in the Zhongshan Angle-Closure Prevention Study: Extended Follow-up of a Randomized Controlled Trial. Ophthalmology. 2023 Aug;130(8):786-794. https://doi.org/10.1016/j.ophtha.2023.03.024
3. Barkana Y, Dorairaj SK, Gerber Y, Liebmann JM, Ritch R. Agreement between gonioscopy and ultrasound biomicroscopy in detecting iridotrabecular apposition. Arch Ophthalmol. 2007 Oct;125(10):1331-5. https://doi.org/10.1001/archopht.125.10.1331
4. Leung CK, Cheung CY, Li H, et al. Dynamic analysis of dark-light changes of the anterior chamber angle with anterior segment OCT. Invest Ophthalmol Vis Sci. 2007 Sep;48(9):4116-22. https://doi.org/10.1167/iovs.07-0010
5. Seager FE, Wang J, Arora KS, Quigley HA. The effect of scleral spur identification methods on structural measurements by anterior segment optical coherence tomography. J Glaucoma. 2014 Jan;23(1):e29-38. https://doi.org/10.1097/IJG.0b013e31829e55ae
6. Quigley HA, Friedman DS, Congdon NG. Possible mechanisms of primary angle-closure and malignant glaucoma. J Glaucoma. 2003 Apr;12(2):167-80. https://doi.org/10.1097/00061198-200304000-00013
7. Silver DM, Quigley HA. Aqueous flow through the iris-lens channel: estimates of differential pressure between the anterior and posterior chambers. J Glaucoma. 2004 Apr;13(2):100-7. https://doi.org/10.1097/00061198-200404000-00004
8. Ishikawa H, Ritch R, Hoh S-T, Liebmann JM. Iris volume decreases during pupillary dilation. Hong Kong J Ophthalmol. 2003;7:6-9.
9. Mak H, Xu G, Leung CK. Imaging the iris with swept-source optical coherence tomography: relationship between iris volume and primary angle closure. Ophthalmology. 2013 Dec;120(12):2517-2524. https://doi.org/10.1016/j.ophtha.2013.05.009
10. Quigley HA, Silver DM, Friedman DS, et al. Iris cross-sectional area decreases with pupil dilation and its dynamic behavior is a risk factor in angle closure. J Glaucoma. 2009 Mar;18(3):173-9. https://doi.org/10.1097/IJG.0b013e31818624ce
11. Aptel F, Chiquet C, Beccat S, Denis P. Biometric evaluation of anterior chamber changes after physiologic pupil dilation using Pentacam and anterior segment optical coherence tomography. Invest Ophthalmol Vis Sci. 2012 Jun 26;53(7):4005-10. https://doi.org/10.1167/iovs.11-9387
12. Narayanaswamy A, Zheng C, Perera SA, et al. Variations in iris volume with physiologic mydriasis in subtypes of primary angle closure glaucoma. Invest Ophthalmol Vis Sci. 2013 Jan 23;54(1):708-13. https://doi.org/10.1167/iovs.12-10844
13. Seager FE, Jefferys JL, Quigley HA. Comparison of dynamic changes in anterior ocular struc-

tures examined with anterior segment optical coherence tomography in a cohort of various origins. Invest Ophthalmol Vis Sci. 2014;55:1672–1683. https://doi.org/10.1167/iovs.13-13641

14. Ganeshrao SB, Mani B, Ulganathan S, Shantha B, Vijaya L. Change in iris parameters with physiological mydriasis. Optom Vis Sci. 2012 Apr;89(4):483-8. https://doi.org/10.1097/OPX.0b013e31824c3731
15. Zhang Y, Li SZ, Li L, He MG, Thomas R, Wang NL. Quantitative analysis of iris changes after physiologic and pharmacologic mydriasis in a rural Chinese population. Invest Ophthalmol Vis Sci. 2014;55:4405–4412. https://doi.org/10.1167/iovs.13-13782
16. Chung C, Dai M, Lin J, Wang Z, Chen H, Huang J. Correlation of iris collagen and in-vivo anterior segment structures in patients in different stages of chronic primary angle-closure in both eyes. Indian J Ophthalmol. 2019;67:1638-44. https://doi.org/10.4103/ijo.IJO_1406_18
17. Lin J, Wang Z, Chung C, Xu J, Dai M, Huang J. Dynamic changes of anterior segment in patients with different stages of primary angle-closure in both eyes and normal subjects. PLoS ONE. 2017;12(5): e0177769. https://doi.org/10.1371/journal.pone.0177769
18. Panda SK, Tan RKY, Tun TA, et al. Changes in Iris Stiffness and Permeability in Primary Angle Closure Glaucoma. Invest Ophthalmol Vis Sci. 2021 Oct 4;62(13):29. https://doi.org/10.1167/iovs.62.13.29
19. Liao C, Quigley H, Jiang Y, et al. Iris volume change with physiologic mydriasis to identify development of angle closure: the Zhongshan Angle Closure Prevention Trial. Br J Ophthalmol. 2024 Feb 21;108(3):366-371. https://doi.org/10.1136/bjo-2022-322931
20. Maul EA, Friedman DS, Chang DS, et al. Choroidal thickness measured by spectral domain optical coherence tomography: factors affecting thickness in glaucoma patients. Ophthalmology. 2011 Aug;118(8):1571-9. https://doi.org/.1016/j.ophtha.2011.01.016
21. Sihota R, Dada T, Aggarwal A, Srinivasan G, Gupta V, Chabra VK. Does an iridotomy provide protection against narrowing of the anterior chamber angle during Valsalva maneuvre in eyes with primary angle-closure. Eye. 2008;22:389–393.
22. Schuman JS, Massicotte EC, Connolly S, et al. Increased intraocular pressure and visual field defects in high resistance wind instrument players. Ophthalmology. 2000;107:127–133.
23. Baskaran M, Raman K, Ramani KK, Roy J, Vijaya L, Badrinath SS. Intraocular pressure changes and ocular biometry during Sirsasana (headstand posture) in yoga practitioners. Ophthalmology. 2006;113:1327–1332.
24. Quigley HA. Angle-closure glaucoma-simpler answers to complex mechanisms: LXVI Edward Jackson Memorial Lecture. Am J Ophthalmol. 2009 Nov;148(5):657-669.e1. https://doi.org/10.1016/j.ajo.2009.08.009
25. Hung L-F, Wallman J, Smith EL. Vision-dependent changes in the choroidal thickness of Macaque monkeys. Invest Ophthalmol Vis Sci. 2000;41:1259-1269.
26. Arora KS, Jefferys JL, Maul EA, Quigley HA. The choroid is thicker in angle closure than in open angle and control eyes. Invest Ophthalmol Vis Sci. 2012 Nov 27;53(12):7813-8. https://

doi.org/10.1167/iovs.12-10483

27. Kumar RS, Quek D, Lee KY, et al. Confirmation of the presence of uveal effusion in Asian eyes with primary angle closure glaucoma: an ultrasound biomicroscopy study. Arch Ophthalmol. 2008 Dec;126(12):1647-51. https://doi.org/10.1001/archophthalmol.2008.514
28. Sakai H, Morine-Shinjyo S, Shinzato M, Nakamura Y, Sakai M, Sawaguchi S. Uveal effusion in primary angle-closure glaucoma. Ophthalmology. 2005 Mar;112(3):413-9. https://doi.org/10.1016/j.ophtha.2004.08.026 Erratum in: Ophthalmology. 2007 Nov;114(11):2012.
29. Arora KS, Jefferys JL, Maul EA, Quigley HA. Choroidal thickness change after water drinking is greater in angle closure than in open angle eyes. Invest Ophthalmol Vis Sci. 2012 Sep 21;53(10):6393-402. https://doi.org/10.1167/iovs.12-10224
30. Dugel PU, Heuer DK, Thach AB, et al. Annular peripheral choroidal detachment simulating aqueous misdirection after glaucoma surgery. Ophthalmology. 1997 Mar;104(3):439-44. https://doi.org/10.1016/s0161-6420(97)30294-2
31. Liebmann JM, Weinreb RN, Ritch R. Angle-closure glaucoma associated with occult annular ciliary body detachment. Arch Ophthalmol. 1998 Jun;116(6):731-5. https://doi.org/doi:10.1001/archopht.116.6.731
32. Kaplowitz K, Yung E, Flynn R, Tsai JC. Current concepts in the treatment of vitreous block, also known as aqueous misdirection. Surv Ophthalmol. 2015 May-Jun;60(3):229-41. https://doi.org/10.1016/j.survophthal.2014.12.004
33. Chen X, Guo X, Xu X, Xiao H, Liu X. Is Thicker Choroid a Risk Factor for Malignant Glaucoma? Ophthalmic Res. 2018;60(3):161-168. https://doi.org/10.1159/000490914
34. Zuo C, Wang D, Guo X, et al. Associations Between the Choroidal Vascularity Index and Malignant Glaucoma After Trabeculectomy for Primary Angle Closure Glaucoma. Front Med (Lausanne). 2021 Dec 8;8:747720. https://doi.org/0.3389/fmed.2021.747720
35. Fatt I. Hydraulic flow conductivity of the vitreous gel. Invest Ophthalmol Vis Sci. 1977 Jun;16(6):565-8. PMID: 863619.
36. Epstein DL, Hashimoto JM, Anderson PJ, Grant WM. Experimental perfusions through the anterior and vitreous chambers with possible relationships to malignant glaucoma. Am J Ophthalmol. 1979 Dec;88(6):1078-86. https://doi.org/10.1016/0002-9394(79)90420-3
37. Quigley HA. Malignant glaucoma and fluid flow rate. Am J Ophthalmol. 1980 Jun;89(6):879-80. https://doi.org/10.1016/0002-9394(80)90190-7
38. Lynch MG, Brown RH, Michels RG, Pollack IP, Stark WJ. Surgical vitrectomy for pseudophakic malignant glaucoma. Am J Ophthalmol. 1986 Aug 15;102(2):149-53. https://doi.org/10.1016/0002-9394(86)90135-2
39. Varma DK, Belovay GW, Tam DY, Ahmed II. Malignant glaucoma after cataract surgery. J Cataract Refract Surg. 2014 Nov;40(11):1843-9. https://doi.org/10.1016/j.jcrs.2014.02.045

Other risk factors in primary angle-closure glaucoma

This section addresses additional risk factors that contribute to the development and progression of PACG, focusing on zonulopathy, vitreous block, ocular collagen abnormalities, autonomic nervous system dysfunction, drugs, and personality characteristics.

Clinical scenarios

Ye Zhang, Ningli Wang

Vitreous block in PACG

Poor vitreous flow conductivity through a mostly solid vitreous gel has been identified as a key contributing factor in PACG pathogenesis.[1] One analysis showed a finite resistance to aqueous movement through the vitreous body.[1,2] When the choroid expands, this resistance becomes particularly significant, creating a pressure differential between the posterior and anterior segments of the eye.[1] This pressure differential can lead to anterior displacement of the lens-iris diaphragm, contributing to angle closure.[1]

Several clinical observations support the role of vitreous block:[1,3]

- Positive pressure during anterior segment surgery, particularly in eyes with PACG after iridotomy.
- Persistence of shallow anterior chamber despite a patent iridotomy.
- Higher incidence of malignant glaucoma in PACG patients following filtration surgery

Understanding the role of vitreous block has important therapeutic considerations because traditional treatments, such as laser peripheral iridotomy, may not adequately address the vitreous component of PACG.[4,5] This may be one factor that helps to explain why some patients continue to experience angle closure despite a patent iridotomy.[6]

Vitreous body block likely plays a role in the pathophysiology of PACG. Recognition of this pathogenic factor may improve patient outcomes through more targeted therapeutic approaches, particularly in cases resistant to conventional treatments.

Ocular collagen abnormalities and PACG

Recent evidence suggests that collagen abnormalities in different ocular tissues, particularly the iris and sclera, may play a role in PACG pathogenesis.[7-10]

Type I and III iris collagen changes

A study of iris tissue from acute PAC and fellow eyes has demonstrated:[7]

- Increased density of type I collagen in the iris stroma.
- Elevated total collagen content.

In contrast, chronic PACG eyes exhibit:[7]

- Looser collagen structure in the iris stroma
- A lower proportion of type I collagen
- More disorganized collagen arrangement

These findings suggest that collagen remodeling in the iris may represent different stages or manifestations of the disease process.[7-8]

Scleral collagen abnormalities

Morphological and ultrastructural studies have revealed significant alterations in scleral collagen organization in nanophthalmic eyes, which may present an extreme form of angle-closure glaucoma.[9-11] Key findings include:

- Increased collagen density compared to normal controls.
- Disorganized arrangement of collagen fibrils.
- Less ordered collagen bundle patterns.

These structural changes may contribute to:

- Altered biomechanical properties of the sclera.
- Impaired fluid dynamics.
- Increased resistance to aqueous outflow.
- Compromised vortex vein function.

SPARC expression

A previous study has identified increased SPARC (secreted protein acidic and rich in cysteine) expression in the iris tissue of PACG patients.[12] SPARC, a matricellular protein involved in collagen assembly and matrix organization, shows:

- Significantly elevated levels in PACG iris tissue.
- Potential role in abnormal collagen deposition and organization.
- Association with ECM modification.

Conclusion

Collagen abnormalities in PACG represent a complex interplay of structural and biochemical changes in multiple ocular tissues. Understanding these alterations provides valuable insights into disease pathogenesis and may lead to novel therapeutic approaches. Continued research in this area is essential for improving patient outcomes in PACG management.

Autonomic nervous system dysfunction in PACG

The autonomic nervous system plays an essential role in regulating IOP and anterior segment dynamics. Recent evidence suggests that autonomic dysfunction, both systemic and ocular, may contribute to the pathogenesis of PACG.[13-21]

Systemic autonomic dysfunction

The relationship between systemic autonomic dysfunction and PACG remains controversial. Some studies have reported significant associations, while others found no clear evidence of systemic autonomic involvement.[13-15]

Early studies suggested that systemic autonomic neuropathy might be present in up to 58% of patients with PACG.[16] Kumar *et al.* found increased sympathetic activity in 61% of PACG subjects and decreased parasympathetic activity in 80% of PACG subjects through tests of galvanic skin resistance, cold pressor response, and various cardiac parameters.[17]

However, more recent investigations using standardized autonomic function tests have yielded conflicting results. A comparative study by Yong *et al.* examining heart rate and sympathetic skin responses found no significant differences in systemic autonomic function between PACG patients and controls.[13] These contradictory findings suggest that the relationship between systemic autonomic dysfunction and PACG requires further investigation with more rigorous methodologies.

Ocular autonomic dysfunction

Evidence for localized autonomic dysfunction in the anterior segment of PACG eyes is more consistent.[15,18-21] Several key findings have been documented:

- Parasympathetic dysfunction:[15,18-21]
    - Reduced light reflex amplitude.
    - Decreased pupillary constriction speed in response to light.
    - Enhanced miotic response to dilute cholinergic agents, possibly indicating denervation hypersensitivity.
    - Prolonged pupil cycle time.
- Sympathetic dysfunction:[15,18-19]
    - Reduced resting pupil diameter in darkness.
    - Exaggerated mydriatic response to adrenergic agents.
    - Abnormal sympathetic control of pupil dilation.

These changes in autonomic function may contribute to PACG pathogenesis through[15]

- Altered pupillary dynamics, leading to increased pupillary block.
- Disrupted aqueous flow regulation.
- Impaired iris mobility and deformability.

Conclusion

While the role of systemic autonomic dysfunction in PACG remains uncertain, there is substantial evidence for localized ocular autonomic dysfunction. Understanding these autonomic abnormalities may lead to improved PACG prevention and treatment strategies. Further research using standardized methodologies and larger patient populations is needed to fully elucidate the relationship between autonomic dysfunction and PACG.

References

1. Quigley HA, Friedman DS, Congdon NG. Possible mechanisms of primary angle closure and malignant glaucoma. J Glaucoma. 2003;12(2):167-180.https://doi.org/10.1097/00061198-200304000-00013
2. Silver DM, Quigley HA. Aqueous flow through the iris-lens channel produces a differential pressure between the anterior and posterior chambers. Presented at the 2002 ARVO Meeting; submitted for publication.
3. Krix-Jachym K, Zarnowski T, Rekas M. Risk Factors of Malignant Glaucoma Occurrence after Glaucoma Surgery. J Ophthalmol. 2017:2017:9616738. https://doi.org/10.1155/2017/9616738
4. Shi Y, Tian J, Han Y, Oatts J, Wang N. Pathogenic role of the vitreous in angle-closure glaucoma with autosomal recessive bestrophinopathy: a case report. BMC Ophthalmol. 2020;20(1):271. https://doi.org/10.1186/s12886-020-01543-5
5. Shi Y, Oatts J, Tian J, et al N. Low-dose transscleral cyclophotocoagulation with subsequent phacoemulsification in the treatment of prolonged acute primary angle closure. Br J Ophthalmol. 2023;107(2): 221-226. https://doi.org/10.1136/bjophthalmol-2021-318880
6. Bao YK, Xu BY, Friedman DS, et al. Biometric Risk Factors for Angle Closure Progression After Laser Peripheral Iridotomy. JAMA Ophthalmol. 2023;141(6):516-524. https://doi.org/10.1001/jamaophthalmol.2023.0937
7. He M, Lu Y, Liu X, Ye T, Foster PJ. Histologic changes of the iris in the development of angle closure in Chinese eyes. J Glaucoma. 2008;17(5):386-392. https://doi.org/10.1097/IJG.0b013e31815c5f69
8. Chung C, Dai M, Lin J, Wang Z, Chen H, Huang J. Correlation of iris collagen and in-vivo anterior segment structures in patients in different stages of chronic primary angle-closure in both eyes. Indian J Ophthalmol. 2019;67(10):1638-1644. https://doi.org/10.4103/ijo.

IJO_1406_18

9. Yue BY, Duvall J, Goldberg MF, Puck A, Tso MO, Sugar J. Nanophthalmic sclera. Morphologic and tissue culture studies. Ophthalmology. 1986;93(4):534-541. https://doi.org/10.1016/S0161-6420(86)33704-7
10. Yue BY, Kurosawa A, Duvall J, Goldberg MF, Tso MO, Sugar J. Nanophthalmic sclera. Fibronectin studies. Ophthalmology. 1988;95(1):56-60. https://doi.org/10.1016/S0161-6420(88)33215-X
11. Trelstad RL, Silbermann NN, Brockhurst RJ. Nanophthalmic sclera. Ultrastructural, histochemical, and biochemical observations. Arch Ophthalmol. 1982;100(12):1935-1938. https://doi.org/10.1001/archopht.1982.01030040915009
12. Chua J, Seet LF, Jiang Y, et al. Increased SPARC expression in primary angle closure glaucoma iris. Mol Vis. 2008;14:1886-1892.
13. Yong VK, Umapathi T, Aung T, et al. Systemic autonomic function in subjects with primary angle-closure glaucoma---a comparative study of symptomatic and asymptomatic disease presentation. Clin Exp Ophthalmol. 2004;32(2):137-1341. https://doi.org/10.1111/j.1442-9071.2004.00791.x
14. Clark CV. The prevalence of autonomic neuropathy in the primary glaucomas. Doc Ophthalmol. 1990;74(4):277-285. https://doi.org/10.1007/BF00145812
15. Zhang X, Liu Y, Wang W, et al. Why does acute primary angle closure happen? Potential risk factors for acute primary angle closure. Surv Ophthalmol. 2017;62(5):635-647. https://doi.org/10.1016/j.survophthal.2017.04.002
16. Mapstone R, Clark CV. The prevalence of autonomic neuropathy in glaucoma. Trans Ophthalmol Soc U K. 1985;104(Pt 3):265-269.
17. Kumar R, Ahuja VM. Glaucoma and concomitant status of autonomic nervous system. Indian J Physiol Pharmacol. 1998;42(1):90-94.
18. Brazier DJ. Iris autonomic function in acute glaucoma. Eye (Lond). 1989: 3 (Pt 3): 288-93.
19. Clark CV. Autonomic denervation hypersensitivity in the primary glaucomas. Eye (Lond). 1989:3(Pt 3): 49-354. https://doi.org/10.1038/eye.1989.40
20. Clark CV, Mapstone R. Pupil cycle time in primary closed-angle glaucoma. Can J Ophthalmol. 1986;21(3):88-91.
21. Zheng C, Cheung CY, Narayanaswamy A, et al. Pupil dynamics in Chinese subjects with angle closure. Graefes Arch Clin Exp Ophthalmol. 2012;250(9):1353-1359. https://doi.org/10.1007/s00417-012-1934-7

Primary angle-closure glaucoma zonulopathy

Chunyan Qiao, Ningli Wang

The zonule of Zinn connects the equatorial region of the lens to the inner side of the ciliary body, functioning to adjust the curvature and position of the lens. Recent evidence suggests that zonulopathy, including zonular laxity and dehiscence, may contribute to the pathogenesis of PACG.

Pathophysiological evidence

Some research suggests that zonular laxity or dehiscence can weaken its regulatory effect on the lens, causing an anterior displacement of the iris-lens diaphragm, leading to a shallow anterior chamber, closure of the angular recess, and elevated IOP, ultimately triggering angle-closure glaucoma. Previous studies have found that zonulopathy among PACG patients is as high as 7.3% to 46.2%, potentially contributing to disease progression. However, further experimental studies are required to confirm the precise mechanisms through which zonulopathy contributes to PACG pathogenesis.

Clinical manifestations

Several clinical observations support the involvement of zonulopathy in PACG:

- Anterior displacement of the iris-lens diaphragm in PACG patients, contributing to a shallow anterior chamber.
- Persistent shallow anterior chamber despite the presence of patent laser peripheral iridotomy.
- Higher incidence of angle closure and its complications in younger PACG patients with zonular abnormalities.

Conclusion

Zonulopathy is a pathogenic factor in PACG that requires consideration in clinical evaluation and treatment planning. Recognizing zonular abnormalities in PACG patients can lead to more targeted and effective treatments, particularly in cases resistant to conventional methods. Future research should focus on understanding the molecular mechanisms of zonulopathy and integrating this knowledge into clinical practice to optimize treatment outcomes.

References

1. Zhang H, Zhang Y, Zhang S, et al. Zonulopathy Identified During Cataract Extraction in Patients With Primary Angle Closure Disease. J Glaucoma. 2023;32(9):783-791. https://doi.

org/10.1097/IJG.0000000000002247

2. Salimi A, Fanous A, Watt H, et al. Prevalence of zonulopathy in primary angle closure disease. Clin Exp Ophthalmol. 2021;49(9):1018-1026. https://doi.org/10.1111/ceo.13983
3. Qiao CY, Zhang H, Zhang Y, et al. Comparison study for the proportion of underdiagnosed zonulopathy in angle closure glaucoma. Zhonghua Yan Ke Za Zhi. 2022;58(11):872-881.
4. Kwon J, Sung KR. Factors Associated With Zonular Instability During Cataract Surgery in Eyes With Acute Angle Closure Attack. Am J Ophthalmol. 2017;183:118-124. https://doi.org/10.1016/j.ajo.2017.09.003
5. Pei XT, Fan ZG, Qing GP, et al. Biometric characteristics of primary angle closure glaucoma with zonular abnormality found during cataract surgery. YanKe. 2021;30(4):264-269.
6. Zhang H, Zhang Y, Zhang S, et al. Lens zonulopathy and primary angle closure glaucoma: what we know and don't know. Eye Science. 2023;38(02):140-147.
7. Zhang C, Guo Y, Huang P. the Mechanism of Lens Factors in Primary Angle Closure Disease. Zhonghua Yan Ke Za Zhi. 2024;60(9): 793-798. https://doi.org/10.3760/cma.j.cn112142-20231208-00276
8. Baskaran M, Yang E, Trikha S, et al. Residual angle closure one year after laser peripheral iridotomy in primary angle closure suspects. Am J Ophthalmol. 2017;183:111-117. https://doi.org/10.1016/j.ajo.2017.08.016
9. Huang J, Huang C. Zonulopathy and Its Relation to Primary Angle Closure Disease: A Review. J Glaucoma. 2024;33(12):931-939. https://doi.org/10.1097/IJG.0000000000002385

Medications

Shuning Li, Ningli Wang

Alpha-adrenergic agonists

- Phenylephrine can be used as a nasal decongestant and can also cause mydriasis via contraction of the iris dilator muscles.

Beta2-adrenergic agonists

- Salbutamol is most commonly used for the treatment of asthma.
- Beta2-receptors induce relaxation of the ciliary muscle, mydriasis, and increased production of aqueous humor in the ciliary muscle epithelium

Anticholinergic agents

Anticholinergic medications generally result in mydriasis.

- Local drugs such as atropine and tropicamide are frequently used as mydriatic medications.
- Benztropine and trihexyphenidyl are used to treat Parkinson's disease.

- Propylamine is used for life-threatening ventricular arrhythmias. Glycopyrrolate reduces airway secretions and reverses neuromuscular block.
- Ipratropium is a bronchodilator that prevents asthma.
- Oxybutynin and tolterodine are used for the treatment of symptoms such as frequent urination, urgent urination or urgent incontinence caused by overexcited bladder.
- Botulinum toxin is injected around the eyes to remove wrinkles.
- Antihistamines, including promethazine and cetirizine, reduce allergies and symptoms of allergic reactions.
- Of all the psychotropic medications, tricyclic antidepressants have the most potent anticholinergic effects.

Cholinergic agents

Cholinergic agents cause the ciliary muscle to contract, which loosens the ciliary body, round the lens, and moves it forward into the anterior chamber.

Sulfonamides

Sulfonamides induce angle-closure glaucoma by causing the ciliary body to expand and the lens-iris diaphragm to move forward.

- Topiramate is often used for seizures and migraines.
- Furosemide and hydrochlorothiazide are diuretics.
- Sulfonylureas treat diabetes mellitus.
- Probenecid is prescribed for arthrolithiasis.

Dopamine D2 receptor agonists

- Cabergoline induces non-pupillary block angle-closure glaucoma associated with choroidal effusion.

Serotonergic agents

Serotonergic [5-hydroxytryptamine (5-HT)] medicines increased aqueous humor production.

- Venlafaxine and escitalopram are used as antidepressants.
- Triptan is used for migraine treatment.
- Aripiprazole, olanzapine, and mirtazapine are used as antipsychotics.

Supplements

- Methylsulfonylmethane is a nutritional supplement used as an anti-inflammatory, antioxidative, and antihistamine medication. It can cause uveal effusion and anterior rotation of the lens–iris diaphragm.

Personality characteristics

Shuning Li, Ningli Wang

Type A behavior pattern

Patients with angle-closure glaucoma are more likely to show type A behavior, characterized by competitiveness, impatience, easily aroused anger, and aggression. This pattern may be linked to reduced estradiol levels in female patients.

Psychological factors

Psychological factors such as anxiety and depression play a significant role in the progression of glaucoma. A history of anxiety or both anxiety and depression in glaucoma suspects was significantly associated with the risk of converting to glaucoma over time.

References

1. Yang MC, Lin KY. Drug-induced Acute Angle-closure Glaucoma: A Review. J Curr Glaucoma Pract. 2019 Sep-Dec;13(3):104-109. https://doi.org/10.5005/jp-journals-10078-1261
2. Razeghinejad MR, Pro MJ, Katz LJ. Non-steroidal drug-induced glaucoma. Eye (Lond). 2011 Aug;25(8):971-80. https://doi.org/10.1038/eye.2011.128
3. Epstein NE, Goldbloom DS. Oral imipramine and acute angle-closure glaucoma. Arch Ophthalmol. 1995 Jun;113(6):698; author reply 699. https://doi.org/10.1001/archopht.1995.01100060020008
4. Rhee DJ, Goldberg MJ, Parrish RK. Bilateral angle-closure glaucoma and ciliary body swelling from topiramate. Arch Ophthalmol. 2001 Nov;119(11):1721-3.
5. Boundaoui ON, Woodruff TE. Presumed Furosemide-associated Bilateral Angle-Closure Glaucoma. J Glaucoma. 2016 Aug;25(8):e748-50. https://doi.org/10.1097/IJG.0000000000000430
6. Kahraman N, Durmaz O, Durna MM. Mirtazapine-induced acute angle closure. Indian J Ophthalmol. 2015 Jun;63(6):539-40. https://doi.org/10.4103/0301-4738.162612
7. Alarfaj MA, Almater AI. Olanzapine-Induced Acute Angle Closure. Am J Case Rep. 2021 Nov 22;22:e934432. https://doi.org/10.12659/AJCR.934432
8. Hwang JC, Khine KT, Lee JC, et al. Methyl-sulfonyl-methane (MSM)-induced acute angle closure. J Glaucoma. 2015;24(4):e28-e30. https://doi.org/10.1097/IJG.0000000000000027

9. Berchuck S, Jammal A, Mukherjee S, Somers T, Medeiros FA. Impact of anxiety and depression on progression to glaucoma among glaucoma suspects. Br J Ophthalmol. 2021 Sep;105(9):1244-1249. https://doi.org/10.1136/bjophthalmol-2020-316617

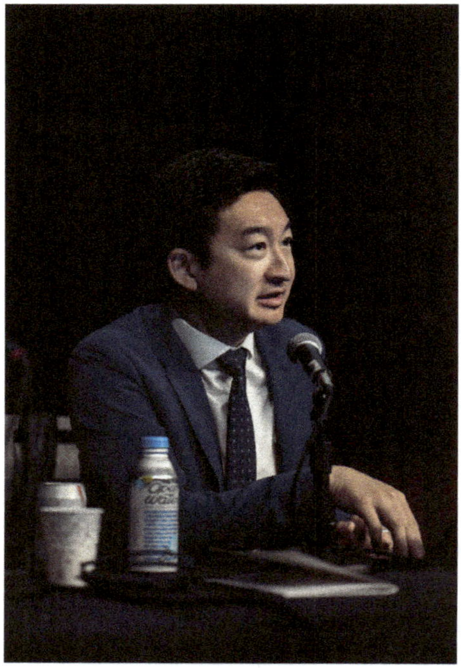

Benjamin Xu

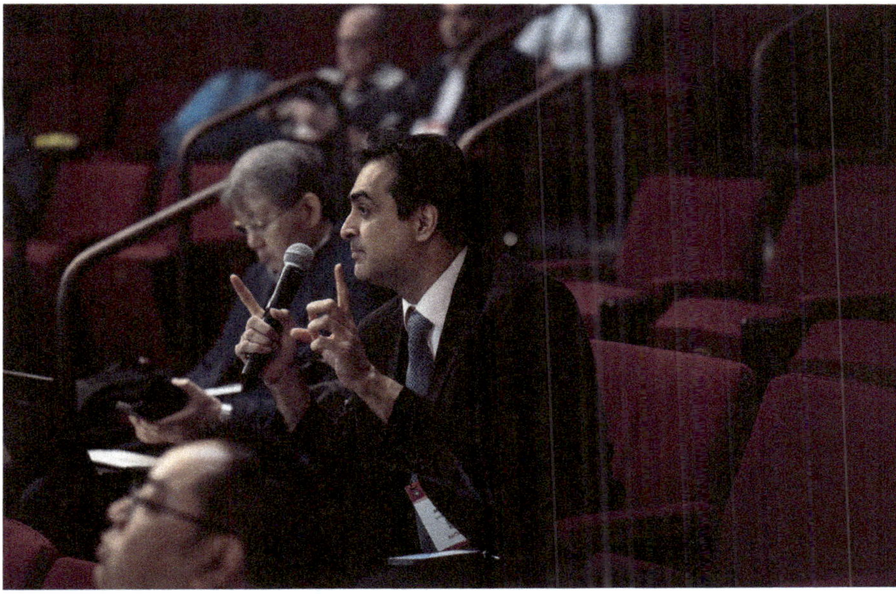

Sasan Moghimi

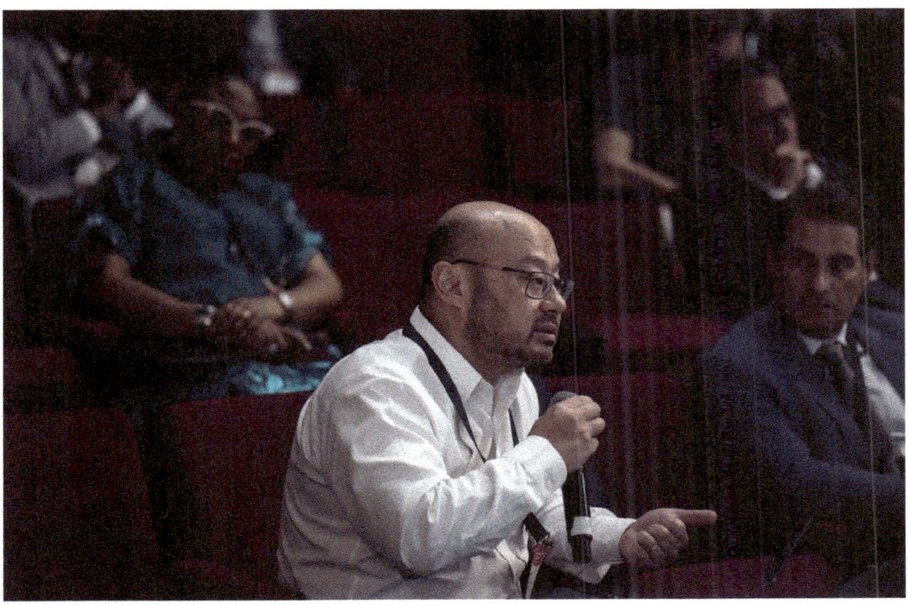

Lisandro Sakata

Section Leaders

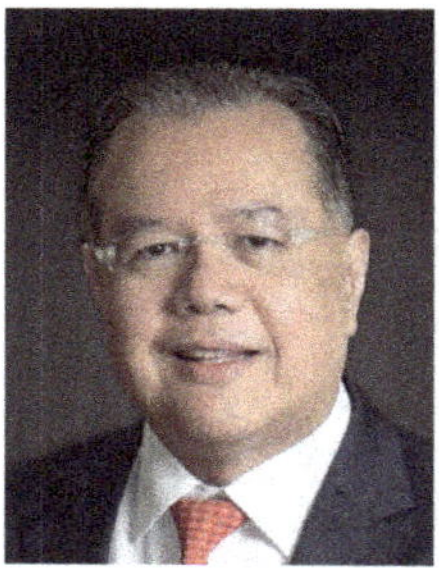

Tin Aung

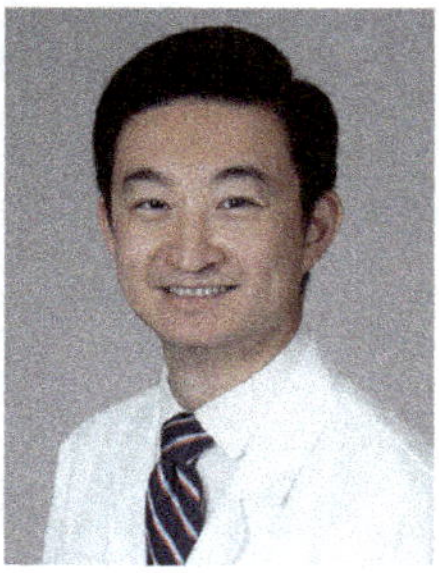

Benjamin Xu

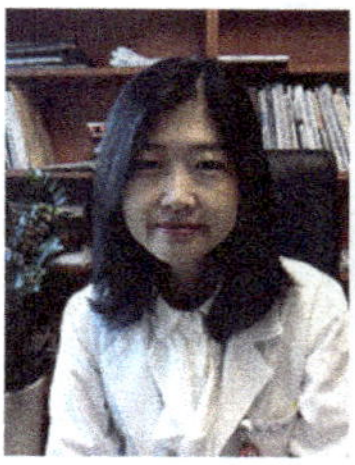

Kyung Rim Sung

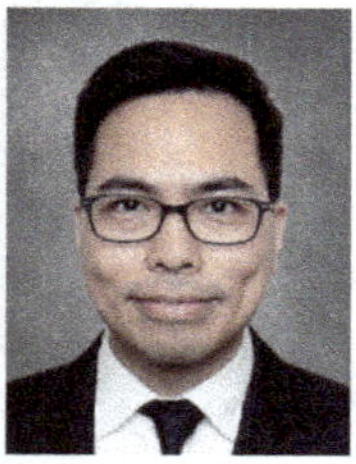

Christopher Leung

3. DIAGNOSIS AND EVALUATION

Tin Aung, Benjamin Xu, Kyung Rim Sung, Christopher Leung

Abbreviations

ACAn: anterior chamber angle
ACAr: anterior chamber area
ACD: anterior chamber depth
ACV: anterior chamber volume
ACW: anterior chamber width
AI: artificial intelligence
AOD: angle opening distance
APAC: acute primary angle closure
ARA: angle recess area
AS-OCT: anterior segment optical coherence tomography
AUC: area under the curve
DRPPT: dark room prone provocative test
IOP: intraocular pressure
ITC: iridotrabecular contact
LACD: limbal anterior chamber depth
LPI: laser peripheral iridotomy
LT: lens thickness
LV: lens vault
PAC: primary angle closure
PACS: primary angle-closure suspect
PACD: primary angle-closure disease
PACG: primary angle closure-glaucoma
PAS: peripheral anterior synechiae
sPAC: spectrum of primary angle closure
TISA: trabecular iris space area
UBM: ultrasound biomicroscopy
ZAP: Zhongshan Angle Closure Prevention trial

Angle Closure and Angle-Closure Glaucoma, pp 1-19
Edited by Robert N. Weinreb, Benjamin Xu, Xiulan Zhang

Consensus statements

1. The definitions of sPAC are based on gonioscopy and clinical findings:
    - Angle closure on gonioscopy is defined as when the posterior, usually pigmented, trabecular meshwork is not visible, possibly indicating the presence of ITC.
    - PACS: 2 or more quadrants of angle closure on gonioscopy.
    - PAC: PACS plus PAS and/or elevated IOP, or an APAC attack.
    - PACG: PACS or PAC plus glaucomatous optic neuropathy.
2. One way of characterizing the spectrum of PAC is:
    - The term PACD includes PAC and PACG.
    - The term sPAC includes PACS and PACD.
3. Gonioscopy is the clinical standard for evaluating the ACAn. However, it is subjective and variable.
    - Gonioscopy is a vital but underutilized part of the eye exam.
    - The patient should be examined in a dark room and with the use of a short, narrow slit-beam to avoid constricting the pupil and artifactually opening the angle.
    - Indentation gonioscopy remains the gold standard for identifying PAS.
    - Tilting of the goniolens can be performed to visualize the angle recess in eyes with a high LV.
4. The Van Herick test of LACD only has moderate sensitivity or specificity in detecting eyes with gonioscopic angle closure and is not a replacement for gonioscopy.
    - LACD can be used for opportunistic case detection when followed by gonioscopy but is less useful for population-based screening as it could generate an unacceptably high number of false positives.
5. AS-OCT and UBM are adjunctive tools to gonioscopy for evaluating the ACAn.
    - Angle closure on AS-OCT and UBM is defined as presence of contact between the anterior iris surface and inner corneal curvature or angle wall anterior to the scleral spur, which indicates the presence of ITC.
    - ITC can be described in terms of circumferential extent and anterior-posterior length (also referred to as height or width). There is no consensus about clinically significant thresholds in extent or length.
6. There may be disagreement between gonioscopy and AS-OCT in detecting angle closure due to differences in definitions.
    - A wide range of factors, including anatomical configurations, examination

  techniques, refraction correction, level of ambient lighting, and pupillary constriction due to light or accommodation, contribute to the disagreement.
- The extent of ITC on AS-OCT is more strongly associated with PACD severity than cumulative gonioscopy grading.

7. Gonioscopy is poorly able to identify which PACS eyes are at high risk for PACD.
   - AS-OCT measurements have been found to be associated with progression from PACS to PAC.
   - No precise ITC or measurement cutoffs have been demonstrated to be clinically significant or widely adopted for routine care.
   - Longitudinal studies assessing the clinical significance of AS-OCT findings alone for risk stratifying PACS eyes are needed.
8. UBM remains the gold standard for evaluating the ciliary body.
   - Newer AS-OCT devices utilizing longer-wavelength swept-source lasers and image averaging provide reproducible visualization and analysis of the ciliary body in some eyes.
9. Plateau iris configuration is characterized by anteriorly positioned ciliary processes causing posterior angulation in the peripheral iris and the absence of the iridociliary sulcus.
   - Plateau iris syndrome is persistence of angle closure despite a patent iridotomy in the presence of plateau iris configuration.
10. Goniophotographs are useful to capture anatomical findings (e.g., iris nevus) but are not commonly used to evaluate the angle recess.
11. There is no consensus about which biometric parameters describing the anterior segment are the most clinically relevant for detecting individuals at high risk for PACG.
    - ACD cutoffs have been tested but are not effective for identifying individuals at high risk for PACG in the community.
    - ACV has better diagnostic performance in detecting angle closure compared to ACAn width parameters, such as AOD.
12. There are no widely accepted provocative tests to identify individuals at high risk for PACG.
    - The DRPPT is unable to risk-stratify PACS for progression to PACD.

Future directions

- There is a need for additional research to:
    - o Identify novel imaging biomarkers to predict angle closure progression.
    - o Establish imaging-based definitions of narrow angles.
    - o Implement AI to facilitate image analysis and widespread clinical adoption.
- Prospective longitudinal studies of individuals with narrow angles, especially those identified using non-invasive imaging, are required to establish clinically meaningful cutoffs and guidelines.

Diagnosis of primary angle-closure disease

Hitomi Saito, Catherine Liu, Chris Leung

PACD is classified into 3 main categories, according to the International Society of Geographical and Epidemiological Ophthalmology (ISGEO).[1]

PACS

PACS is diagnosed when there is contact between the peripheral iris and the posterior trabecular meshwork, with no other ocular abnormalities. The pigmented posterior trabecular meshwork is not visible on gonioscopy for at least 180°. While originally requiring 270° of ITC for diagnosis, recent studies have adopted a more lenient criterion of 180° of appositional contact.[2] The intraocular pressure (IOP) must be ≤ 21 mmHg and there should be no PAS, with the optic nerve head appearing healthy.

Gonioscopy remains the standard method of assessing the ACAn to detect angle closure. By visualizing the angle structures and the width of the angle, the likelihood of closure can be assessed using grading systems, such as the Spaeth classification[3] and the Shaffer classification.[4] A Spaeth classification grade < 3 or a Shaffer classification grade < 2 is generally indicative of angle closure. Other methods of angle evaluation include AS-OCT, UBM, and goniophotography.

PACS eyes typically show no abnormalities beyond angle narrowing. This stage of PACD is generally asymptomatic. The 5-year conversion rate from PACS to PAC is relatively low, at approximately 6%, with a narrow baseline angle width being the strongest predictor of conversion.[6]

PAC

PAC is diagnosed when there are signs of trabecular meshwork apposition by the peripheral iris, without any evidence of glaucomatous optic neuropathy; however, evidence of obstruction of aqueous humor outflow must be present. Indicators of aqueous outflow obstruction include elevated IOP (> 21 mmHg), iris whorling, excessive pigment deposition on the trabecular meshwork, and presence of PAS. PAS is confirmed when the peripheral iris is adherent to the angle and cannot be separated through indentation gonioscopy. The extent of PAS can vary, appearing either localized or widespread, and may manifest as either pinpoint or broad adhesions.

Most PAC cases are asymptomatic; however, some patients may experience temporary blurring of vision or ocular pain during episodes of IOP elevation. These episodes may occur at night or when the patient assumes a downward head position. Provocative tests, such as dark room or mydriatic provocative tests, may be conducted to detect these temporary IOP elevations. Nevertheless, the results must be interpreted with caution, as these tests have low sensitivity in predicting which PAC eyes are at risk of progressing to PACD.[7]

PACG

PACG is diagnosed when PAC is associated with evidence of glaucomatous optic neuropathy. This condition indicates that optic nerve damage has occurred as a result of IOP elevation with optic nerve head and/or visual field abnormalities indicative of glaucoma.

APAC

APAC is characterized by a sudden and significant elevation in IOP due to angle closure. Patients with APAC typically present with ocular pain, eye redness, nausea, vomiting, and/or intermittent blurring of vision or halos around lights. IOP is usually severely elevated. Clinical signs include marked conjunctival injection, corneal edema, a mid-dilated unreactive pupil, shallow anterior chamber, and the presence of a closed angle on gonioscopy. If not treated promptly, APAC can lead to ischemic optic nerve damage with permanent visual impairment.

References

1. Foster PJ, Buhrmann R, Quigley HA, Johnson GJ. The definition and classification of glaucoma in prevalence surveys. Br J Ophthalmol. 2002;86:238-242. https://doi.org/10.1136/bjo.86.2.238

2. Teo ZL, Soh ZD, Tham YC, et al. Six-Year Incidence and Risk Factors for Primary Angle-Closure Disease: The Singapore Epidemiology of Eye Diseases Study. Ophthalmology. 2022;129:792-802. https://doi.org/10.1016/j.ophtha.2022.03.009
3. Spaeth GL. The normal development of the human anterior chamber angle: a new system of descriptive grading. Trans Ophthalmol Soc U K (1962). 1971;91:709-739.
4. Shaffer RN. Primary glaucomas. Gonioscopy, ophthalmoscopy and perimetry. Trans Am Acad Ophthalmol Otolaryngol. 1960;64:112-127.
5. Lai I, Mak H, Lai G, Yu M, Lam DS, Leung CK. Anterior chamber angle imaging with swept-source optical coherence tomography: measuring peripheral anterior synechia in glaucoma. Ophthalmology. 2013;120:1144-1149. https://doi.org/10.1016/j.ophtha.2012.12.006
6. Zhang Y, Thomas R, Zhang Q, Li SZ, Wang NL. Progression of Primary Angle Closure Suspect to Primary Angle Closure and Associated Risk Factors: The Handan Eye Study. Invest Ophthalmol Vis Sci. 2021;62:2. https://doi.org/10.1167/iovs.62.7.2
7. Wilensky JT, Kaufman PL, Frohlichstein D, et al. Follow-up of angle-closure glaucoma suspects. Am J Ophthalmol. 1993;115:338-346. https://doi.org/10.1016/S0002-9394(14)73585-8

New diagnostic criteria based on anterior segment optical coherence tomography

Poemen Chan, Syril Dorairaj, Paul Foster, Xiulan Zhang, Chris Leung

ITC assessment using AS-OCT: implications for the definition of angle closure

The assessment of ITC using AS-OCT represents a significant advancement in the understanding of angle closure. AS-OCT offers a more precise assessment of the circumferential extent of ITC compared to gonioscopy. The technology enables detailed examination of the ACAn over 360°, providing objective data on the extent and length of ITC. This level of detail is helpful for identifying risk factors associated with PACD and for developing tailored management strategies.

Definitions of ITC

ITC is defined as contact between the iris and angle wall anterior to the scleral spur, a landmark that is identifiable on AS-OCT and relative to which the location of the trabecular meshwork can be determined.[1-5] Some studies have used manufacturer-provided software to evaluate ITC by measuring the total area of ITC, including the height and extent, obtained from circumferential scans and the ITC index, the percentage of scans showing ITC relative to the total number of scans analyzed for each eye.[1,2,6-14] Two additional parameters related to ITC have also been described:

- Short iridoangle contact (or short ITC), which refers to a short segment of contact between the iris and angle wall just anterior to the scleral spur.
- Steep iris profile, characterized by a pronounced convex contour of the anterior surface of the iris while maintaining an open ACAn.[15]

The AS-OCT definitions of angle closure vary across studies (Table 1). Some studies define angle closure based on AS-OCT detection of ≥ 2 quadrants with ITC.[15-18] Others use a specific number of consecutive B-scans with detectable ITC, ranging from 3 consecutive B-scans (out of 128 B-scans, equating to 8.4° of ITC)[19] to 5 consecutive B-scan of short ITC (14°).[20] One study considered several thresholds of the extent of angle closure by specifying whether the ITC was present in ≥ 35%, ≥ 50%, and ≥ 75% of the angle circumference.[21]

ITC has also been defined using AOD500 or TISA500, measured at a distance of 500 µm from the scleral spur:[22]

- AOD500 = 0 mm: This indicates that there is no measurable distance between the posterior corneoscleral junction and the anterior iris surface at a distance of 500 µm anterior to the scleral spur.
- TISA500 = 0 mm^2: This indicates that there is no measurable area between the trabecular meshwork and the iris over a distance of 500 µm anterior to the scleral spur.

The threshold of contact between the peripheral iris and the corneoscleral wall measuring 500 µm from the scleral spur was established based on anatomical studies suggesting that the trabecular meshwork length is approximately 575 µm in eyes with gonioscopic angle closure.[23]

Disparity between AS-OCT and gonioscopy assessment

Using AOD500 and TISA500-based definitions, a significant percentage of eyes classified as having angle closure based on gonioscopy do not exhibit ITC when assessed with AS-OCT. Specifically, while all eyes with gonioscopic angle closure showed non-visible posterior trabecular meshwork for at least 180°, 15.3% to 17.6% of these eyes had no evidence of ITC for the same extent on AS-OCT.[1] This discrepancy indicates that gonioscopy may overestimate the extent of angle closure compared to AS-OCT.

Risk assessment for PAC and PACG

ITC assessment via AS-OCT may be more reliable than gonioscopy for evaluating the risk of PAC and PACG. The extent of ITC measured by AS-OCT correlates significantly with the odds of PAC/PACG diagnosis, with each 10° increase in ITC associated with a 5% increase in these odds. In contrast, cumulative gonioscopy scores did not show a similar correlation, suggesting that the extent of ITC as measured by AS-OCT may be a more clinically relevant measure than traditional gonioscopic grading.[22]

Treatment recommendations

Current treatment recommendations for PACD primarily rely on studies that have utilized gonioscopy for angle assessment. The role of AS-OCT in the clinical management of PACD remains to be fully explored. Longitudinal studies are needed to determine how AS-OCT can influence treatment decisions, particularly regarding the need for laser iridotomy or cataract surgery in patients diagnosed with PACS.

In conclusion, while AS-OCT represents a promising tool for assessing ITC and evaluating angle closure more accurately than gonioscopy, further research is necessary to integrate this technology into clinical practice. The potential benefits of AS-OCT could lead to improved patient outcomes by facilitating better-informed treatment decisions based on precise anatomical assessments.

Table 1. Definitions of angle closure and ITC in AS-OCT studies

Authors	AS-OCT models	Definitions of ITC
Lavanya et al., 2008[18]	Visante, (Carl Zeiss Meditec, Dublin, CA)	Closed angle: AS-OCT-detected contact between the iris and any part of the angle wall anterior to the scleral spur. Eye with closed angle: AS-OCT detected ≥ 2 quadrants (nasal, temporal, superior, and inferior) were closed. Individual with closed angle: Either eye has ≥ 2 quadrants of closed angle.
Nolan et al., 2007[17]	A prototype of AS-OCT (Carl Zeiss Meditec, Dublin, CA)	Closed angle: Visible contact between the peripheral iris and any part of the angle wall anterior to the scleral spur. Eye with closed angle: ≥ 1 of the temporal, inferior, and nasal quadrants were found to be closed.
Porporato et al., 2019[21]	SS-OCT (CASIA SS-1000; Tomey Corporation, Nagoya, Japan)	Closed angle: Contact between the iris and any part of the angle wall anterior to the scleral spur.
Choi et al., 2024[6]	SS AS-OCT (CASIA 2, Tomey Corporation, Nagoya, Japan)	ITC: Contact between the iris and the corneal endothelium in front of the scleral spur. ITC index and area: Percentage of the circumference and the total area where there was contact between the iris and the inner surface of the cornea in the anterior part of the scleral spur.
Zhang et al., 2023[22]	SS-OCT (CASIA2, Tomey Corporation, Nagoya, Japan)	ITC of an angle location (ITC500): Defined by 2 criteria: (1) AOD500 = 0 mm, and (2) TISA500 = 0 mm^2 (i.e., visible contact between the peripheral iris and the corneoscleral wall for at least 500 μm from the scleral spur). Extent of ITC: Estimated form the number of angle locations with AOD500 = 0 mm or TISA500 = 0 mm^2 (each eye had 36 angle locations measured; each angle location spanned ~10°).

Authors	AS-OCT models	Definitions of ITC
Song et al., 2023[7]	SS-OCT (CASIA2, Tomey Corporation, Nagoya, Japan)	ITC index: Percentage of scans showing contact above the scleral spur. ITC area: Total area of contact between the iris and anterior angle wall above the scleral spur.
Porporato et al., 2023[8]	SS-OCT (CASIA SS-1000; Tomey Corporation, Nagoya, Japan)	ITC index: Percentage of scans (out of 8) that had any presence of ITC above the scleral spur. ITC area: Total area of contact (height and extent) between the iris and the anterior angle wall above the scleral spur, obtained from the circumferential scans.
Song et al., 2024[9]	SS-OCT (CASIA2, Tomey Corporation, Nagoya, Japan)	ITC index: Percentage of scans showing contact above the scleral spur. ITC area: Total area of contact between the iris and anterior angle wall above the scleral spur (determined by averaging 8 AS-OCT meridional scans).
Tang et al., 2023[10]	SS-OCT (CASIA2, Tomey Corporation, Nagoya, Japan)	ITC index: Percentage of scans showing contact above the scleral spur. ITC area: Contact area between the iris and anterior angle wall above the scleral spur.
Tan et al., 2024[24]	SS-OCT (CASIA, Tomey Corporation, Nagoya, Japan)	ITC definition not mentioned
Yu et al., 2022[12]	SS-OCT (CASIA2, Tomey Corporation, Nagoya, Japan)	ITC index: Percentage of ITC areas to all measured areas (8 x AS-OCT meridional scans).
Chen et al., 2022[11]		ITC index: Ratio of angle closure in degrees to the total angle with visible scleral spur and end point in degrees. ITC area: Area of the extent of circumferential contact of peripheral iris to the angle wall.
Ho et al., 2013[1]	SS-OCT (CASIA SS-1000; Tomey Corporation, Nagoya, Japan)	ITC detection: Based on the CASIA software (effectively, whenever there is iris contact with the anterior angle wall above the scleral spur). ITC index: Ratio of angle closure in degrees to the total angle with visible scleral spur and end point in degrees (essentially represents the extent of angle closure as a percentage). ITC area ("invisible range"): Circumferential extent (in degrees) throughout which either the scleral spur or end point could not be determined in the meridional frames. A minimum of 7 points needed to be identified for each eye for the calculation of ITC index (as per the manufacturer), and this criterion was used for quality control.
Tun et al., 2015[25]	SS-OCT (CASIA SS-1000; Tomey Corporation, Nagoya, Japan)	ITC area: Area of the extent of circumferential contact of the peripheral iris to the angle wall.
Gupta et al., 2020[2]	SS-OCT (CASIA SS-1000; Tomey Corporation, Nagoya, Japan)	ITC endpoint: Identified as the most anterior point of contact of the iris to the angle wall. ITC index (by native CASIA software): Quantitative measure of the extent of angle closure across 360° of the angles, expressed as a percentage (128 frames/eyes).
Porporato et al., 2021[3]	SS-OCT (CASIA SS-1000; Tomey Corporation, Nagoya, Japan)	Closed angle on SS-OCT: Contact between the iris and any part of the angle wall anterior to the scleral spur. 128 consecutive meridional scans.
Porporato et al., 2020[26]	SS-OCT (CASIA SS-1000; Tomey Corporation, Nagoya, Japan)	Short ITC: Considered closed if the 5 adjacent scans had ITC from scleral spur to Schwalbe's line. A steep iris profile was present when there was a pronounced convex profile of the anterior surface of the iris with an open angle.
Sakata et al., 2008[15]	Visante, (Carl Zeiss Meditec, Dublin, CA)	Short irido-angle contact was present when there was contact between the iris and angle wall just above the scleral spur, but the contact distance was short. A steep iris profile was present when there was a pronounced convex profile of the anterior surface of the iris with an open ACAn.
Cho et al., 2017[13,14]	SS-OCT (CASIA SS-1000; Tomey Corporation, Nagoya, Japan)	ITC index (by native CASIA software): Quantitative measure of the extent of angle closure across 360° of the angles, expressed as a percentage.

Authors	AS-OCT models	Definitions of ITC
Baskaran et al., 2015[16]	Visante, (Carl Zeiss Meditec, Dublin, CA)	Number of quadrants with presence of ITC.
Moghimi et al., 2016[4]	Visante, (Carl Zeiss Meditec, Dublin, CA)	ITC: Iridotrabecular contact anterior to the scleral spur. AS-OCT images were assessed grossly for the presence and extent of ITC.
Mishima et al., 2013[5]	SS-OCT (CASIA SS-1000; Tomey Corporation, Nagoya, Japan)	Quadrant-based study, where: ITC: EP located more anteriorly than the scleral spur. ITC-positive quadrant: At least 1 ITC in the quadrant. ITC in eye: At least 1 quadrant of ITC in an eye. The following parameters of ITC were calculated: Unobservable range (UR): Range of angles in degrees that could not be analyzed because of low image quality that prevented scleral spur or end point from being identified or the absence of the angle image, mainly due to the upper or lower eyelid). ITC range: Ratio of angle degree of ITC excluding the UR. The SS-1000 CASIA software also determined the values of these parameters in each quadrant.
Fukuda et al., 2012[19]	SS-OCT (CASIA SS-1000; Tomey Corporation, Nagoya, Japan)	When the EP was located more proximally than SS in 3 consecutive B-scan images, it was supposed that there was ITC at that position. 128 image scan, 2.8° each; 8.4° of ITC = closed angle.
Lai et al., 2013[27]	SS-OCT (CASIA SS-1000; Tomey Corporation, Nagoya, Japan)	Extent of PAS in each meridian was measured by the built-in software after manual detection of the scleral spur and the anterior irido-angle adhesion (the iris end point). Used all 128 angle meridians.

AS-OCT: anterior segment optical coherence tomography; EP: end point; ITC: iridotrabecular contact: PAS: peripheral anterior synechiae; SS-OCT: swept source optical coherence tomography

References

1. Ho SW, Baskaran M, Zheng C, et al. Swept source optical coherence tomography measurement of the iris-trabecular contact (ITC) index: a new parameter for angle closure. Graefes Arch Clin Exp Ophthalmol. Apr 2013;251(4):1205-11. https://doi.org/10.1007/s00417-012-2158-6
2. Gupta B, Angmo D, Yadav S, Dada T, Gupta V, Sihota R. Quantification of Iridotrabecular Contact in Primary Angle-Closure Disease. J Glaucoma. Aug 2020;29(8):681-688. https://doi.org/10.1097/IJG.0000000000001572
3. Porporato N, Baskaran M, Perera S, et al. Evaluation of meridional scans for angle closure assessment with anterior segment swept-source optical coherence tomography. Br J Ophthalmol. Jan 2021;105(1):131-134. https://doi.org/10.1136/bjophthalmol-2019-315461
4. Moghimi S, Chen R, Johari M, et al. Changes in Anterior Segment Morphology After Laser Peripheral Iridotomy in Acute Primary Angle Closure. Am J Ophthalmol. Jun 2016;166:133-140. https://doi.org/10.1016/j.ajo.2016.03.032
5. Mishima K, Tomidokoro A, Suramethakul P, et al. Iridotrabecular contact observed using anterior segment three-dimensional OCT in eyes with a shallow peripheral anterior chamber. Invest Ophthalmol Vis Sci. Jul 10 2013;54(7):4628-35. https://doi.org/10.1167/iovs.12-11230
6. Choi HI, Song WK, Sung KR. Changes in Iridotrabecular Contact and Intraocular Pressure after Phacoemulsification in Primary Angle-Closure Disease Spectrum. Korean J Ophthalmol. Oct 2024;38(5):342-353. https://doi.org/10.3341/kjo.2024.0014

7. Song WK, Sung KR, Kim KE. Assessment of Iridotrabecular Contact and Its Association With Intraocular Pressure After Phacoemulsification in Primary Angle Closure. Am J Ophthalmol. May 2023;249:1-11. https://doi.org/10.1016/j.ajo.2022.12.023
8. Porporato N, Chong R, Xu BY, et al. Angle closure extent, anterior segment dimensions and intraocular pressure. Br J Ophthalmol. Jul 2023;107(7):927-934. https://doi.org/10.1136/bjophthalmol-2021-320453
9. Song WK, Sung KR, Kim KE. Anterior Chamber Angle and Intraocular Pressure Control After Phacoemulsification in Primary Angle Closure With Different Mechanisms. J Glaucoma. Oct 1 2024;33(10):748-757. https://doi.org/10.1097/IJG.0000000000002454
10. Tang C, Sun T, Sun Z, et al. Evaluation of biometric indicators of anterior segment parameters after ICL implantation by swept-source optical coherence tomography. BMC Ophthalmol. May 2 2023;23(1):193. https://doi.org/10.1186/s12886-023-02942-0
11. Chen X, Wang X, Tang Y, Sun X, Chen Y. Optical coherence tomography analysis of anterior segment parameters before and after laser peripheral iridotomy in primary angle-closure suspects by using CASIA2. BMC Ophthalmol. Mar 28 2022;22(1):144. https://doi.org/10.1186/s12886-022-02366-2
12. Yu B, Wang K, Zhang X, Xing X. Biometric indicators of anterior segment parameters before and after laser peripheral iridotomy by swept-source optical coherent tomography. BMC Ophthalmol. May 16 2022;22(1):222. https://doi.org/10.1186/s12886-022-02448-1
13. Cho HK, Kee C, Yang H, et al. Comparison of circumferential peripheral angle closure using iridotrabecular contact index after laser iridotomy versus combined laser iridotomy and iridoplasty. Acta Ophthalmol. Nov 2017;95(7):e539-e547. https://doi.org/10.1111/aos.13450
14. Cho HK, Ahn D, Kee C. Evaluation of circumferential angle closure using iridotrabecular contact index after laser iridotomy by swept-source optical coherence tomography. Acta Ophthalmol. May 2017;95(3):e190-e196. https://doi.org/10.1111/aos.13190
15. Sakata LM, Lavanya R, Friedman DS, et al. Comparison of gonioscopy and anterior segment ocular coherence tomography in detecting angle closure in different quadrants of the anterior chamber angle. Ophthalmology. May 2008;115(5):769-74. https://doi.org/10.1016/j.ophtha.2007.06.030
16. Baskaran M, Iyer JV, Narayanaswamy AK, et al. Anterior Segment Imaging Predicts Incident Gonioscopic Angle Closure. Ophthalmology. Dec 2015;122(12):2380-4. https://doi.org/10.1016/j.ophtha.2015.07.030
17. Nolan WP, See JL, Chew PT, et al. Detection of primary angle closure using anterior segment optical coherence tomography in Asian eyes. Ophthalmology. Jan 2007;114(1):33-9. https://doi.org/10.1016/j.ophtha.2006.05.073
18. Lavanya R, Foster PJ, Sakata LM, et al. Screening for narrow angles in the singapore population: evaluation of new noncontact screening methods. Ophthalmology. Oct 2008;115(10):1720-7, 1727 e1-2. https://doi.org/10.1016/j.ophtha.2008.03.015

19. Fukuda R, Usui T, Tomidokoro A, et al. Noninvasive observations of peripheral angle in eyes after penetrating keratoplasty using anterior segment fourier-domain optical coherence tomography. Cornea. Mar 2012;31(3):259-63. https://doi.org/10.1097/ICO.0b013e318226daa9
20. Porporato N, Baskaran M, Tun TA, et al. Assessment of Circumferential Angle Closure with Swept-Source Optical Coherence Tomography: A Community Based Study. Am J Ophthalmol. Mar 2019;199:133-139. https://doi.org/10.1016/j.ajo.2018.11.015
21. Porporato N, Baskaran M, Tun TA, et al. Understanding diagnostic disagreement in angle closure assessment between anterior segment optical coherence tomography and gonioscopy. Br J Ophthalmol. Jun 2020;104(6):795-799. https://doi.org/10.1136/bjophthalmol-2019-314672
22. Zhang X, Guo PY, Lin C, et al. Assessment of Iris Trabecular Contact in Eyes with Gonioscopic Angle-Closure. Ophthalmology. Jan 2023;130(1):111-119. https://doi.org/10.1016/j.ophtha.2022.08.017
23. Choi W, Lee MW, Kang HG, et al. Comparison of the trabecular meshwork length between open and closed angle with evaluation of the scleral spur location. Sci Rep. May 2 2019;9(1):6857. https://doi.org/10.1038/s41598-019-43315-2
24. Tan SS, Tun TA, Aung T, Nongpiur ME. Comparison of intraocular pressure and anterior segment parameters in subjects with asymmetrical primary angle closure disease. Clin Exp Ophthalmol. Sep-Oct 2024;52(7):724-731. https://doi.org/10.1111/ceo.14402
25. Tun TA, Baskaran M, Perera SA, Htoon HM, Aung T, Husain R. Swept-source optical coherence tomography assessment of iris-trabecular contact after phacoemulsification with or without goniosynechialysis in eyes with primary angle closure glaucoma. Br J Ophthalmol. Jul 2015;99(7):927-31. https://doi.org/10.1136/bjophthalmol-2014-306223
26. Porporato N, Baskaran M, Tun TA, et al. Understanding diagnostic disagreement in angle closure assessment between anterior segment optical coherence tomography and gonioscopy. Br J Ophthalmol. Jun 2020;104(6):795-799. https://doi.org/10.1136/bjophthalmol-2019-314672
27. Lai I, Mak H, Lai G, Yu M, Lam DS, Leung CK. Anterior chamber angle imaging with swept-source optical coherence tomography: measuring peripheral anterior synechia in glaucoma. Ophthalmology. Jun 2013;120(6):1144-9. https://doi.org/10.1016/j.ophtha.2012.12.006

Gonioscopy

Sanjay Asrani, Tin Aung

Despite its many shortcomings, gonioscopy remains the so-called gold standard for evaluating the ACAn and for assessing a patient's risk for angle-closure glaucoma. The method's advantages include its speed, simplicity, and low cost (requiring a relatively inexpensive instrument, the goniolens). Its disadvantages include the subjective nature of the assessment, the need for skill and interpretation by the examiner, and the need to contact the patient's eye and its associated discomfort.

Because PACD may be more prevalent—and more subtle—than many clinicians realize, gonioscopy should be performed on all persons with a diagnosis of, or suspicion of glaucoma, or risk factors for angle closure, including patients whose peripheral anterior chamber depth appears shallow with the van Herick technique. Risk factors for narrow angles are an age greater than 55 years, a family history of glaucoma, hyperopia, incipient cataract, diabetes and a history of retinal vein occlusion. Additionally, gonioscopy should be performed on patients undergoing repeated intravitreal injections and patients undergoing hemodialysis.

Ideally, gonioscopy should be performed on all patients, but especially when the peripheral anterior chamber depth is estimated to be shallow (*i.e.*, approximately one-fourth of the corneal thickness by van Herick slit lamp examination), careful gonioscopic examination of the angle is required. This is best accomplished with a Zeiss/Sussman 4-mirror lens or similar indentation goniolens. The Goldmann gonioscopy lens can also be used, but its ability to do compression gonioscopy may be limited. However, the Goldmann lens does provide a more magnified view of the angle structures. The patient should be examined in a dark room and with the use of a short, narrow slit-beam to avoid constricting the pupil and artifactually opening the angle. Additionally, the initial impression of gonioscopy should be disregarded, as the pupil constricts with accommodation and light, resulting in the angle appearing open initially. However, waiting approximately 10–15 seconds allows the pupil to relax and resume its resting state, thus allowing for aqueous humor to collect behind the root of the iris with resumption of relative pupillary block and consequently a much narrower angle. The gonioscopic findings after 10 seconds may be significantly different than those observed at the start of gonioscopy. The examiner also should take care to avoid extra pressure on the cornea so that the angle does not deepen artifactually.

The presence of $\geq 180°$ of appositional angle closure (*i.e.*, trabecular meshwork not visible) with the eye in primary gaze (or with a minimal shift of gaze in case of a steep iris insertion), constitutes an occludable angle. The configuration of the iris should also be observed. A volcano cone-like shape may suggest the mechanism to be phacomorphic angle closure due to the high LV; if the iris contour is rounded ("iris bombe"), it is more likely to be pupillary block. If the iris is flat but the angle structures are not seen, then it could be plateau iris syndrome or creeping chronic angle closure. Irregularly shaped convexities at the root of the iris could indicate peripheral iris epithelial cysts or other pathology of the iris or ciliary body.

Numerous grading systems have been proposed to standardize documentation of the gonioscopic angle appearance and correlate with the potential for angle closure. Scheie (Table 1) proposed a system based on the extent of the ACAn structures that can be visualized.[1] He observed a high risk of angle closure in eyes with grade III or IV angles. Shaffer suggested using the angular width of the angle recess as the criterion for grading the angle and attempted to correlate this with the potential for angle closure.[2]

Table 1. Scheie's gonioscopic classification of the ACAn according to the extent of the visible angle structures

Classification	Gonioscopic appearance
Wide open	All structures visible
Grade I narrow	Hard to see over iris root into recess
Grade II narrow	Ciliary body band obscured
Grade III narrow	All structures including posterior trabecular meshwork obscured
Grade IV narrow (closed)	Only Schwalbe's line visible

Spaeth suggested an evaluation of 3 variables: angular width of the angle recess, configuration of the peripheral iris, and apparent insertion of the iris root.[3] Whichever system the clinician uses to document the appearance of the ACAn, it is important to pay close attention to these 3 aspects.

It is important to use compression gonioscopy to determine whether closed areas of the angle are appositional or synechial. This is determined by indenting the central cornea with a Sussman or Zeiss goniolens. This forces aqueous into the peripheral portion of the anterior chamber, which deepens it and facilitates visualization of the angle.

During gonioscopy, additional features of the angle should also be studied and documented, such as the pigmentation characteristics of the trabecular meshwork and the location and angular extent of PAS. Heterogeneity of the trabecular meshwork pigmentation may indicate the possibility of intermittent angle closure. Intermittent angle closure is seen especially in patients who have large pupils and or a phacomorphic component. Eyes with intermittent ITC, even in the absence of PAS, may develop impaired outflow facility and IOP elevation due to damage to the trabecular meshwork.

Trabeculectomy specimens from subjects with chronic angle closure and absence of synechiae show severe changes in the architecture and arrangement of the trabecular fibers characterized by irregularity and reduction of their spaces, with clusters of juxtacanalicular trabecular cells containing melanin granules.[4,5] Iris tissue remnants adhered to the uveal trabecular meshwork were also observed, indicating that pre-synechial ITC could lead to irreversible changes in the trabecular meshwork.

A major issue with gonioscopy is its underutilization and incorrect interpretation, even amongst glaucoma specialists. One study of Medicare patients in the United States found that a significant proportion of ophthalmologists (approximately 50%) do not perform gonioscopy in their routine examination or even in the examination of glaucoma patients.[6] In a study of 922 glaucoma and glaucoma suspect patients at an academic medical center, 52% of patients never had evaluation by gonioscopy. In the majority of cases when gonioscopy was performed, it was done once throughout the entire duration of the patient's care.[7] In a study of over 3,000 patients who had experienced an acute attack of narrow angle glaucoma, 796 patients had consulted an optometrist or ophthalmologist in the 2 years prior to the attack. Fewer than 33% had undergone gonioscopy and only 42% of these had received a diagnosis of an anatomic narrow angle.[8] In one study, iridotomy at any stage of the PACD spectrum showed a significant decrease in ITC.[9] Even in patients with PACG, iridotomy is effective in exposing parts of the trabecular meshwork that had contact earlier. Greater baseline ITC and post-laser ITC were biomarkers for higher IOP and greater visual field damage.

Gonioscopy is one of the vital tests for any form of glaucoma since it allows not only the evaluation of the width of the angle but also the extent and type of pigmentation of the trabecular meshwork. Gonioscopy can help determine if the angle closure is primary or secondary. Asymmetric and heavy pigmentation of the trabecular meshwork could indicate the possibility of an iris or ciliary body melanoma. Dense homogenous pigment of the trabecular meshwork is suggestive of pigment dispersion. Mild asymmetric pigmentation could indicate the possibility of pseudoexfoliation or intermittent ITC. It also permits the detection of angle recession, neovascularization, and clues to the possibility of underlying uveitis in the presence of broad anterior synechiae if the angle is not narrow in configuration. The clinical skill of gonioscopy as well as its interpretation is currently even more necessary. This is due to the increased frequency of the laser trabeculoplasty procedures and angle surgeries, both of which require correct identification of the trabecular meshwork.

References

1. Scheie HG. Width and pigmentation of the angle of the anterior chamber; a system of grading by gonioscopy. Arch Ophthalmol. 1957;58(4):510-512. https://doi.org/10.1001/archopht.1957.00940010526005
2. Shaffer RN. Primary glaucomas. Gonioscopy, ophthalmoscopy and perimetry. Trans Am Acad Ophthalmol Otolaryngol. 1960;64:112-127.
3. Spaeth GL. The normal development of the human anterior chamber angle: a new system of descriptive grading. Trans Ophthalmol Soc UK. 1971;91:709-739.
4. Sihota R, Lakshimaiah NC, Walia KB, Sharma S, Pailoor J, Agarawal HC. The trabecular meshwork in acute and chronic angle closure glaucoma. Indian J Ophthalmol. 2001;49:255-259.
5. Sihota R, Goyal A, Kaur J, Gupta V, Nag TC. Scanning electron microscopy of the trabecular meshwork: understanding the pathogenesis of primary angle closure glaucoma. Indian J Ophthalmol. 2012;60:183-188. https://doi.org/10.4103/0301-4738.95868
6. Coleman AL, Yu F, Evans SJ. Use of gonioscopy in Medicare beneficiaries before glaucoma surgery. J Glaucoma. 2006;15(6):486e93. https://doi.org/10.1097/01.ijg.0000212287.62798.8f
7. To LK, Carrabba NV, Kalathuru CG, Chuang AZ, Smith L, Feldman RM. Risk Factors for Diagnostic Change from Glaucoma Suspect to Primary Open-Angle Glaucoma and Vice Versa over Two Years. Ophthalmology Glaucoma. 2024. https://doi.org/10.1016/j.ogla.2024.12.006
8. Wu, AM, Stein, JD, Shah M. Potentially Missed Opportunities in Prevention of Acute Angle-Closure Crisis. JAMA Ophthalmol 2022 Jun 1;140(6):598-603. https://doi.org/10.1001/jamaophthalmol.2022.1231
9. Gupta, B, Angmo, D, Yadav, SM, Dada, T, Gupta, V, Sihota. Quantification of Iridotrabecular Contact in Primary Angle-Closure Disease. J Glaucoma. 2020 29;8:681-688. https://doi.org/10.1097/IJG.0000000000001572

Anterior segment optical coherence tomography

Reconciling disagreement between gonioscopy and AS-OCT

Robert Feldman, Tin Aung

Gonioscopy has long been considered the gold standard for assessment of the ACAn in glaucoma.[1,2] However, gonioscopy is a difficult skill to learn and interobserver variability leads to inconsistent assessments.[3] Several factors lead to this variability: the type of gonioscope used, the examiner's technique, ambient light levels, the brightness of the light used to visualize the angle, patient cooperation and the grading system employed. The variability has also resulted in the adoption of various gonioscopy grading systems and updates of those systems over time, which leads to variability in reporting of grading even within the same system.

More recently, AS-OCT has become available. In contrast to posterior segment OCT, these platforms use longer wavelengths of light (≥ 1300 nm) to image the ACAn, allowing better visualization of the angle recess. These devices rapidly image the entire 360° of the angle. Some systems are capable of automated detection of the scleral spur, which enables reproducible quantitative measurements of the ACAn morphology.[4-6] Measurements such as AOD, TISA, trabecular iris circumference volume (TICV), ITC, and LV have been reported to be useful in predicting angle-closure disease and AS-OCT ITC has been suggested as a measure of closure.[7-10] However, ACAns do generally appear qualitatively narrower on AS-OCT than gonioscopy.[11]

The AS-OCT imaging measurements do not directly correlate with the grading scales of gonioscopy, but agreement has been fair to very good when distinguishing between open and closed angles.[12] One study found extensive agreement between the estimated iridocorneal angle measurement using the Shaffer grading system and the measurement of the iridocorneal angle using AS-OCT image.[13] At present, the clinical use of AS-OCT in PACD is mostly limited to qualitative interpretation rather than using device-specific measurements given that, to date, no measurements have been definitively validated to correlate with disease progression. Increased knowledge regarding measurements such as ITC/AOD/TISA and its correlation to gonioscopy and to clinical outcomes are promising.[10,14-20] Another limitation to widespread clinical adoption is the challenge of identifying the scleral spur in narrow and closed angle eyes, which can be prone to error,[6,21,22] in the very population in which accurate measurements are needed most. Measurements with AS-OCT are based on identifying the scleral spur as the pivotal and stable landmark from which currently utilized angle measurements are based. It is unclear if there are changes in the scleral spur position with accommodation (anterior rotation) or with aging, which would alter the measurements.

Gonioscopy and AS-OCT offer different perspectives: gonioscopy measures the en face view while AS-OCT provides radial cross-sectional images, making the tests complimentary. AS-OCT is useful in providing quantitative angle measurements at the initial visit that can be tracked precisely over time to assess for change, while gonioscopy remains valuable for the initial evaluation, especially for grading of angle pigmentation and PAS, but lacks the precision for sequential follow-up in angle grading. A third means of evaluating the angle, UBM can be used to adjudicate differences. It is especially useful for detecting plateau iris configuration and will be discussed further in another section.

The interpretation of an angle on AS-OCT and gonioscopy may be discordant. In a cross-sectional study of over 2,000 subjects, using gonioscopy as the reference standard, investigators observed false-positive classification as angle closure in 14.7% with AS-OCT and false-negative calls in 2%. Compared to subjects for which gonioscopy and AS-OCT classified subjects as having angle closure, multivariable analysis showed deeper anterior chamber depth (adjusted OR 9.31, 95% CI 1.45 to 59.714, $p < 0.05$) and higher LV (adjusted OR 0.038, 95% CI 0.004 to 0.314, $p < 0.05$) were factors significantly associated with discordancy. Compared to subjects for which both modalities classified subjects as having open angles, false negatives (eyes classified as closed by gonioscopy but open with AS-OCT) had shallower ACD (2.2 vs 2.7 mm, $p < 0.001$) and narrower ACW (11.6 vs 11.8 mm, $p < 0.001$). The investigators observed short ITC in 52.57% and irregular ITC in 39% of the false-positive cases, while 66.7% of the false negatives had steep iris profiles and 33.3% irregular ITC with iris rolls.[23] Also, it should be noted that studies typically exclude images in which it is difficult to identify angle structures. There is little in the literature to help reconcile cases of disagreement.

Why would the angle be closed on gonioscopy and open on AS-OCT?

- Gonioscopic technique: The difficulty of gonioscopic technique may be responsible. There is an iris configuration called bowed iris on gonioscopy and steep iris profile on AS-OCT where the mid peripheral iris extends anteriorly due to the pressure gradient between the anterior and posterior chambers and intrinsic structural characteristics of the iris and, possibly, the ciliary body. This may prevent the clinician from being able to see the peripheral angle "over the hill," giving the appearance of a closed angle even if the peripheral angle is open. There may also be a steep iris insertion that can be missed as the peripheral iris appears to insert into the angle, but there is a space between the iris and the trabecular meshwork. Also, the angle may appear closed because the gonioscopy lens is too peripheral and may press the angle closed. This is more likely to happen if a larger lens is used, the patient is looking far off axis, or if the gonioscope is tilted too far off axis.
- Iris processes and PAS: Other considerations are iris processes and PAS. Iris processes may look like a closed angle on gonioscopy when it is open, although in some cases iris processes may be more easily identifiable on gonioscopy. Iris processes are not as densely compact as PAS and aqueous can flow through them to the trabecular meshwork. It can also be helpful to view the next slice on AS-OCT as there may be variability in the appearance of processes along their length whereas PAS are more consistently dense.

- Effects of accommodation: During accommodation, the pupil constricts, which can result in decreasing pupillary block and deepening the peripheral angle. Although the AS-OCT devices attempt to reduce accommodation with a distant fixation target, the eyes are often rotated inward during imaging due to convergence, which suggests accommodation may be occurring as part of the synkinetic near response. On the other hand, accommodation may also rotate the lens iris diaphragm forward, which in other cases could narrow the angle. Inward rotation of the eye is easily detected on gonioscopy.

Why would the angle be open on gonioscopy and closed on AS-OCT?

- The angle may appear narrower on AS-OCT due to less light exposure or image refraction correction. The angles typically appear more closed (ITC) on AS-OCT than on gonioscopy (non-visible trabecular meshwork), as demonstrated by the high sensitivity but lower specificity of AS-OCT in angle closure (many false positives).[10,23-25] It is important to note that studies supporting this observation were conducted with gonioscopy as the gold standard, not a disease diagnosis as the gold standard. Lastly, AS-OCT and gonioscopy use light to image/view the anterior segment but with differing mechanisms. Gonioscopy uses a mirror to overcome total internal reflection, while AS-OCT mostly avoids light refraction by the structures being imaged, relying instead on reflectivity. However, the AS-OCT light still encounters interfaces between different refractive surfaces of structures such as air, tear film (lipid and aqueous components), cornea (even the layers), aqueous humor, and iris stroma, etc. AS-OCT devices use a standard refraction correction, but this correction is not individualized. For example, tear film composition may vary across the cornea with different mixes centrally and peripherally. Furthermore, an effect may be seen at the ACAn in which the peripheral angle is imaged through the limbus, not the cornea. The way in which the variability of the refractive index of aqueous humor that may occur in angle closure affects measurements by AS-OCT is also unknown. The effects of this standardized refraction correction are poorly studied, and the correction value can differ between manufacturers of AS-OCT devices.[7] It is unknown whether there is a relationship between refraction correction and short ITC a finding reported associated with disagreement.[23] Lastly, the grading systems used are not necessarily evaluating the same information to determine closure: where gonioscopy relies on a non-visible posterior trabecular meshwork, AS-OCT relies on ITC, which again may be related to the en face versus cross-sectional evaluation. and may thus not be reconcilable.

- The angle may appear more open with gonioscopy than with AS-OCT for several reasons related to the technique used during gonioscopy.
  - Inadvertent compression: When using a lens designed for dynamic gonioscopy (*i.e.*, Sussman, Zeiss 4-mirror gonioprism), any pressure on the cornea will cause the angle to open. Although careful technique can mitigate this, it cannot be entirely eliminated. The presence of corneal striae typically indicates excessive pressure is being applied; however, the angle anatomy may change with even less pressure than required to cause striae to appear.
  - Lighting: It is difficult to eliminate all light that causes pupil constriction during gonioscopy, which can result in angle opening. There are 2 types of lighting to consider: background illumination and slit-lamp lighting. Background illumination, such as from computer monitors, can cause pupil constriction and should be minimized by performing gonioscopy in the dark. Slit-lamp lighting, which cannot be eliminated, can be reduced by turning the illumination down to its lowest setting while still allowing for angle visualization, and ensuring the beam is short enough to only pass through the mirror and not the pupil. In eyes with lighter-colored irides or eyes with thin or atrophic irides, even minimal light can still reach the retina and cause pupil constriction despite the best technique.
  - Accommodation on AS-OCT: As stated above, the iris-lens diaphragm may shift forward, resulting in a narrower angle on AS-OCT. Note that pupils are likely larger on AS-OCT performed in the dark than gonioscopy, although it is difficult to measure pupil size during gonioscopy for direct comparison.[26]
- Special considerations
  - Plateau iris configuration can be difficult to assess on gonioscopy (steep insertion and double hump sign) or AS-OCT (steep insertion with limited iris bow) and currently requires UBM for diagnosis, which is described elsewhere.

Overall, when faced with discordance between gonioscopy and AS-OCT, it is important to consider the factors outlined above. If the angle appears more open with AS-OCT than with gonioscopy, consider AS-OCT as the gold standard; when AS-OCT is more closed than gonioscopy, consider assessing ITC vertical extension, as short ITC lengths may be artifactual and possibly related to device refraction correction.

References

1. Fu H, Li F, Sun X, et al. AGE challenge: Angle Closure Glaucoma Evaluation in Anterior Segment Optical Coherence Tomography. Med Image Anal. 2020 Dec;66:101798. https://doi.org/10.1016/j.media.2020.101798
2. Barbour-Hastie C, Deol SS, Peroni A, Gillan S, Trucco E, Tatham AJ. Feasibility of Automated Gonioscopy Imaging in Clinical Practice. J Glaucoma. 2023 Mar 1;32(3):159-164. https://doi.org/10.1097/IJG.0000000000002162
3. Riva I, Micheletti E, Oddone F, et al. Anterior Chamber Angle Assessment Techniques: A Review. J Clin Med. 2020 Nov 25;9(12):3814. https://doi.org/10.3390/jcm9123814
4. Xu BY, Chiang M, Pardeshi AA, Moghimi S, Varma R. Deep Neural Network for Scleral Spur Detection in Anterior Segment OCT Images: The Chinese American Eye Study. Transl Vis Sci Technol. 2020 Mar 30;9(2):18. https://doi.org/10.1167/tvst.9.2.18
5. Bolo K, Apolo Aroca G, Pardeshi AA, et al. Automated expert-level scleral spur detection and quantitative biometric analysis on the ANTERION anterior segment OCT system. Br J Ophthalmol. 2024 May 21;108(5):702-709. https://doi.org/10.1136/bjo-2022-322328
6. Cumba RJ, Radhakrishnan S, Bell NP, et al. Reproducibility of scleral spur identification and angle measurements using Fourier domain anterior segment optical coherence tomography. J Ophthalmol. 2012;2012:487309. https://doi.org/10.1155/2012/487309
7. Radhakrishnan S, Goldsmith J, Huang D, et al. Comparison of optical coherence tomography and ultrasound biomicroscopy for detection of narrow anterior chamber angles. Arch Ophthalmol. 2005 Aug;123(8):1053-9. https://doi.org/10.1001/archopht.123.8.1053
8. Rigi M, Blieden LS, Nguyen D, et al. Trabecular-iris circumference volume in open angle eyes using swept-source Fourier domain anterior segment optical coherence tomography. J Ophthalmol. 2014;2014:590978. https://doi.org/10.1155/2014/590978
9. Ho SW, Baskaran M, Zheng C, et al. Swept source optical coherence tomography measurement of the iris-trabecular contact (ITC) index: a new parameter for angle closure. Graefes Arch Clin Exp Ophthalmol. 2013 Apr;251(4):1205-11. https://doi.org/10.1007/s00417-012-2158-6
10. Melese EK, Chan JD, Blieden LS, et al. Determination and Validation of Thresholds of Anterior Chamber Parameters by Dedicated Anterior Segment Optical Coherence Tomography. Am J Ophthalmol. 2016 Sep;169:208-217. https://doi.org/10.1016/j.ajo.2016.06.032
11. Nolan WP, See JL, Chew PT, et al. Detection of primary angle closure using anterior segment optical coherence tomography in Asian eyes. Ophthalmology. 2007 Jan;114(1):33-9. https://doi.org/10.1016/j.ophtha.2006.05.073
12. Tay EL, Yong VK, Lim BA, Sia S, Wong EP, Yip LW. Agreement of angle closure assessments between gonioscopy, anterior segment optical coherence tomography and spectral domain optical coherence tomography. Int J Ophthalmol. 2015 Apr 18;8(2):342-6. https://doi.org/10.3980/j.issn.2222-3959.2015.02.23

13. Lune A, Prabhudesai A. A Comparative Study of Anterior Segment Optical Coherence Tomography and Gonioscopy in Detection of Narrow, Occludable Angles. Cureus. 2024 Sep 21;16(9):e69879. https://doi.org/10.7759/cureus.69879
14. Guo PY, Zhang X, Li F, et al. Diagnostic criteria of anterior segment swept-source optical coherence tomography to detect gonioscopic angle closure. Br J Ophthalmol. 2024 Jul 23;108(8):1130-1136. https://doi.org/10.1136/bjo-2023-323860
15. Hong KL, Xu BY, Wang W, et al. Short-Term Ocular Biometric Changes as Predictors of Long-Term Angle Closure Progression. JAMA Ophthalmol. 2025 May 29:e251007. https://doi.org/10.1001/jamaophthalmol.2025.1007
16. Gedde SJ, Chopra V, Vinod K. Contemplating the Laser Question for Primary Angle Closure Suspect. JAMA Ophthalmol. 2025 May 29. https://doi.org/10.1001/jamaophthalmol.2025.1494
17. Porporato N, Chong R, Xu BY, et al. Angle closure extent, anterior segment dimensions and intraocular pressure. Br J Ophthalmol. 2023 Jul;107(7):927-934. https://doi.org/10.1136/bjophthalmol-2021-320453
18. Xu BY, Friedman DS, Foster PJ, et al. Ocular Biometric Risk Factors for Progression of Primary Angle Closure Disease: The Zhongshan Angle Closure Prevention Trial. Ophthalmology. 2022 Mar;129(3):267-275. https://doi.org/10.1016/j.ophtha.2021.10.003
19. Xu BY, Friedman DS, Foster PJ, et al. Anatomic Changes and Predictors of Angle Widening after Laser Peripheral Iridotomy: The Zhongshan Angle Closure Prevention Trial. Ophthalmology. 2021 Aug;128(8):1161-1168. https://doi.org/10.1016/j.ophtha.2021.01.021
20. Bao YK, Xu BY, Friedman DS, et al. Biometric Risk Factors for Angle Closure Progression After Laser Peripheral Iridotomy. JAMA Ophthalmol. 2023 Jun 1;141(6):516-524. https://doi.org/10.1001/jamaophthalmol.2023.0937
21. Sakata LM, Lavanya R, Friedman DS, et al. Assessment of the scleral spur in anterior segment optical coherence tomography images. Arch Ophthalmol. 2008 Feb;126(2):181-5. https://doi.org/10.1001/archophthalmol.2007.46
22. Liu S, Li H, Dorairaj S, et al. Assessment of scleral spur visibility with anterior segment optical coherence tomography. J Glaucoma. 2010 Feb;19(2):132-5. https://doi.org/10.1097/IJG.0b013e3181a98ce4
23. Porporato N, Baskaran M, Tun TA, et al. Understanding diagnostic disagreement in angle closure assessment between anterior segment optical coherence tomography and gonioscopy. Br J Ophthalmol. 2020 Jun;104(6):795-799. https://doi.org/10.1136/bjophthalmol-2019-314672
24. Grewal DS, Brar GS, Jain R, Grewal SP. Comparison of Scheimpflug imaging and spectral domain anterior segment optical coherence tomography for detection of narrow anterior chamber angles. Eye (Lond). 2011 May;25(5):603-11. https://doi.org/10.1038/eye.2011.14
25. Narayanaswamy A, Sakata LM, He MG, et al. Diagnostic performance of anterior chamber angle measurements for detecting eyes with narrow angles: an anterior segment OCT study. Arch Ophthalmol. 2010 Oct;128(10):1321-7. https://doi.org/10.1001/archophthalmol.2010.231

26. Hao H, Zhao Y, Yan Q, et al. Angle-closure assessment in anterior segment OCT images via deep learning. Med Image Anal. 2021 Apr;69:101956. https://doi.org/10.1016/j.media.2021.101956

The role of iridotrabecular contact in diagnosis and management

Natalia Porporato, Tin Aung

Definition of ITC in AS-OCT

ITC observed in AS-OCT is defined as the visible contact between the peripheral iris and any part of the angle wall, including the trabecular meshwork (if visible), located anterior to the scleral spur (Fig. 1).[1] It can also be estimated by quantitative parameters that evaluate the space area between the iris and the angle wall (TISA) at 500 or 750 um anterior to the scleral spur, *i.e.*, TISA500 or TISA750 equal to 0 or very close to 0 indicates ITC.

Characteristics of ITC in AS-OCT

As with gonioscopy, ITC in AS-OCT can be measured in its circumferential and vertical extension. AS-OCT provides more variability of ITC within a quadrant or clock hour section.

- Circumferential extent: Proportion of cross-sectional scans in which ITC is present. As shown in Figure 2[2] and demonstrated in the literature,[3] gonioscopy and gonioscopic-based imaging techniques significantly underrepresent anatomic variations of the ACAn compared with AS-OCT.
- Vertical extent: Also referred to as length, width, or height, represents the anatomically anterior-posterior extension of the ITC from the scleral spur to Schwalbe's line (Fig. 3).[4]

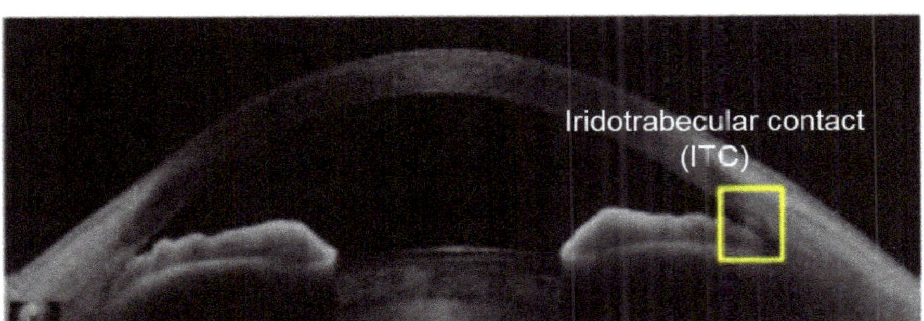

Fig. 1. Horizontal AS-OCT scan showing ITC. Reproduced from Porporato *et al.*[2]

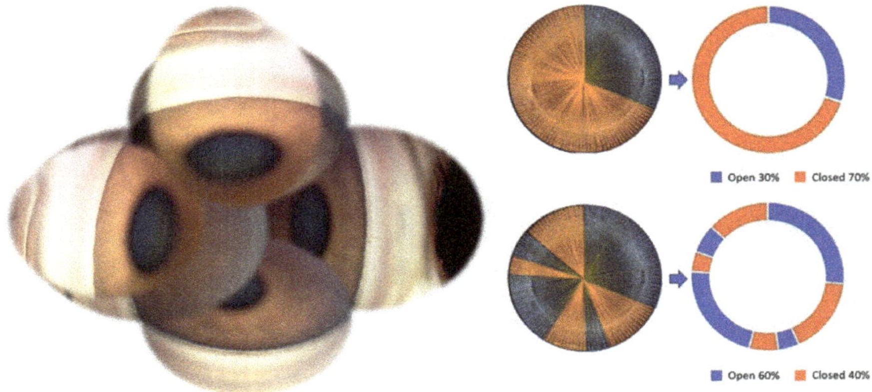

Fig. 2. Frontal view of goniophotographs showing 4 quadrants open based on the visibility of the posterior trabecular meshwork *(right)* compared to regions of iridotrabecular contact (ITC) based on AS-OCT imaging *(left)*. Reproduced from Porporato *et al.*[2]

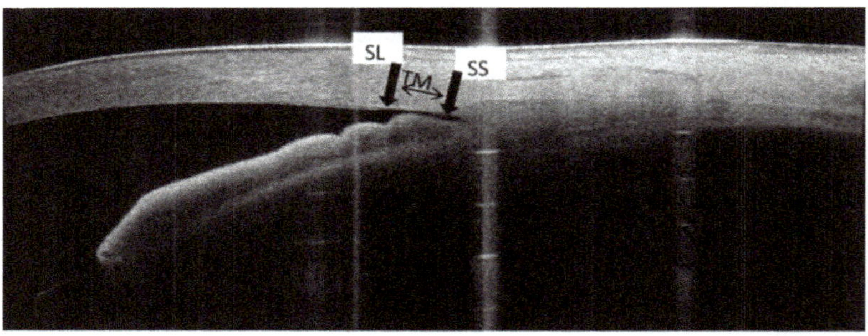

Fig. 3. Swept–source OCT images showing Schwalbe's line (SL), scleral spur (SS), and trabecular meshwork (TM). Reproduced from Tun *et al.*[4]

Diagnostic approaches in AS-OCT

Based on gonioscopic standards, several diagnostic methods using AS-OCT have been proposed:

- Quadrant-wise: Assessing ITC in specific angle quadrants corresponding to nasal-temporal (horizontal scan) and superior-inferior (vertical scan).[5]
- Circumferential evaluation: Measuring ITC across the entire 360° circumference.[6]
- Single scan: The single scan at 80° to 260° has demonstrated the highest diagnostic performance for gonioscopic angle closure (*i.e.*, gonioscopic PACS diagnosis).[7]
- Single or combined quantitative parameters: Using one or more quantitative parameters, such as AOD750,[8] TISA500,[9] or a combination of AOD750 and LV.[10]

Challenges in diagnostic thresholds

The variability in ITC detected on AS-OCT—across circumferential and vertical dimensions—poses challenges for standardization against gonioscopic criteria. While gonioscopy is the current clinical standard for diagnosing angle closure, aligning AS-OCT criteria with gonioscopic standards has proven difficult. A commonly accepted gonioscopic threshold is 180° of contact, but that criteria may prove too simplistic. AS-OCT provides multiple quantifiable measurements beyond ITC to account for the variability in angle parameters that may better predict the development and progression of angle closure.[11]

Management of ITC

AS-OCT is an objective and reproducible tool for monitoring angle closure, as it provides quantifiable data on the status of the ACAn for ongoing evaluation. The management of ITC depends on the underlying mechanism, as different causes of angle closure necessitate tailored interventions. Appositional ITC, commonly caused by pupillary block, is typically managed with LPI or lens extraction, which restores aqueous humor flow by creating an alternative pathway. In cases of synechial ITC, characterized by permanent adhesions between the iris and angle structures, surgical interventions, such as lens extraction with or without goniosynechialysis, may be required to reopen the angle. For patients with a plateau iris configuration, additional laser or surgical procedures may be necessary to prevent recurrence of angle closure after LPI. A thorough understanding of the mechanism of ITC is critical for guiding appropriate management and avoiding unnecessary or ineffective treatments.[12,13]

References

1. Nolan WP, See JL, Chew PTK, et al. Detection of Primary Angle Closure Using Anterior Segment Optical Coherence Tomography in Asian Eyes. Ophthalmology. 2007;114(1):33-39. https://doi.org/10.1016/j.ophtha.2006.05.073
2. Porporato N, Baskaran M, Husain R, Aung T. Recent advances in anterior chamber angle imaging. Eye. 2020;34(1):51-59. https://doi.org/10.1038/s41433-019-0555-0
3. Xu BY, Pardeshi AA, Burkemper B, et al. Differences in Anterior Chamber Angle Assessments Between Gonioscopy, EyeCam, and Anterior Segment OCT: The Chinese American Eye Study. Transl Vis Sci Technol. 2019;8(2):5-5. https://doi.org/10.1167/tvst.8.2.5
4. Tun TA, Baskaran M, Zheng C, et al. Assessment of trabecular meshwork width using swept source optical coherence tomography. Graefes Arch Clin Exp Ophthalmol. 2013;251(6):1587-1592. https://doi.org/10.1007/s00417-013-2285-8

5. Sakata LM, Lavanya R, Friedman DS, et al. Comparison of Gonioscopy and Anterior Segment Ocular Coherence Tomography in Detecting Angle Closure in Different Quadrants of the Anterior Chamber Angle. Ophthalmology. 2008;115(5):769-774. https://doi.org/10.1016/j.ophtha.2007.06.030
6. Porporato N, Baskaran M, Tun TA, et al. Assessment of Circumferential Angle Closure with Swept-Source Optical Coherence Tomography: a Community Based Study. Am J Ophthalmol. 2019;199:133-139. https://doi.org/10.1016/j.ajo.2018.11.015
7. Porporato N, Baskaran M, Perera S, et al. Evaluation of meridional scans for angle closure assessment with anterior segment swept-source optical coherence tomography. Br J Ophthalmol. Published online March 9, 2020:bjophthalmol-2019-315461. https://doi.org/10.1136/bjophthalmol-2019-315461
8. Narayanaswamy A, Sakata LM, He MG, et al. Diagnostic performance of anterior chamber angle measurements for detecting eyes with narrow angles: an anterior segment OCT study. Arch Ophthalmol Chic Ill 1960. 2010;128(10):1321-1327. https://doi.org/10.1001/archophthalmol.2010.231
9. Xu BY, Friedman DS, Foster PJ, et al. Ocular Biometric Risk Factors for Progression of Primary Angle Closure Disease. Ophthalmology. 2022;129(3):267-275. https://doi.org/10.1016/j.ophtha.2021.10.003
10. Nongpiur ME, Aboobakar IF, Baskaran M, et al. Association of Baseline Anterior Segment Parameters With the Development of Incident Gonioscopic Angle Closure. JAMA Ophthalmol. 2017;135(3):252-258. https://doi.org/10.1001/jamaophthalmol.2016.5847
11. Foster PJ, Buhrmann R, Quigley HA, Johnson GJ. The definition and classification of glaucoma in prevalence surveys. Br J Ophthalmol. 2002;86(2):238-242. https://doi.org/10.1136/bjo.86.2.238
12. Weinreb RN, Aung T, Medeiros FA. The Pathophysiology and Treatment of Glaucoma: A Review. JAMA. 2014;311(18):1901-1911. https://doi.org/10.1001/jama.2014.3192
13. Nongpiur ME, Gong T, Lee HK, et al. Subgrouping of Primary Angle-Closure Suspects Based on Anterior Segment Optical Coherence Tomography Parameters. Ophthalmology. 2013;120(12):2525-2531. https://doi.org/.1016/j.ophtha.2013.05.028

Risk stratification of angle-closure eyes

Tin A Tun, Tin Aung

Diagnosis and evaluation of PACD

AS-OCT is utilized to qualitatively and quantitatively assess various anatomical structures, such as the anterior chamber, angle, iris, lens, and choroid along with physiological/dynamic factors for objective angle evaluation and monitoring of angle closure progression and prognosis.

Angle closure progression

Recent randomized controlled trials indicate that the risk of progression from PACS to PAC or PACG is relatively low.[1,2] Therefore, widespread prophylactic LPI for asymptomatic PACS cases at a population level is not recommended based on gonioscopic grading alone without consideration of other specific risk factors for angle-closure glaucoma. Identifying which PACS cases are at higher risk of severe progression is increasingly important but challenging.

Predictive and prognostic modelling can aid in identifying high-risk cases and guiding clinical management. Multivariable regression models and/or AI identify important predictors and assign weights to achieve high specificity and sensitivity. These predictors may include demographic, clinical, ocular, imaging, and genetic factors.

Stepwise logistic regression has been found to be the most stable algorithm, exhibiting the least variability and achieving an AUC of 0.95 for gonioscopic angle closure detection using AS-OCT-derived parameters (ACW, ACAr, ACV, LV, iris thickness [IT750], and iris area [IArea]) from a single meridional scan (0° to 180°).[3] Gonioscopic angle closure is defined as the absence of visibility of the posterior pigmented trabecular meshwork for at least 180° on non-indentation gonioscopy with the eye in the primary position. Among 6 predictors, ACV and ACAr were larger contributors to angle closure than LV or IT750. The algorithm was also validated on an independent sample of 200 subjects, yielding consistent results.[3] A score and probability estimate[4] were developed using these 6 parameters:

Score = -29.0 – 0.3 x (ACV) + 3.2 x (ACW) + 7.3 x (IT750) - 2.2 x (IArea) + 1.5 x (ACAr) + 0.1 (LV).

A horizontal (0° to 180°) B-scan across the nasal and temporal quadrants showed the highest predictive value compared to the average of all 8 meridians.[5] A model using 3 parameters (ACAr, LV, and iris curvature [Icurv]) demonstrated a similar AUC to that of the model using the full set of parameters for angle closure detection.[5]

At baseline, a narrower AOD, Icurv, and older age were associated with a higher risk of progression from untreated PACS to PAC after 6 years.[6] Specifically, older age (≥ 59 years), AOD < 0.042 mm, and Icurv < 0.34 mm increased the odds of progression. Progressors also exhibited higher IOP and thicker lens.[6]

After LPI treatment, baseline factors such as older age, narrower TISA (TISA500 $\leq$ 0.05 mm^2), and/or smaller cumulative gonioscopy scores were linked to angle closure progression.[7] Thus, eyes with these high-risk features may be considered for earlier treatment and/or more frequent monitoring by eye care providers.

Predicting the efficacy of interventions for PACD

Although a multicenter randomized controlled trial found that clear-lens extraction in eyes with PACG and PAC with IOP greater than 30 mmHg was more effective and cost-efficient than LPI, this intervention may involve intra- and postoperative complications.[8] A risk stratification model may help identify cases that would benefit most from such interventions. AS-OCT not only provides information on the status of the ACAn, similar to gonioscopy, but also offers cross-sectional images of the anterior segment, allowing assessment of the thickness, curvature, and area of the iris. Using this information, risk stratification based on AS-OCT can be achieved. For example, LPI treatment was most effective in cases with pupillary block compared to those with plateau iris and thick peripheral iris.[9,10] Greater AOD, IArea, pupil diameter, and less Icurv were linked to higher odds of poor angle widening after LPI.[11] Temporal or nasal LPI locations were also associated with poor angle widening.

Blindness occurs in approximately 10% of glaucoma cases, highlighting the critical need to identify those at high risk. By utilizing risk stratification models, healthcare providers can effectively distribute resources, control the disease burden, and prevent both under-treatment and over-treatment. This approach also helps reduce negative consequences, such as high costs, diminished quality of life, and unsatisfactory patient experiences. Despite their potential benefits, evidence-based risk stratification models for glaucoma care have not been adopted on a global scale. Therefore, it is essential to justify and validate their value in routine clinical settings.

References

1. He M, Jiang Y, Huang S, et al. Laser peripheral iridotomy for the prevention of angle closure: a single-centre, randomised controlled trial. Lancet. 2019;393:1609-1618. https://doi.org/10.1016/S0140-6736(18)32607-2
2. Baskaran M, Kumar RS, Friedman DS, et al. The Singapore Asymptomatic Narrow Angles Laser Iridotomy Study: Five-Year Results of a Randomized Controlled Trial. Ophthalmology. 2022;129:147-158. https://doi.org/10.1016/j.ophtha.2021.08.017

3. Nongpiur ME, Haaland BA, Friedman DS, et al. Classification algorithms based on anterior segment optical coherence tomography measurements for detection of angle closure. Ophthalmology. 2013;120:48-54. https://doi.org/10.1016/j.ophtha.2012.07.005
4. Nongpiur ME, Haaland BA, Perera SA, et al. Development of a score and probability estimate for detecting angle closure based on anterior segment optical coherence tomography. Am J Ophthalmol. 2014;157:32-38 e31. https://doi.org/10.1016/j.ajo.2013.09.012
5. Tan SS, Tun TA, Sultana R, et al. Diagnostic accuracy of swept source optical coherence tomography classification algorithms for detection of gonioscopic angle closure. Br J Ophthalmol. 2022;106:1716-1721. https://doi.org/10.1136/bjophthalmol-2021-319165
6. Xu BY, Friedman DS, Foster PJ, et al. Ocular Biometric Risk Factors for Progression of Primary Angle Closure Disease: The Zhongshan Angle Closure Prevention Trial. Ophthalmology. 2022;129:267-275. https://doi.org/10.1016/j.ophtha.2021.10.003
7. Bao YK, Xu BY, Friedman DS, et al. Biometric Risk Factors for Angle Closure Progression After Laser Peripheral Iridotomy. JAMA Ophthalmol. 2023;141:516-524. https://doi.org/10.1001/jamaophthalmol.2023.0937
8. Azuara-Blanco A, Burr J, Ramsay C, et al. Effectiveness of early lens extraction for the treatment of primary angle-closure glaucoma (EAGLE): a randomised controlled trial. Lancet. 2016;388:1389-1397. https://doi.org/10.1016/S0140-6736(16)30956-4
9. Kwon J, Sung KR, Han S. Long-term Changes in Anterior Segment Characteristics of Eyes With Different Primary Angle-Closure Mechanisms. Am J Ophthalmol. 2018;191:54-63. https://doi.org/10.1016/j.ajo.2018.04.005
10. Tun TA, Sawicki A, Wilkos-Kuc A, Aung T, Zarnowski T. Changes in Anterior Segment Parameters After Laser Peripheral Iridotomy in Caucasian Eyes With Different Primary Angle Closure Mechanisms. J Glaucoma. 2023 Oct 1;32(10):820-825. https://doi.org/10.1097/IJG.0000000000002282
11. Xu BY, Friedman DS, Foster PJ, et al. Anatomic Changes and Predictors of Angle Widening after Laser Peripheral Iridotomy: The Zhongshan Angle Closure Prevention Trial. Ophthalmology. 2021;128:1161-1168. https://doi.org/10.1016/j.ophtha.2021.01.021

Ciliary body

Alex Huang, Benjamin Xu

The ciliary body is important for a number of anterior segment physiologic processes (including, but not limited to, aqueous humor production, trabecular aqueous humor outflow regulation, and accommodation) and anterior segment diseases (including, but not limited to, plateau iris, hypotony, and presbyopia).[1]

Composed of muscles of different orientation, vasculature, and the ciliary epithelium, the ciliary body is difficult to evaluate because of its location behind the opaque sclera and iris.

The ciliary body can be imaged using multiple approaches. First, it can be directly visualized using the Apple-Miyake[2] approach or the endoscopic photocoagulation[3] probe from Endo Optiks. The latter has the benefit of being diagnostic and therapeutic for some diseases via its 810 nm diode laser.[3] The disadvantage is that these approaches require intraocular surgery. For non-invasive imaging, UBM[4] uses high-frequency ultrasound to improve image resolution (~20 microns). While the imaging penetration (~4-5 mm) is reduced compared to traditional ultrasound, this depth of penetration is sufficient for the ciliary body. Limitations of UBM include the requirement of an immersion method or direct contact of the transducer onto the eye. Also, the imaging device is hand-held and dependent on operator skill. Thus, reproducibility is variable as subjects must hold the exact same eye position while the operator holds the probe at the exact same location, tilt, and rotation to be able to image the exact same anatomical location across different sessions.

OCT has revolutionized eye care and vision research as a non-invasive tool that provides histology-level image quality.[5] AS-OCT is a logical solution for imaging the ciliary muscle. AS-OCT is both non-invasive and non-contact. However, the challenge is that OCT assesses the reflectance patterns of light waves, which can be blocked by the sclera and iris. This problem is particularly acute for spectral-domain OCTs that operate at a ~850 nm laser illumination. One simple solution is to increase the illumination wavelength to ~1050–1300 nm. Available options include the swept-source CASIA1 and 2 (Tomey Corporation, Nagoya, Japan)[6] and ANTERION[7,8] (Heidelberg Engineering, Heidelberg, Germany). The Visante[9] (Carl Zeiss Meditec, Jena, Germany) is an older time-domain option that is still found in clinics and research labs, but is no longer marketed, has no replacement parts available, nor is supported by the manufacturer. Increased illumination wavelength improves the depth of imaging to visualize the ciliary body; however, axial resolution decreases. To improve the signal-to-noise ratio, tracking and image averaging are used by the ANTERION.[10] Thus, ANTERION imaging of the ciliary muscle, when visible, has shown good reproducibility.[10] It has also been used to show that posterior ciliary muscle contraction is an early biomarker for presbyopia and that myopes, in particular, have paradoxically larger ciliary muscles that retain contractile capability longer.[11]

In the future, the next step may be to apply AI deep learning to AS-OCT ciliary body imaging. For instance, clinical interpretation of ciliary body plateau iris configuration[12] using the Visante shows poor interobserver agreement.[13] Thus, starting with UBM imaging as the gold standard, "label transfer" and "style transfer" techniques have been used to develop a successful AI model to detect plateau iris (AUC = 0.95) from Visante AS-OCT images.[14] However, as discussed above, the Visante is slowly disappearing. Therefore, re-developing the AI algorithms using current AS-OCTs or applying "label" and "style" transfer methods from current AI algorithms to current AS-OCTs will be important to achieve wider clinical applicability.

References

1. Delamere NA. Ciliary Body and Ciliary Epithelium. Adv Organ Biol. Jan 01 2005;10:127-148. https://doi.org/10.1016/S1569-2590(05)10005-6
2. Pereira FA, Werner L, Milverton EJ, Coroneo MT. Miyake-Apple posterior video analysis/photographic technique. J Cataract Refract Surg. Mar 2009;35(3):577-87. https://doi.org/10.1016/j.jcrs.2008.11.059
3. Francis BA, Pouw A, Jenkins D, et al. Endoscopic Cycloplasty (ECPL) and Lens Extraction in the Treatment of Severe Plateau Iris Syndrome. J Glaucoma. Mar 2016;25(3):e128-33. https://doi.org/10.1097/IJG.0000000000000156
4. Pavlin CJ, Sherar MD, Foster FS. Subsurface ultrasound microscopic imaging of the intact eye. Ophthalmology. Feb 1990;97(2):244-50. https://doi.org/10.1016/s0161-6420(90)32598-8
5. Huang D, Swanson EA, Lin CP, et al. Optical coherence tomography. Science. Nov 1991;254(5035):1178-81.
6. Xu BY, Liang S, Pardeshi AA, et al. Differences in Ocular Biometric Measurements among Subtypes of Primary Angle Closure Disease: The Chinese American Eye Study. Ophthalmol Glaucoma. 2021;4(2):224-231. https://doi.org/10.1016/j.ogla.2020.09.008
7. Pardeshi AA, Song AE, Lazkani N, Xie X, Huang A, Xu BY. Intradevice Repeatability and Interdevice Agreement of Ocular Biometric Measurements: A Comparison of Two Swept-Source Anterior Segment OCT Devices. Transl Vis Sci Technol. Aug 2020;9(9):14. https://doi.org/10.1167/tvst.9.9.14
8. Bolo K, Apolo Aroca G, Pardeshi AA, et al. Automated expert-level scleral spur detection and quantitative biometric analysis on the ANTERION anterior segment OCT system. Br J Ophthalmol. May 21 2024;108(5):702-709. https://doi.org/10.1136/bjo-2022-322328
9. Kaphle D, Schmid KL, Davies LN, Suheimat M, Atchison DA. Ciliary Muscle Dimension Changes With Accommodation Vary in Myopia and Emmetropia. Invest Ophthalmol Vis Sci. Jun 01 2022;63(6):24. https://doi.org/10.1167/iovs.63.6.24
10. Xie X, Corradetti G, Song A, et al. Age- and refraction-related changes in anterior segment anatomical structures measured by swept-source anterior segment OCT. PLoS One. 2020;15(10):e0240110. https://doi.org/10.1371/journal.pone.0240110

11. Xie X, Sultan W, Corradetti G, et al. Assessing accommodative presbyopic biometric changes of the entire anterior segment using single swept-source OCT image acquisitions. Eye (Lond). Feb 25 2021. https://doi.org/10.1038/s41433-020-01363-3
12. Tabatabaei SM, Fakhraie G, Ansari S, Hamzeh N, Safizadeh M, Beikmarzehei A. Plateau Iris: A Review. J Curr Ophthalmol. 2023;35(1):11-16. https://doi.org/10.4103/joco.joco_319_22
13. Wanichwecharungruang B, Pattanapongpaiboon W, Kongsomboon K, Parivisutt N, Annopawong K, Seresirikachorn K. Diagnostic performance of anterior segment optical coherence tomography in detecting plateau iris. BMJ Open Ophthalmol. 2022;7(1):e000931. https://doi.org/10.1136/bmjophth-2021-000931
14. Wanichwecharungruang B, Kaothanthong N, Pattanapongpaiboon W, et al. Deep Learning for Anterior Segment Optical Coherence Tomography to Predict the Presence of Plateau Iris. Transl Vis Sci Technol. Jan 2021;10(1):7. https://doi.org/10.1167/tvst.10.1.7

Ultrasound biomicroscopy

Ko Eun Kim, Kyung Rim Sung

With the recent advent of AS-OCT, which allows for the non-contact and non-invasive assessment of anterior segment structures, UBM has become less frequently used due to its more cumbersome examination process. Unlike AS-OCT, UBM requires topical anesthesia and a trained examiner to obtain high-quality images. However, UBM plays a unique role in the diagnosis of PAC, enabling visualization of areas behind the iris, which are blocked from the OCT signal, by using ultrasound. Like AS-OCT, UBM enables both qualitative and quantitative assessments of the anterior segment structure. Thus, UBM examination is highly recommended for an accurate diagnosis of PAC, especially to determine the underlying mechanism of PAC.

The mechanism of PAC can be divided into pupillary block and non-pupillary block mechanisms. Pupillary block is considered a key element in the pathogenesis of PAC. However, other factors, such as the relative position and thickness of the ciliary body, iris configuration, the location of iris insertion into the ciliary body, iris volume, and lens position also contribute to PAC. Among non-pupillary block mechanisms, plateau iris configuration is the most frequently observed condition. In studies utilizing UBM, approximately one-third of eyes with angle closure demonstrated plateau iris.[1] However, the diagnostic criteria for plateau iris are not well defined, and many investigators rely on qualitative and variable criteria, including anteriorly directed ciliary process, a steep rise in the iris root

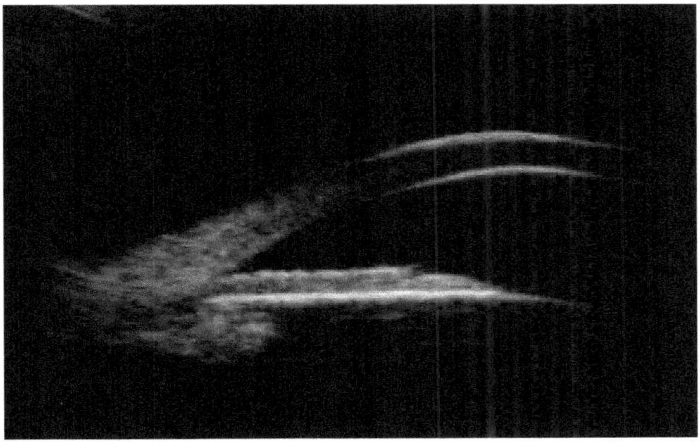

Fig. 1. Plateau iris with flat iris plane and a relatively deeper ACAn. An anteriorly displaced ciliary body with absent ciliary sulcus is observed.

from its insertion, a central flat iris plane, absence of a ciliary sulcus, and iridocorneal touch.

To better elucidate the mechanism of PAC, the relationship between the iris and the ciliary body, the size of the ciliary body, and the presence of a ciliary sulcus or other features not visible with AS-OCT should be evaluated. In a study comparing the effectiveness of AS-OCT and UBM in detecting plateau iris, UBM confirmed plateau iris by revealing iris root indentation caused by the ciliary body, while AS-OCT could only show indirect signs of plateau iris (Fig. 1).[2] One study quantitatively measured ciliary body size, trabecular-ciliary process angle (TCA), and trabecular-ciliary process distance (TCPD) using UBM and subclassified PAC eyes alongside AS-OCT-derived parameters.[3] The study revealed that the 2 clusters identified through AS-OCT and UBM parameters showed distinct features in TCA and TCPD determined by UBM, as well as iris curvature assessed by AS-OCT. Among the clusters, the group with a more anteriorly positioned ciliary process and substantially narrower TCA (which displayed a flatter iris and middle-to-apical iris insertion) showed significantly less IOP reduction after LPI. This finding corroborated previous reports that eyes with a plateau iris shape respond less effectively to LPI than those with pupillary block.

Additionally, the study confirmed that a more anteriorly located ciliary body is associated with an increased risk of progressive angle closure following LPI.[4] This result highlights the importance of quantitative analysis of UBM images using multiple parameters, which can provide critical insights to differentiate plateau iris from PB. With this differential diagnosis, clinicians can offer more personalized treatment plans for patients with angle closure.

Overall, UBM remains a valuable tool in the field of angle-closure glaucoma. It helps elucidate the mechanisms behind elevated IOP, identify the causes of secondary glaucoma (such as pigment dispersion syndrome, lens-induced glaucoma, ciliary block, cysts, and solid tumors of the anterior segment), and assess the outcomes of various interventions, including LPI.

References

1. Kumar RS, Baskaran M, Chew PT, et al. Prevalence of plateau iris in primary angle closure suspects an ultrasound biomicroscopy study. Ophthalmology. 2008;115:430-434. https://doi.org/10.1016/j.ophtha.2007.07.026
2. Parc C, Laloum J, Berges O. Comparison of optical coherence tomography and ultrasound biomicroscopy for detection of plateau iris. J Fr Ophtalmol. 2010;33:266.e1-e3. https://doi.org/10.1016/j.jfo.2010.01.010
3. Kwon J, Sung KR, Han S, et al. Subclassification of Primary Angle Closure Using Anterior Segment Optical Coherence Tomography and Ultrasound Biomicroscopic Parameters. Ophthalmology. 2017;124:1039-1047. https://doi.org/10.1016/j.ophtha.2017.02.025
4. Yao BQ, Wu LL, Zhang C, et al. Ultrasound biomicroscopic features associated with angle closure in fellow eyes of acute primary angle closure after laser iridotomy. Ophthalmology. 2009;116:444-448.e2. https://doi.org/10.1016/j.ophtha.2008.10.019

Goniophotographs

Ko Eun Kim, Kyung Rim Sung

Goniophotographs obtained through slit-lamp gonioscopy are helpful for assessing the anatomy and pathology of the ACAn, even with advancements in imaging techniques. This section aims to establish standardized diagnostic criteria for interpreting goniophotographs, ensuring consistency and accuracy in clinical evaluations.

Identification of anatomical landmarks to evaluate the ACAn

Figure 1 presents the anatomical landmarks used to evaluate the ACAn.

- Schwalbe's line: The most anterior structure, marking the boundary between the corneal endothelium and trabecular meshwork.
- Trabecular meshwork: Divided into 2 sections
    - Anterior portion (non-pigmented): Between Schwalbe's line and the anterior edge of the Schlemm's canal.

  - o Posterior portion (pigmented): Between the anterior edge of Schlemm's canal and the scleral spur.
- Scleral spur: Critical landmark that separates the trabecular meshwork from the ciliary body band.
- Ciliary body band: Dark or grayish band whose width may vary depending on the angle configuration.
- Peripheral iris contour: The iris configuration may be flat, concave, or convex.

Standardized grading systems, most notably those by Shaffer, Scheie, and Spaeth, should be used to evaluate the angle.

Diagnostic criteria for angle closure based on goniophotographs

The field of view in goniophotography varies depending on the device and lens used, ranging from 22.5° sectors to 360° panoramic views. Establishing a consensus on the number of goniophotographs required to adequately assess angle closure remains challenging. The number of images should be sufficient to ensure comprehensive coverage without redundancy or overlap.

- Open angle: All structures from Schwalbe's line to the ciliary body band are visible.
- Occludable angle: The absence of visible trabecular meshwork in 2 or more quadrants of the whole angle (Fig. 2).

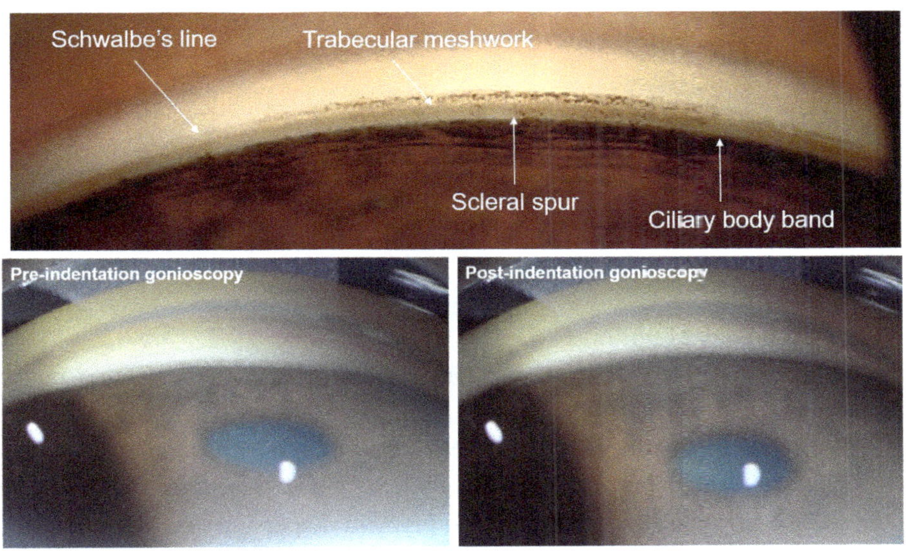

Fig. 1. Normal iridocorneal angle as seen in gonioscopy.

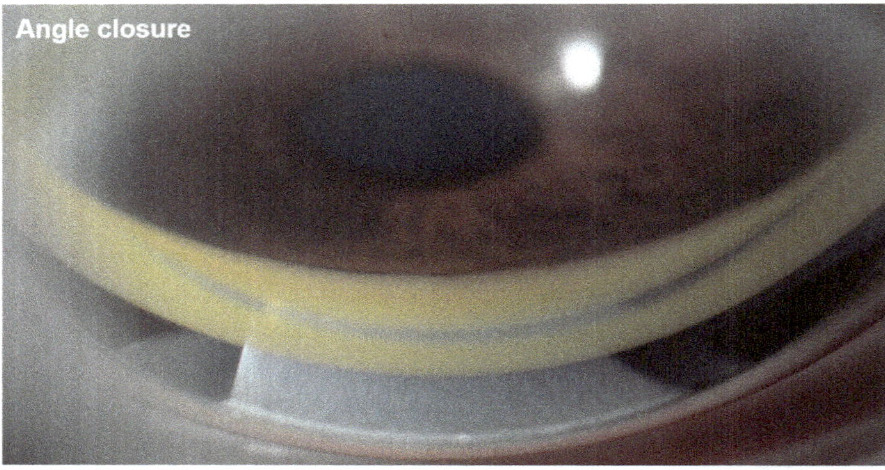

Fig. 2. Goniophotograph with non-visible trabecular meshwork.

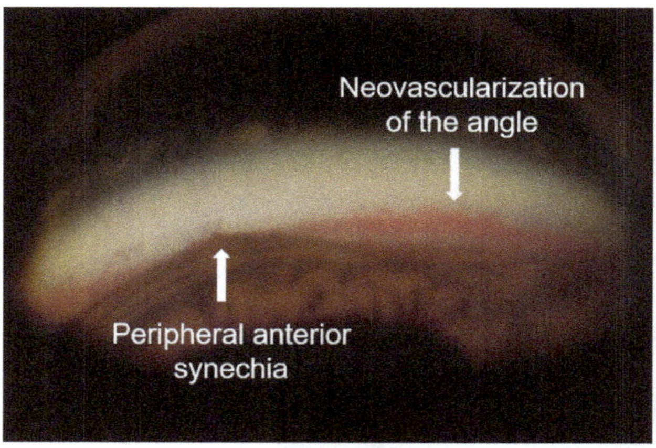

Fig. 3. Goniophotograph showing periperipheral anterior synechia and neovascularization of the angle.

Other pathological findings

In addition to angle classification, goniophotographs can reveal other ocular conditions affecting the angle:

- PAS: Abnormal adhesions between the iris and the corneal angle (Fig. 3).
- Pigment dispersion: Excess pigmentation in the trabecular meshwork or along Schwalbe's line may indicate pigment dispersion syndrome or pseudoexfoliation syndrome. Additionally, heterogeneous pigmentation of the trabecular meshwork may suggest the possibility of intermittent angle closure.

- <u>Neovascularization:</u> New vessel growth within the angle, suggesting neovascular glaucoma (Fig. 3).

Recent advances in goniophotographs

Automated 360° goniophotography

The Gonioscope GS-1 (NIDEK, Gamagori, Japan) is an automated gonioscope with a 16-mirror lens that captures 360° images of the eye.[1,2] It attaches to an anesthetized eye using gel, similar to traditional slit-lamp gonioscopy. The system automatically adjusts focus across different focal planes, with the option for manual adjustments simultaneously. The final image is presented as a linear or circular montage of the entire 360° iridocorneal angle.

Assessment of goniophotographs using AI

Researchers have explored the application of AI in assessing goniophotographs to assist in differentiating between open angle and closed angle status. Chiang *et al.* reported that a convolutional neural network classifier based on the ResNet-50 architecture outperformed both individual graders and collective assessment in evaluating ACAn status.[3] While AI tools may have limitations in assessing poor-quality images and complex cases, potentially leading to poor segmentation or incorrect identification, they can facilitate remote detection and reduce the challenges associated with manual interpretation.

Conclusion

This diagnostic consensus establishes clear, standardized criteria for interpreting goniophotographs in evaluating the ACAn, enabling clinicians to achieve a more consistent and reliable approach to diagnosing angle status. Risk stratification based on standardized grading systems helps identify patients at various stages of angle closure risk, guiding appropriate management and intervention strategies. Additionally, recognizing pathological findings further enhances the utility of goniophotographs in diagnosing a range of ocular conditions. However, caution is needed when interpreting goniophotographs, as they tend to have low inter-observer and inter-operator agreement. These guidelines support a comprehensive approach to ACAn evaluation, ultimately contributing to improved patient outcomes in clinical practice.

References

1. Shi Y, Yang X, Marion KM, et al. Novel and semiautomated 360-degree gonioscopic anterior chamber angle imaging in under 60 seconds. Ophthalmol Glaucoma. 2019;2(4):215-23. https://doi.org/10.1016/j.ogla.2019.04.002
2. Madu CT, Phelps T, Schuman JS, et al. Automated 360-degree goniophotography with the NIDEK Gonioscope GS-1 for glaucoma. PLoS One. 2023;18(3):e0270941. https://doi.org/10.1371/journal.pone.0270941
3. Chiang M, Guth D, Pardeshi AA, et al. Glaucoma expert-level detection of angle closure in goniophotographs with convolutional neural networks: the Chinese American Eye Study. Am J Ophthalmol. 2021;226:100-7. https://doi.org/10.1016/j.ajo.2021.02.004

Population-based screening for primary angle-closure disease

Benjamin Xu

LACD

Theodoros Filippopoulos, Benjamin Xu

Gonioscopy is the clinical standard method for the assessment of ACAn configuration and classification of eyes along the sPAC. Gonioscopy should be performed on both eyes in all individuals with suspected angle closure. However, gonioscopy requires skill, is subjective, and is often underutilized in clinical settings.[1,2] Non-contact screening methods for the detection of eyes with narrow ACAns—such as the original van Herick test (4 grades)[3] or the assessment of LACD, often referred to as the modified van Herick test (7 grades) as proposed by Foster *et al.*[4]—have emerged as potential alternatives to gonioscopy. These tests are performed at the slit lamp under high magnification with the illumination column being offset by 60° from the axis of the microscope. A narrow, vertical, bright light beam is directed perpendicular towards the temporal limbus, and the LACD at the most peripheral point of the cornea is expressed as a fraction of the peripheral corneal thickness.[4,5]

Most studies evaluating the diagnostic performance of such tests have been performed in Asian populations, many of which employed a case-control study design and some of which have utilized enriched populations with a significantly higher prevalence of PACS and/or PACD cases compared to what is encountered in the general population. A recent Cochrane review of 16 studies reported that a LACD threshold ≤ 25% (with % denoting the percentage of peripheral corneal thickness) provided an 83% sensitivity for an 88% specificity in identifying occludable angles.[6] Based on these figures, the authors concluded that performing LACD on 1,000 individuals with a 10% population prevalence of occludable angles would miss 17 cases and incorrectly classify 108 cases without angle closure.[6] The above figures have been derived from a substantial number of studies and individuals but have been performed both on enriched populations where the diagnostic performance is generally higher and in cohorts that have emerged from population-based screening. For example, in an Asian-enriched population that included subjects from both the ZAP Trial and the Liwan Eye Study, a LACD ≤ 25% yielded a 94% sensitivity for an 88% specificity in identifying PACS status (AUROC = 0.94), while PACS cases and control cases demonstrated an average ± SD LACD of 22% ± 9% and 54% ± 25%, respectively.[7] A similar diagnostic performance with the same cutoff (LACD ≤ 25%) has been documented in an Asian-enriched population (85% sensitivity for a 90% specificity) in identifying subjects with a Shaefer grade ≤ 1 for more than 180° of the angle[8] and in a mixed-race, enriched population (80% sensitivity for a 92% specificity) in identifying eyes with ITC ≥ 270° by gonioscopy.[9] Conversely, during screening of the general population, the diagnostic performance drops and stricter thresholds have been proposed to achieve a reasonable specificity. Foster *et al.* reported 84% sensitivity for a 86% specificity in identifying subjects with ITC ≥ 270° in a population-based sample of 1,717 subjects from Mongolia with a cutoff of ≤ 15%.[4] A cutoff of ≤ 25% yielded a much lower specificity (66%) in this study. Nolan *et al.* reported 83% sensitivity for a 88% specificity utilizing a cutoff of ≤ 15% in identifying subjects with ITC ≥ 270° among a representative sample of 1,090 Chinese-Singaporean individuals.[5] Finally, in the ZAP Trial, screening of the general population with a LACD threshold ≤ 25% achieved an adjusted 93% sensitivity for only a 62% specificity to detect PACS status, resulting in a very low positive predictive value even under the assumption of a relatively high disease prevalence.[10]

It therefore can be concluded that LACD can be used for opportunistic case detection, *i.e.*, patients presenting to the comprehensive ophthalmologist with hypermetropia, a positive family history of angle closure, or a shallow anterior chamber. However, LACD is less useful for population-based screening, as it would generate an unacceptably high number of false positives given the low prevalence of the disease and cases detected by LACD would require gonioscopic confirmation by trained glaucoma professionals. Such an approach has been tested on the field in the Inuit population, where screening with LACD and central

ACD was subsequently confirmed by gonioscopy before proceeding with LPI or surgical iridectomy accordingly. This approach resulted in significant morbidity reduction in this high-risk population.[11-13] It should also be noted that LACD thresholds of ≤ 25% are encountered at a relatively low prevalence of approximately 2% in predominantly white populations,[14] possibly due to higher rates of cataract surgery utilization in these populations.[15,16] Finally, if the stakes are high, such as in individuals requiring dilated fundus examination, which has been the most frequent precipitating factor for APAC in the ZAP trial,[17] more sensitive thresholds could be utilized for referring patients for gonioscopy. Foster *et al.* reported a 100% sensitivity with a LACD threshold of ≤ 40%.[4] A prospective trial comparing the diagnostic performance and cost-effectiveness of LACD assessment by trained optometrists versus gonioscopy by trained glaucoma specialists is currently underway in patients referred to tertiary care centers.[18]

The role of ACD in diagnosing PACS status and PACD

Theodoros Filippopoulos

Indirect gonioscopy is the clinical standard method for diagnostic ACAn assessment and patient classification but requires expertise, is subjective, and is often underutilized.[1,19,20] Furthermore, the ZAP Trial[17] and the Singapore Asymptomatic Narrow Angles Laser Iridotomy Study (ANA-LIS)[21] have demonstrated that current gonioscopic classification[22] is weakly predictive of angle closure outcomes among PACS.[23] As a consequence, several ocular biometric parameters derived from imaging devices such AS-OCT, A-scan ultrasound biometry, optical biometry, Scheimpflug imaging, and UBM are currently being investigated not only as potential surrogate indicators of PACD but also in an effort to risk stratify progression along the sPAC[24,25] and to predict outcomes after interventions such as LPI.[26] Racial and ethnic differences in PACS/PACD prevalence were previously attributed to biometric differences, although recent work suggests these differences may be small among patients of Asian, European, or African ancestry.[27-30] However, gender-related differences in some ocular biometric parameters may explain in part the higher PACG prevalence among women.[23,31]

Among these parameters, ACD has been extensively studied in Asian populations, for which normative databases exist;[32] is readily available to clinicians, as it can be measured with various devices; demonstrates, in contrast to gonioscopy, excellent repeatability and reproducibility;[23,24,33,34] and does not require manual identification of any anatomic landmark as opposed to other AS-OCT-derived ocular biometric parameters.[35] Although different imaging modalities provide highly correlated measurements,[36,37] these are not interchangeable,[38,39] even among devices with similar technology, *i.e.*, AS-OCT.[40]

As a strong component of angle width, ACD reflects the contribution of both relative lens position and size-to-angle crowding.[23,41] PACG prevalence increases exponentially with increasing age[42,43] as the crystalline lens exhibits bidirectional growth,[27,44,45] while cataract surgery rates inversely affect cumulative PACS/PACD incidence.[16] Cross-sectional and longitudinal studies indicate that ACD decreases by approximately 0.1 mm per decade[13,32,34,44,46] and this in turn affects several other ocular biometric parameters.[47] As a consequence, prevalence and/or incidence across the sPAC also increase exponentially with diminishing ACD,[16,41,48] which makes ACD an appealing diagnostic biomarker from a mathematical standpoint. In models investigating risk factors for PACG, the effect of age becomes negligible when adjusted for ACD.[20] Further, patients with a unilateral APAC attack demonstrate lower mean ACD in affected eyes compared to fellow unaffected eyes.[49]

Although the contribution of shallow ACD in the pathogenesis of PACD has long been recognized,[50,51] criteria incorporating ACD as a screening tool have only recently been utilized in Greenland, in an ethnic group with a very high prevalence of angle closure-related blindness.[46] Shallow ACD is a significant risk factor for angle closure in Asian and Caucasian populations alike, even after adjusting for confounding factors such as age, gender, axial length, ACW, and iris convexity[28] or LT, gender, axial length, LACD, and lens position.[52] Congdon *et al.* reported a 77% sensitivity for an 87% specificity with an ACD threshold of 2.7 mm measured by ultrasound in a population-based cohort from rural Taiwan in identifying patients with at least 1 eye that would classify as PAC with current nomenclature. Nolan *et al.* reported a 76% sensitivity for a 74% specificity using an ACD threshold of 2.5 mm measured by ultrasound in a population-based cohort from Singapore in identifying individuals with ITC ≥ 270° by gonioscopy (AUROC = 0.81).[5] Similarly, a 2.6-mm ACD threshold measured by ultrasound was associated with a 78% sensitivity for an 82% specificity after excluding cases that had undergone cataract surgery or LPI in discriminating between eyes with PACD or PACS (defined as ITC ≥ 270°) over controls in the Chinese American Eye Study.[41]

Optical methods usually measure higher ACD values compared to ultrasound if corneal thickness is incorporated, such as in optical biometry, and lower measurements if measuring true ACD (*i.e.*, endothelium to anterior lens capsule) as with AS-OCT or Scheimpflug technology. In the ZAP trial, for example, investigators recruited PACS patients through population-based screening and reported a mean ACD of 2.6 mm by UBM and 2.2 by AS-OCT in the same cohort of patients.[17,53] Investigators determined that an ACD screening threshold of 2.2 mm measured by optical means provided an 85% sensitivity for an 84% specificity in identifying subjects with ITC ≥ 270° (AUROC = 0.91).[34] As a matter of fact, an ACD threshold of 2.3 mm in this large population-based cohort in Mongolia would identify almost every case of PACD or PACS.[13,34] This threshold has been subsequently confirmed with the current PACS definition (ITC ≥ 180°) and the utilization of swept-source AS-OCT, with ACD alone achieving an AUROC = 0.94 in differentiating PACD/PACS cases from controls[54] in an enriched Asian population. Although ACD thresholds cannot resolve PACS, PAC, or PACG,[54,55] neither can other AS-OCT-derived ocular biometric parameters,[33] at least at a population-based level.

Therefore, such ACD thresholds (2.6 mm by ultrasound, 2.2 mm by AS-OCT, and 2.2 mm + central corneal thickness by optical biometry[56,57]) can be helpful for opportunistic screening (case detection) of PACS status or PACD due to the low disease prevalence and moderate specificity of this screening method. However, suspect cases identified by the above thresholds would have to be confirmed with gonioscopy and classified accordingly. Finally, it must be noted that clinic patients with more severe phenotypes, such as APAC and PACG, are an order of magnitude shallower compared to population-based PACS cohorts and frequently demonstrate ACDs below 2.0 mm by AS-OCT.[39] Therefore, shallower ACD measurements in this range could help in identifying individuals at increasing risk for progression along the sPAC.

The role of other ocular biometric parameters in diagnosing PACS status and PACD

If sequential images are obtained circumferentially, AS-OCT non-contact imaging of the angle can identify— qualitatively or quantitatively— appositional contact between the peripheral iris and the trabecular meshwork as well as measure several ocular biometric parameters once the scleral spur is manually identified. Compared to gonioscopy and UBM, the advantages of AS-OCT imaging include that it can be performed in a sitting position in complete darkness, that the longer wavelength utilized only minimally affects pupil diameter, and that it provides high-resolution images.[58] Its disadvantages are the cost and bulkiness of the equipment, which makes it less appealing for population-based screening, suboptimal imaging of the structures behind the iris, and challenges in identifying the scleral spur, a crucial anatomic landmark, which cannot be identified in up to one-third of cases.[59-61]

Qualitative AS-OCT assessment of the angle tends to identify more closed angles than gonioscopy.[56,58,62,63] Angle closure with AS-OCT in this context is defined as any contact between the peripheral iris and structures anterior to the scleral spur. Such a methodology demonstrated a 98% sensitivity in identifying PACS/PACD but only a 55% specificity in an enriched Asian cohort.[62] Due to low specificity, qualitative AS-OCT angle assessment of a cohort in Singapore with a high PACD prevalence demonstrated inferior diagnostic performance compared to central ACD or LACD.[56]

AS-OCT instruments and Scheimpflug cameras also allow cross-sectional imaging of the entire anterior segment in a single scan and provide parameters such as ACAr and ACV, which do not rely on manual identification of any anatomic landmark. In cross-sectional studies, these parameters also decline significantly with age and are significantly smaller in women.57 Both ACAr and ACV were associated with high odds ratios, 53 and 40 per 1 standard deviation decrease in such parameters, respectively, in identifying PACS subjects after adjusting for age, sex, ACD, axial length, and pupil size in a high prevalence, community-based sample of elderly Singaporeans and demonstrated a 90% sensitivity for an 85% specificity, which is superior to ACD in this population.[57] A similarly high diagnostic performance (AUROC = 0.988) for ACV was confirmed in an enriched population distinguishing sPAC from eyes with open angles with a threshold of < 98 mm^3, outperforming all other ocular biometric parameters.[64]

AS-OCT and UBM also provide lens-related parameters, such as LV, which is defined as the perpendicular distance between the anterior pole of the crystalline lens and a horizontal line connecting the 2 scleral spurs and incorporates both LT and relative lens position (RLP) in a single parameter.[31,55] LV decreases with age, even after LPI.[47] Increased LV is significantly associated with angle closure (PAC, PACG, or previous APAC) in eyes with a patent LPI, conveying an odds ratio of 48 when comparing the highest with the lowest quartile after adjusting for age, gender, ACD, LT, and RLP; specifically, LV thresholds achieved a sensitivity and specificity of 88% in this enriched Chinese population.[31] The role of LV has been subsequently confirmed in an independent Japanese cohort with similar diagnostic performance.[65]

While several angle-specific AS-OCT parameters exist, there is currently no consensus on the most useful one in characterizing the ACAn. Such parameters obviously differ significantly between PACS/PACD patients and controls.[61] Some of these parameters demonstrated significant correlation with IOP below certain thresholds in previously undiagnosed and untreated Chinese-American subjects with PACS or PACD with ARA at 750 μm from the scleral spur (ARA750), exhibiting the highest Spearman correlation coefficient ($r = -0.68$).[66] Among angle-specific AS-OCT parameters, angle opening distance at 750 μm from the sceral spur (AOD750) demonstrated the highest AUROC of 0.90 at a threshold of 225 μm in distinguishing PACS or PACD from controls in a cohort of patients seen at a general medical clinic with a relatively high proportion of such eyes.[59] Other studies have demonstrated comparable performances for AOD, ARA, TISA at 500 or 750 μm from the scleral spur (AUROC 0.97 for AOD500, ARA500, and TISA500) in a predominantly Caucasian cohort independently if AS-OCT or UBM is used to perform these measurements.[58] Several of these parameters (AOD, ARA, TISA) at various distances from the scleral spur have similar diagnostic performances, likely due to their collinear behavior as many of them are closely interrelated or directly derived from one another.[25] Of note, angle-specific ocular biometric parameters such as AOD or TISA provided by different imaging, *i.e.*, AS-OCT or UBM, cannot be used interchangeably.[58]

Another interesting approach is to utilize more than 1 parameter as a screening tool. Nongpiur *et al.* utilized 6 AS-OCT provided parameters combined, such as ACW, ACAr, ACV, LV, iris thickness (IT750), and iris area (Iarea), and achieved a high diagnostic performance with AUROC of 0.96 in identifying eyes with PAC or PACG in an enriched population of Chinese individuals.[61]

Finally, a fairly novel approach is to utilize thresholds derived from age- and angle location-specific normative databases for various AS-OCT parameters. With this methodology, a cutoff below the 10th percentile for AOD500 for 90° of the angle achieved the best performance, with AUROC of 0.93 at 88% sensitivity for an 85% specificity, in identifying eyes with gonioscopic angle closure (PACS or PACD) and outperformed the criterion of any ITC in an enriched study population.[63]

In conclusion, AS-OCT-derived ocular biometric parameters, especially if used in combination, are useful at this stage for opportunistic screening (case detection) in clinic, for patient education, and to confirm the clinician's gonioscopic impression. However, these parameters are not yet ready for population-based screening due to practical reasons and insufficient specificity in low-prevalence settings. However, by overcoming the subjective nature of gonioscopy, parameters such as AOD750, LV, and ACAr/ACV may hold promise in the near future for disease classification and risk assessment with the advent of AI-guided automated detection algorithms that do not require manual identification of the scleral spur.[67,68] Furthermore, the evaluation of the dynamic behavior of such parameters in response to variable lighting conditions may also be useful in the future but is not well-suited for population-based screening and is currently only used in experimental settings.[69]

Ocular biometric risk factors for progression along the sPAC

Several ocular biometric parameters appear to also have a role in predicting progression along the sPAC. The Liwan Eye Study has demonstrated that shallow ACD is the strongest risk factor for incident PACS status or PACD. An ACD threshold of 2.6 mm measured by ultrasound was associated with a 74% sensitivity but only a 57% specificity in predicting incident PACS status or PACD over 10 years after excluding patients who had undergone bilateral cataract surgery.[70] Aung *et al.* demonstrated that the risk of incident synechial closure (PAC) rises exponentially below an ACD threshold of 2.4 mm measured by optical means in a Mongolian population with limited access to health care services.[48] Among several prediction models derived from the ZAP trial, IOP at baseline, central ACD, and limbal ACD emerged as the most important risk factors predicting progression from PACS status in untreated eyes, although with moderate performance (AUROC = 0.70).[71] In another multivariate model developed in the untreated cohort of the ZAP trial, narrower horizontal AOD500 and flatter horizontal iris curvature along with age were associated with progression, again with modest performance (AUROC = 0.73),[24] while cumulative Shaffer gonioscopy score was not predictive of progression in a model adjusted for age, ACD, and iris curvature. The optimal ACD threshold by ultrasound was calculated at the level of 2.44 mm in this study, whereas substitution of LACD by more sophisticated AS-OCT parameters did not substantially improve the model's performance.[72] The performance of such progression prediction models was only superseded with the inclusion of physiologic parameters, such as iris volume change in response to dark and light, which may be impractical for widespread clinical use.[73]

Angle-specific AS-OCT parameters can aid in assessing the response to treatment. AOD750 and iris thickness (IT750) at 750 μm from the scleral spur predicted angle widening after LPI among Asian PACS eyes.[26] Furthermore, TISA500 ≤ 0.05 mm^2 and cumulative Shaffer gonioscopy score ≤ 6 two weeks after LPI were significant risk factors associated with progression towards more severe disease phenotypes in LPI-treated ZAP Trial participants.[25] If such measures of angle width are included in a multivariate analysis model, the effect of age becomes insignificant in determining the risk of progression.

In the future, it may be possible to further risk stratify patients with narrow angles based on demographic, anatomic, and physiologic criteria, and determine who would benefit most from early interventions such as LPI or cataract surgery.

References

1. Lee JH, Yoo K, Lung K, Apolo G, Toy B, Sanvicente C, Xu B. Patterns and disparities in recorded gonioscopy during initial glaucoma evaluations in the United States. Am J Ophthalmol. 2024;264:90-98. https://doi.org/10.1016/j.ajo.2024.02.032
2. Wu AM, Stein JD, Shah M. Potentially missed opportunities in prevention of acute angle-closure crisis. JAMA Ophthalmol. 2022;140(6):598-603. https://doi.org/10.1001/jamaophthalmol.2022.1231
3. Van Herick W, Shaffer RN, Schwartz A. Estimation of width of angle of anterior chamber. Incidence and significance of the narrow angle. Am J Ophthalmol. 1969;68(4):626-629. https://doi.org/10.1016/0002-9394(69)91241-0
4. Foster PJ, Buhrmann R, Quigley HA, Johnson GJ. Detection of gonioscopically occludable angles and primary angle closure glaucoma by estimation of limbal chamber depth in Asians: modified grading scheme. Br J Ophthalmol. 2000;84(2):186-192. https://doi.org/10.1136/bjo.84.2.186
5. Nolan WP, Aung T, Machin D, Bhooberos J, Seah SKL, Foster PJ. Detection of narrow angles and established angle closure in Chinese residents of Singapore: potential screening tests. Am J Ophthalmol. 2006;141(5):896-901. https://doi.org/10.1016/j.ajo.2005.12.008
6. Jindal A, Rao HL, Kapoor KG, Kumar RS, Sreelatha OK, Sharma T, Foster PJ. Non-contact tests for identifying people at risk of primary angle closure glaucoma. Cochrane Database Syst Rev. 2020;5(5):CD012947. https://doi.org/10.1002/14651858.CD012947.pub2
7. Andrews J, Foster PJ, Devereux JG, Wormald R, Foster RS. Comparing approaches to screening for angle closure in older Chinese adults. Eye (Lond). 2012;26(1):96-100. https://doi.org/10.1038/eye.2011.244
8. Baskaran M, Nongpiur ME, Wilensky JT, He M, Friedman DS, Aung T. Comparison of the scanning peripheral anterior chamber depth analyzer and the modified van Herick grading system in the assessment of angle closure. Ophthalmology. 2007;114(3):501-506. https://doi.org/10.1016/j.ophtha.2006.08.019
9. Dabasia PL, Thomas R, George R, Baskaran M, He M, Aung T. Noncontact screening methods for the detection of narrow anterior chamber angles. Invest Ophthalmol Vis Sci. 2015;56(6):3929-3935. https://doi.org/10.1167/iovs.15-16727
10. Halawa OA, Ishii Y, Leonidi A, Aung T, Webers CAB. Population-based utility of van Herick grading for angle-closure detection. Ophthalmology. 2021;128(12):1779-1782. https://doi.org/10.1016/j.ophtha.2021.06.010
11. Alsbirk PH. Early detection of primary angle-closure glaucoma. Limbal and axial chamber depth screening in a high risk population (Greenland Eskimos). Acta Ophthalmol (Copenh). 1988;66(5):556-564. https://doi.org/10.1111/j.1755-3768.1988.tb04380.x
12. Alsbirk PH. Strategy for decentralised prevention of angle closure glaucoma in Greenland. Int J Circumpolar Health. 2004;63 Suppl 2:315-319. https://doi.org/10.3402/ijch.v63i0.17927

13. Johnson GJ, Foster PJ. Can we prevent angle-closure glaucoma? Eye (Lond). 2005;19(10):1119-1124. https://doi.org/10.1038/sj.eye.6701970
14. Wolfs RC, De Jong PT, Vingerling JR, Hofman A, Grobbee DE; Rotterdam Study Group. Risk of acute angle-closure glaucoma after diagnostic mydriasis in nonselected subjects: the Rotterdam Study. Invest Ophthalmol Vis Sci. 1997;38(12):2683-2687.
15. Keenan TD, Quigley HA, Zhang Q, et al. Trends in rates of primary angle closure glaucoma and cataract surgery in England from 1968 to 2004. J Glaucoma. 2009;18(3):201-205. https://doi.org/10.1097/IJG.0b013e318181540a
16. Vijaya L, George R, Arvind H, et al. Six-year incidence of angle-closure disease in a South Indian population: the Chennai Eye Disease Incidence Study. Am J Ophthalmol. 2013;156(6):1308-1315.e2. https://doi.org/10.1016/j.ajo.2013.07.027
17. He M, Foster PJ, Ge J, et al. Laser peripheral iridotomy for the prevention of angle closure: a single-centre, randomised controlled trial. Lancet. 2019;393(10181):1609-1618. https://doi.org/10.1016/S0140-6736(18)32607-2
18. Azuara-Blanco A, Marshall H, Sidhartha A, et al. Technologies for the diagnosis of angle closure glaucoma (ACE): protocol of a prospective, multicentre, cross-sectional diagnostic study. BMJ Open. 2023;13(10):e073975. https://doi.org/10.1136/bmjopen-2023-073975
19. Coleman AL, Yu F, Evans SJ. Use of gonioscopy in Medicare beneficiaries before glaucoma surgery. J Glaucoma. 2006;15(6):486-493. https://doi.org/10.1097/01.ijg.0000212287.62798.8f
20. Congdon NG, Quigley HA, Hung PT, Lin SC, Kangakian T, Tielsch J. Screening techniques for angle-closure glaucoma in rural Taiwan. Acta Ophthalmol Scand. 1996;74(2):113-119. https://doi.org/10.1111/j.1600-0420.1996.tb00053.x
21. Baskaran M, Li X, Nongpiur ME, Chan E, Aung T, Friedman DS. The Singapore Asymptomatic Narrow Angles Laser Iridotomy Study: five-year results of a randomized controlled trial. Ophthalmology. 2022;129(2):147-158. https://doi.org/10.1016/j.ophtha.2021.08.017
22. Foster PJ, Buhrmann R, Quigley HA, Johnson GJ. The definition and classification of glaucoma in prevalence surveys. Br J Ophthalmol. 2002;86(2):238-242. https://doi.org/10.1136/bjo.86.2.238
23. Xu BY, Lin SC, Oliva MS, et al. Ocular biometric determinants of anterior chamber angle width in Chinese Americans: the Chinese American Eye Study. Am J Ophthalmol. 2020;220:19-26. https://doi.org/10.1016/j.ajo.2020.07.030
24. Xu BY, Nongpiur ME, Aung T, et al. Ocular biometric risk factors for progression of primary angle closure disease: the Zhongshan Angle Closure Prevention Trial. Ophthalmology. 2022;129(3):267-275. https://doi.org/10.1016/j.ophtha.2021.10.003
25. Bao YK, Chan E, Nongpiur ME, Huang J, Aung T, Friedman DS. Biometric risk factors for angle closure progression after laser peripheral iridotomy. JAMA Ophthalmol. 2023;141(6):516-524. https://doi.org/10.1001/jamaophthalmol.2023.0937
26. Sung KR, Lee KS, Hong JW. Baseline anterior segment parameters associated with the long-

term outcome of laser peripheral iridotomy. Curr Eye Res. 2015;40(11):1128-1133. https://doi.org/10.3109/02713683.2014.986334

27. Wojciechowski R, Yazar S, Munoz B, West SK, Friedman DS, Aung T, et al. Age, gender, biometry, refractive error, and the anterior chamber angle among Alaskan Eskimos. Ophthalmology. 2003;110(2):365-375. https://doi.org/10.1016/S0161-6420(02)01748-7
28. Leung CK, Huang G, Weinreb RN, et al. Comparisons of anterior segment biometry between Chinese and Caucasians using anterior segment optical coherence tomography. Br J Ophthalmol. 2010;94(9):1184-1189. https://doi.org/10.1136/bjo.2009.167296
29. Congdon NG, Wang JJ, Klein BE, et al. Biometry and primary angle-closure glaucoma among Chinese, white, and black populations. Ophthalmology. 1997;104(9):1489-1495. https://doi.org/10.1016/S0161-6420(97)30112-2
30. Quigley HA. Angle-closure glaucoma - simpler answers to complex mechanisms: LXVI Edward Jackson Memorial Lecture. Am J Ophthalmol. 2009;148(5):657-669.e1. https://doi.org/10.1016/j.ajo.2009.08.009
31. Nongpiur ME, He M, Amerasinghe N, et al. Lens vault, thickness, and position in Chinese subjects with angle closure. Ophthalmology. 2011;118(3):474-479. https://doi.org/10.1016/j.ophtha.2010.07.025
32. Xu L, Wang Y, Jonas JB, et al. Anterior chamber depth and chamber angle and their associations with ocular and general parameters: the Beijing Eye Study. Am J Ophthalmol. 2008;145(5):929-936. https://doi.org/10.1016/j.ajo.2008.01.004
33. Xu BY, Chan E, Nongpiur ME, et al. Differences in ocular biometric measurements among subtypes of primary angle closure disease: the Chinese American Eye Study. Ophthalmol Glaucoma. 2021;4(2):224-231. https://doi.org/10.1016/j.ogla.2020.09.008
34. Devereux JG, Foster PJ, Vallabh NA, et al. Anterior chamber depth measurement as a screening tool for primary angle-closure glaucoma in an East Asian population. Arch Ophthalmol. 2000;118(2):257-263. https://doi.org/10.1001/archopht.118.2.257
35. Zhao T, He M, Friedman DS, et al. Repeatability and reproducibility of anterior chamber angle measurement with swept-source optical coherence tomography in patients with primary angle closure suspect. Curr Eye Res. 2021;46(12):1853-1860. https://doi.org/10.1080/02713683.2021.1942069
36. Zhang Q, Jin W, Wang Q. Repeatability, reproducibility, and agreement of central anterior chamber depth measurements in pseudophakic and phakic eyes: optical coherence tomography versus ultrasound biomicroscopy. J Cataract Refract Surg. 2010;36(6):941-946. https://doi.org/10.1016/j.jcrs.2009.12.038
37. Nakakura S, Hirasawa H, Hayashi K, et al. Comparison of anterior chamber depth measurements by 3-dimensional optical coherence tomography, partial coherence interferometry biometry, Scheimpflug rotating camera imaging, and ultrasound biomicroscopy. J Cataract Refract Surg. 2012;38(7):1207-1213. https://doi.org/10.1016/j.jcrs.2012.02.036

38. Dada T, Krishna R, Somashekar R, et al. Comparison of anterior segment optical coherence tomography and ultrasound biomicroscopy for assessment of the anterior segment. J Cataract Refract Surg. 2007;33(5):837-840. https://doi.org/10.1016/j.jcrs.2007.01.021
39. Filippopoulos T, Singh K, Friedman DS, et al. Rethinking prophylactic laser peripheral iridotomy in primary angle-closure suspects: a review. Ophthalmol Glaucoma. 2023;6(6):657-667. https://doi.org/10.1016/j.ogla.2023.06.004
40. Shan J, DeBoer C, Xu BY. Anterior segment optical coherence tomography: applications for clinical care and scientific research. Asia Pac J Ophthalmol (Phila). 2019;8(2):146-157.
41. Zhou S, Liao C, Zhao P, et al. Refractive error and anterior chamber depth as risk factors in primary angle closure disease: the Chinese American Eye Study. J Glaucoma. 2023;32(4):257-264. https://doi.org/10.1097/IJG.0000000000002154
42. Sekimitsu S, Fukuchi T, Araie M, et al. Interaction of background genetic risk, psychotropic medications, and primary angle closure glaucoma in the UK Biobank. PLoS One. 2022;17(6):e0270530. https://doi.org/10.1371/journal.pone.0270530
43. Sawaguchi S, Sakai H, Iwase A, et al. Prevalence of primary angle closure and primary angle-closure glaucoma in a southwestern rural population of Japan: the Kumejima Study. Ophthalmology. 2012;119(6):1134-1142. https://doi.org/10.1016/j.ophtha.2011.12.038
44. Klein BE, Klein R, Moss SE. Correlates of lens thickness: the Beaver Dam Eye Study. Invest Ophthalmol Vis Sci. 1998;39(8):1507-1510.
45. Shajari M, Pourreza HE, Askarizadeh F, et al. Anterior chamber angle, volume, and depth in a normative cohort - a retrospective cross-sectional study. Curr Eye Res. 2019;44(6):632-637. https://doi.org/10.1080/02713683.2019.1576205
46. Alsbirk PH. Anatomical risk factors in primary angle-closure glaucoma. A ten-year follow-up survey based on limbal and axial anterior chamber depths in a high-risk population. Int Ophthalmol. 1992;16(4-5):265-272. https://doi.org/10.1007/BF00917973
47. Kwak J, Boey PY, Tan Tock H, et al. Progressive changes in the anterior segment and their impact on the anterior chamber angle in primary angle closure disease. Am J Ophthalmol. 2024;257:57-65. https://doi.org/10.1016/j.ajo.2023.08.016
48. Aung T, Seah SKL, Machin D, et al. Anterior chamber depth and the risk of primary angle closure in 2 East Asian populations. Arch Ophthalmol. 2005;123(4):527-532. https://doi.org/10.1001/archopht.123.4.527
49. Atalay E, Aydin U, Pinarci EY, et etc. Biometric factors associated with acute primary angle closure: comparison of the affected and fellow eye. Invest Ophthalmol Vis Sci. 2016;57(13):5320-5325. https://doi.org/10.1167/iovs.16-20006
50. Lowe RF. Aetiology of the anatomical basis for primary angle-closure glaucoma. Biometrical comparisons between normal eyes and eyes with primary angle-closure glaucoma. Br J Ophthalmol. 1970;54(3):161-169. https://doi.org/10.1136/bjo.54.3.161
51. Tornquist R. Chamber depth in primary acute glaucoma. Br J Ophthalmol. 1956;40(7):421-

429. https://doi.org/10.1136/bjo.40.7.421

52. Zhang Y, Li M, Li L, et al. Development of angle closure and associated risk factors: the Handan Eye Study. Acta Ophthalmol. 2022;100(1):e253-e261. https://doi.org/10.1111/aos.14887
53. Jiang Y, Nongpiur ME, Aung T, et al. Longitudinal changes of angle configuration in primary angle-closure suspects: the Zhongshan Angle-Closure Prevention Trial. Ophthalmology. 2014;121(9):1699-1705. https://doi.org/10.1016/j.ophtha.2014.03.039
54. Ma P, Chan E, Ung AL, et al. Evaluation of the diagnostic performance of swept-source anterior segment optical coherence tomography in primary angle closure disease. Am J Ophthalmol. 2022;233:68-77. https://doi.org/10.1016/j.ajo.2021.06.033
55. Vryonis N, Loewen RT, Samuelson T, et al. Anterior chamber morphology before and after laser peripheral iridotomy determined by Scheimpflug technology in white patients with narrow angles. J Glaucoma. 2013;22(9):679-683. https://doi.org/10.1097/IJG.0b013e318264b908
56. Lavanya R, Jeganathan VSE, Zheng Y, Wong TY, Foster PJ, Aung T. Screening for narrow angles in the Singapore population: evaluation of new noncontact screening methods. Ophthalmology. 2008;115(10):1720-1727.e1-2. https://doi.org/10.1016/j.ophtha.2008.03.015
57. Wu RY, Friedman DS, Kong X, et al. Association of narrow angles with anterior chamber area and volume measured with anterior-segment optical coherence tomography. Arch Ophthalmol. 2011;129(5):569-574. https://doi.org/10.1001/archophthalmol.2011.68
58. Radhakrishnan S, Rollins AM, Roth DB, et al. Comparison of optical coherence tomography and ultrasound biomicroscopy for detection of narrow anterior chamber angles. Arch Ophthalmol. 2005;123(8):1053-1059. https://doi.org/10.1001/archopht.123.8.1053
59. Narayanaswamy A, Perera SA, Zheng Y, et al. Diagnostic performance of anterior chamber angle measurements for detecting eyes with narrow angles: an anterior segment OCT study. Arch Ophthalmol. 2010;128(10):1321-1327. https://doi.org/10.1001/archophthalmol.2010.231
60. Sakata LM, Lavanya R, Friedman DS, et al. Assessment of the scleral spur in anterior segment optical coherence tomography images. Arch Ophthalmol. 2008;126(2):181-185. https://doi.org/10.1001/archophthalmol.2007.46
61. Nongpiur ME, Aung T, Perera SA, et al. Classification algorithms based on anterior segment optical coherence tomography measurements for detection of angle closure. Ophthalmology. 2013;120(1):48-54. https://doi.org/10.1016/j.ophtha.2012.07.005
62. Nolan WP, Aung T, Selvendran S, et al. Detection of primary angle closure using anterior segment optical coherence tomography in Asian eyes. Ophthalmology. 2007;114(1):33-39. https://doi.org/10.1016/j.ophtha.2006.05.073
63. Guo PY, Kwong CH, Lau NN, et al. Diagnostic criteria of anterior segment swept-source optical coherence tomography to detect gonioscopic angle closure. Br J Ophthalmol. 2024;108(8):1130-1136. https://doi.org/10.1136/bjo-2023-323860
64. Li F, Xu BY, Zheng Y, et al. Volumetric parameters-based differentiation of narrow angle from open angle and classification of angle configurations: an SS-OCT study. Br J Ophthalmol.

2020;104(1):92-97. https://doi.org/10.1136/bjophthalmol-2018-313386

65. Ozaki M, Yoshida A, Miyadera K, et al. Increased lens vault as a risk factor for angle closure: confirmation in a Japanese population. Graefes Arch Clin Exp Ophthalmol. 2012;250(12):1863-1868. https://doi.org/10.1007/s00417-012-2011-y
66. Xu BY, Chan E, Zheng Y, et al. Correlation between intraocular pressure and angle configuration measured by OCT: the Chinese American Eye Study. Ophthalmol Glaucoma. 2018;1(3):158-166. https://doi.org/10.1016/j.ogla.2018.09.001
67. Xu BY, Perera SA, Zheng Y, et al. Deep learning classifiers for automated detection of gonioscopic angle closure based on anterior segment OCT images. Am J Ophthalmol. 2019;208:273-280. https://doi.org/10.1016/j.ajo.2019.08.004
68. Yao H, Zhong X, Huang LJ, et al. Primary angle-closed diseases recognition through artificial intelligence-based anterior segment-optical coherence tomography imaging. Graefes Arch Clin Exp Ophthalmol. 2025;263(4):1081-1087. https://doi.org/10.1007/s00417-024-06709-1
69. Zhang Y, Jiang Y, Nongpiur ME, et al. Dynamic iris changes as a risk factor in primary angle closure disease. Invest Ophthalmol Vis Sci. 2016;57(1):218-225. https://doi.org/10.1167/iovs.15-17651
70. Wang L, Zhuang W, Lin J, et al. Ten-year incidence of primary angle closure in elderly Chinese: the Liwan Eye Study. Br J Ophthalmol. 2019;103(3):355-360. https://doi.org/10.1136/bjophthalmol-2017-311808
71. Yuan Y, Nongpiur ME, Aung T, et al. Fourteen-year outcome of angle-closure prevention with laser iridotomy in the Zhongshan Angle-Closure Prevention Study: extended follow-up of a randomized controlled trial. Ophthalmology. 2023;130(8):786-794. https://doi.org/10.1016/j.ophtha.2023.03.024
72. Yuan Y, Huynh TT, Kapetanakis VV, et al. Long-term risk and prediction of progression in primary angle closure suspect. JAMA Ophthalmol. 2024;142(3):216-223. https://doi.org/10.1001/jamaophthalmol.2023.5286
73. Liao C, Perera SA, Zheng Y, et al. Iris volume change with physiologic mydriasis to identify development of angle closure: the Zhongshan Angle Closure Prevention Trial. Br J Ophthalmol. 2024;108(3):366-371. https://doi.org/10.1136/bjo-2022-322981

Provocative testing

Clemens Strohmaier, Benjamin Xu

Provocation testing for glaucoma is commonly used with the intention to assess the risk of IOP increase in patients identified as PACS.[1] Different provocation stimuli have been proposed, including the dark room test,[2] the prone position test,[3] a combination of dark room and prone position,[4] and medically induced mydriasis.[5] A perfect test for the assessment of angle-closure subjects would inform the clinician with high sensitivity and specificity about the clinical significance of the identified risk factors (most commonly a shallow anterior chamber) and the future risk for the development of angle-closure disease. Currently, such a diagnostic provocative test does not exist.

When considering the diagnostic performance of any of these tests, it is important to consider the clinical setting that the test is being performed in, *e.g.*, general population screening vs a high-risk cohort or primary open-angle glaucoma patients vs angle-closure suspects.

As could be expected, those preconditions cause highly variable numbers regarding diagnostic performance. In its initial description, the prone test was positive (> 8 mmHg increase in IOP) in 70% of patients with angle-closure glaucoma, 49% of angle-closure suspects, 7% of open-angle glaucoma patients, and 4% of normal eyes.[3] Sihota *et al.* examined family members of primary angle-closure patients using a dark room prone position test (DRPPT). Of those affected with PACG (36.9%), 70.3% showed a positive DRPPT.[6] This is higher than the numbers reported by Yamada *et al.*, who investigated PACS, PAC, and PACG patients and reported a positive DRPPT in 32% of the individuals.[7] Interestingly, in the former study, an ACD of 2.07 mm was identified as the cutoff for excellent sensitivity, which was undercut by both the test-positive (1.77 mm) and test-negative (1.96 mm) in the latter study. This further highlights the need to carefully consider the study cohort when assessing any diagnostic test performance. A recent investigation by Friedman *et al.* showed no significant difference between open-angle glaucoma patients and PACS using a modified DRPPT in 889 Chinese PACS and 89 Chinese open-angle glaucoma patients.[8]

Even more important than the number of immediate positive patients in any test environment is the predictive value for future angle-closure disease. Only a few studies have reported such numbers. Wilensky *et al.* followed a cohort of 129 patients with an ACD of less than 2 mm or a chamber angle considered narrow for up to 5 years.[9] The dark room provocative test was positive in 25 eyes of 17 patients (19%). Six of those 25 eyes (24% of those with a positive test) developed acute or non-acute angle-closure disease compared to 32 eyes with a negative test (25% of the total cohort). Friedman et. al. investigated the predictive value of a modified DRPPT in the ZAP trial cohort, a population-based screening trial in China.[8,10] In a multivariate analysis, they found no statistical association between the DRPPT result and the incidence of angle closure in the ZAP trial.

In summary, the current evidence is inconclusive regarding the interpretation of provocative testing in many clinical situations. More research, especially on potential confounders (AS-OCT parameters, ethnicity, etc.) is needed.

References

1. European Glaucoma Society Terminology and Guidelines for Glaucoma, 5th Edition. Br J Ophthalmol. 2021;105(Suppl 1):1-169. https://doi.org/10.1136/bjophthalmol-2021-egsguidelines
2. Higgitt AC. The Dark-Room Test. Br J Ophthalmol. 1954;38(4):242-247. https://doi.org/10.1136/bjo.38.4.242
3. Hyams SW, Friedman Z, Neumann E. Elevated Intraocular Pressure in the Prone Position. Am J Ophthalmol. 1968;66(4):661-672. https://doi.org/10.1016/0002-9394(68)91287-7
4. Harris LS, Galin MA. Prone Provocative Testing for Narrow Angle Glaucoma. Arch Ophthalmol. 1972;87(5):493-496. https://doi.org/10.1001/archopht.1972.01000020495001
5. Mills DW, Becker B. The dilatation provocative test. Trans Can Opthalmolog Soc. 1963;26:196-209.
6. Sihota R, Mohan S, Dada T, Gupta V, Pandey RM, Ghate D. An evaluation of the darkroom prone provocative test in family members of primary angle closure glaucoma patients. Eye (Lond). 2007;21(7):984-989. https://doi.org/10.1038/SJ.EYE.6702375
7. Yamada R, Hirose F, Matsuki T, Kameda T, Kurimoto Y. Comparison of Mydriatic Provocative and Dark Room Prone Provocative Tests for Anterior Chamber Angle Configuration. J Glaucoma. 2016;25(6):482-486. https://doi.org/10.1097/IJG.0000000000000310
8. Friedman DS, Chang DST, Jiang Y, et al. Darkroom prone provocative testing in primary angle closure suspects and those with open angles. Br J Ophthalmol. 2019;103(12):1834-1839. https://doi.org/10.1136/BJOPHTHALMOL-2018-313362
9. Wilensky JT, Kaufman PL, Frohlichstein D, et al. Follow-up of Angle-closure Glaucoma Suspects. Am J Ophthalmol. 1993;115(3):338-346. https://doi.org/10.1016/S0002-9394(14)73585-8
10. Jiang Y, Friedman DS, He M, Huang S, Kong X, Foster PJ. Design and Methodology of a Randomized Controlled Trial of Laser Iridotomy for the Prevention of Angle Closure in Southern China: The Zhongshan Angle Closure Prevention Trial. Ophthalmic Epidemiol. 2010;17(5):321-332. https://doi.org/10.3109/09286586.2010.508353

Artificial intelligence: automated detection of gonioscopic angle closure, iridotrabecular contact, and peripheral anterior synechiae

Fei Li, Benjamin Xu

AI leverages algorithms to simulate intelligent behavior and has increasingly been applied in ophthalmology, driven by advancements in digital health technologies.[1] The integration of AI into the screening of PACD represents a significant breakthrough, addressing challenges associated with large-scale detection and improving access to healthcare. Traditional diagnostic methods, including gonioscopy, UBM, and AS-OCT, are operator-dependent, prone to subjectivity, and limited by variability between examiners. The standard method to identify angle closure and assess eyes at risk is through examination using a gonioscope. However, the clinical expertise and instrumentation required make gonioscopy less suitable for widespread screening.[2] AI-powered models overcome these barriers by providing fast, accurate, and consistent evaluations, making them ideal for population screening programs. Key AI-based advancements include the automated detection of gonioscopic angle closure, ITC, PAS, and scleral spur identification. These technologies not only enhance diagnostic accuracy but also facilitate early intervention, ensuring patients are identified in time to prevent irreversible vision loss.

Automated PACD detection based on AS-OCT scans

AS-OCT is widely recognized for its non-contact, high-resolution imaging of the anterior segment, making it particularly suited for large-scale screening.[3-7] AI models for AS-OCT automate key processes, enhancing diagnostic efficiency. Recent advances in machine learning and deep learning have substantially enhanced the capabilities of AS-OCT imaging in identifying angle closure. Since 2013, AI models using expert interpretation of AS-OCT images as a reference standard have been able to distinguish between open angles and angle closure with high accuracy, achieving AUC values exceeding 0.95.[8] These developments have the potential to improve population-based screening programs aimed at early detection and management of glaucoma, potentially curbing the progression of this sight-threatening condition. Another significant innovation in this field is the development of a 3D deep learning-based automated diagnostic system, which has demonstrated robust diagnostic capabilities in identifying narrow iridocorneal angles and PAS.[9]

Automated PACD detection based on goniophotographs

Gonioscopy is a reference standard for assessing the iridocorneal angle of the eye. However, the process is subjective, time-consuming, and varies significantly among clinicians. Goniophotography allows for the capture and analysis of detailed images of the angle. Integrating AI into goniophotograph analysis offers a promising advancement, enhancing the speed and reliability of screenings and making it more feasible for widespread application.[10] AI models have the capability to effectively distinguish between open angles and angle closure in goniophotographs with impressively high specificity and sensitivity rates—reaching up to 92.6% and 97.8%, respectively.[11] Furthermore, innovative software designed for analyzing angle closure in EyeCam (Clarity Medical Systems, Pleasanton, CA, USA) goniophotographs has demonstrated remarkable diagnostic consistency with traditional manual grading methods, achieving a kappa coefficient as high as 0.88. These advancements underscore the potential of AI to enhance the precision and reliability of glaucoma screenings.

Automated localization of scleral spur

The scleral spur serves as a vital anatomical marker in evaluating the angle anatomy in glaucoma patients. AS-OCT image analysis typically begins with identifying this landmark. However, approximately 20%–30% of images fail to accurately depict bilateral scleral spurs, especially in cases of angle-closure glaucoma.[12] AI algorithms have achieved high accuracy in localizing the scleral spur on AS-OCT images, which is essential for accurate measurement of the angle and subsequent glaucoma management. A deep convolutional neural network has been utilized for scleral spur localization and for segmenting AS-OCT images.[13] This network achieved a Dice coefficient of 95.7% in segmenting essential structures. Moreover, AI models can perform these segmentations and measurements in less than 2 seconds per scan. This efficiency supports a comprehensive and objective assessment of the anterior segment. In another application, a convolutional neural network based on the ResNet-18 architecture has proven effective in detecting the scleral spur in AS-OCT images.[14] This model has shown precision with mean absolute prediction errors close to those seen in human intra-grader variability for both X and Y coordinates. Such capabilities indicate that deep neural networks can provide reliable, automated assessments of AS-OCT images, enhancing both qualitative and quantitative analysis necessary for optimal ophthalmic care.

Automated anterior segment analysis based on UBM

Similar to AS-OCT, UBM is a valuable imaging modality that provides high-resolution cross-sectional images of the anterior segment of the eye.[15] The integration of AI algorithms in analyzing UBM images shows great promise in automating and standardizing the interpretation process, thereby enhancing efficiency, accuracy, and reproducibility. AI has proven effective in automating the localization and classification of the ACAn using UBM images, crucial for diagnosing PACG. Yu *et al.* developed a model that has demonstrated a high success rate, achieving 95% accuracy in pinpointing the angle recess and an overall classification accuracy of 77.8% for the ACAn.[16] This innovative approach not only enhances accuracy but also significantly reduces the time and level of expertise traditionally required for assessments. Using advanced convolutional neural networks, the AI system achieved an impressive 98.18% accuracy in classifying the ACAn. It also reliably measured various angle parameters, such as the trabecular-iris angle and AOD, with precision comparable to that of manual methods.[17] Such results highlight AI's potential to streamline and refine the accuracy of glaucoma diagnostics within clinical settings.

Economic implications of AI-assisted screening for PACD

While advancements in AI-driven diagnostic tools for PACD are promising, the economic viability of these screenings remains under scrutiny. A study conducted in Changjiang County, China, explored the economic impact of implementing AI-assisted glaucoma screening programs. This research utilized a Markov model to predict disease progression and associated healthcare costs over a 15-year period, focusing exclusively on PACG. The findings indicated that while AI-assisted screening significantly reduces the risks and prevalence of PACG, the high initial costs of screening are not fully offset by the reduction in disease progression, even though visual blindness decreased by 33.3%.[18] The study highlights the challenge of managing budgetary concerns when adopting new screening technologies, suggesting that while AI screening effectively reduces disease burden, further analysis on its cost-effectiveness is necessary. This insight is critical for policymakers and healthcare providers considering the broad implementation of AI-driven screening tools in community settings, balancing clinical benefits against economic sustainability. Moreover, experts suggest that glaucoma screening might only be economically justified when combined with other major ocular disease screenings, such as for cataract, diabetic retinopathy, and age-related macular degeneration. Such integrated approaches, especially when enhanced by AI, could lead to significant economies of scale, enhancing the overall yield and improving clinical outcomes.[19]

References

1. McCarthy J, Minsky ML, Rochester N, Shannon CE. A Proposal for the Dartmouth Summer Research Project on Artificial Intelligence, August 31, 1955. AI Magazine. 2006;27(4):12.
2. Thomas R, Parikh R, Paul P, Muliyil J. Population-based screening versus case detection. Indian J Ophthalmol. 2002;50(3):233-7.
3. Qian CX, Hassanaly S, Harissi-Dagher M. Anterior segment optical coherence tomography in the long-term follow-up and detection of glaucoma in Boston type I keratoprosthesis. Ophthalmology. 2015;122(2):317-25. https://doi.org/10.1016/j.ophtha.2014.08.007
4. Sng CCA, Aquino MCD, Liao J, Ang M, Zheng C, Loon SC, et al. Pretreatment anterior segment imaging during acute primary angle closure: insights into angle closure mechanisms in the acute phase. Ophthalmology. 2014;121(1):119-25. https://doi.org/10.1016/j.ophtha.2013.08.004
5. Salim S. The role of anterior segment optical coherence tomography in glaucoma. J Ophthalmol. 2012;2012:476801. https://doi.org/10.1155/2012/476801
6. Huang W, Li X, Gao X, Zhang X. The anterior and posterior biometric characteristics in primary angle-closure disease: Data based on anterior segment optical coherence tomography and swept-source optical coherence tomography. Indian J Ophthalmol. 2021;69(4):865-70. https://doi.org/10.4103/ijo.IJO_936_20
7. Zhang X, Guo PY, Lin C, Li F, Nguyen A, Sakata R, et al. Assessment of Iris Trabecular Contact in Eyes with Gonioscopic Angle-Closure. Ophthalmology. 2023;130(1):111-9. https://doi.org/10.1016/j.ophtha.2022.08.017
8. Fu H, Baskaran M, Xu Y, et al. A Deep Learning System for Automated Angle-Closure Detection in Anterior Segment Optical Coherence Tomography Images. Am J Ophthalmol. 2019;203:37-45. https://doi.org/10.1016/j.ajo.2019.02.028
9. Li F, Yang Y, Sun X, et al. Digital Gonioscopy Based on Three-dimensional Anterior-Segment OCT: An International Multicenter Study. Ophthalmology. 2022;129(1):45-53. https://doi.org/10.1016/j.ophtha.2021.09.018
10. Sakata LM, Lavanya R, Friedman DS, et al. Comparison of gonioscopy and anterior segment ocular coherence tomography in detecting angle closure in different quadrants of the anterior chamber angle. Ophthalmology. 2008;115(5):769-74. https://doi.org/10.1016/j.ophtha.2007.06.030
11. Cheng J, Liu J, Lee BH, et al. Closed angle glaucoma detection in RetCam images. Annu Int Conf IEEE Eng Med Biol Soc. 2010;2010:4096-9. https://doi.org/10.1109/IEMBS.2010.5627290
12. Sakata LM, Lavanya R, Friedman DS, et al. Assessment of the scleral spur in anterior segment optical coherence tomography images. Arch Ophthalmol. 2008;126(2):181-5. https://doi.org/10.1001/archophthalmol.2007.46

13. Pham TH, Devalla SK, Ang A, et al. Deep learning algorithms to isolate and quantify the structures of the anterior segment in optical coherence tomography images. Br J Ophthalmol. 2021;105(9):1231-7. https://doi.org/10.1136/bjophthalmol-2019-315723
14. Xu BY, Chiang M, Pardeshi AA, Moghimi S, Varma R. Deep Neural Network for Scleral Spur Detection in Anterior Segment OCT Images: The Chinese American Eye Study. Transl Vis Sci Technol. 2020;9(2):18. https://doi.org/10.1167/tvst.9.2.18
15. Kottaridou E, Hatoum A. Imaging of Anterior Segment Tumours: A Comparison of Ultrasound Biomicroscopy Versus Anterior Segment Optical Coherence Tomography. Cureus. 2024;16(1):e52578. https://doi.org/10.7759/cureus.52578
16. Yu J, Li W, Chen Q, et al. Automatic Classification of Anterior Chamber Angle Based on Ultrasound Biomicroscopy Images. Ophthalmic Res. 2021;64(5):732-9. https://doi.org/10.1159/000510924
17. Wang W, Wang L, Wang X, Zhou S, Lin S, Yang J. A Deep Learning System for Automatic Assessment of Anterior Chamber Angle in Ultrasound Biomicroscopy Images. Transl Vis Sci Technol. 2021;10(11):21. https://doi.org/10.1167/tvst.10.11.21
18. Xiao X, Xue L, Ye L, Li H, He Y. Health care cost and benefits of artificial intelligence-assisted population-based glaucoma screening for the elderly in remote areas of China: a cost-offset analysis. BMC public health. 2021;21(1):1065. https://doi.org/10.1186/s12889-021-11097-w
19. Bhartiya S. Glaucoma Screening: Is AI the Answer? J Curr Glaucoma Pract. 2022;16(2):71-3. https://doi.org/10.5005/jp-journals-10078-1380

Future directions

Benjamin Xu, Tin Aung

Recent scientific and technological advances offer a promising horizon for enhancing diagnostic precision and early detection of PACD. This section explores future directions in the diagnostic landscape, highlighting the roles of advanced imaging, AI, risk stratification, biomarker discovery, and public health strategies.

Advancements in imaging technologies

The future of angle closure diagnostics is increasingly hinged on advancements shifting toward imaging technologies such as AS-OCT. Current research aims to refine these technologies and make them more accessible and more easily implementable by incorporating AI algorithms capable of identifying critical anatomical landmarks and ensuring precise and reproducible assessments. However, there is a need to reduce the cost of devices and improve their interoperability, developments that could democratize access to these advanced technologies, especially in resource-limited settings.

AI in diagnostic processes

AI is set to revolutionize PACD diagnostics by providing objective, reproducible, scalable, point-of-care solutions. Current AI algorithms are already able to detect gonioscopic angle closure, ITC, and PAS in AS-OCT images with expert-level performance. Future efforts should focus on integrating AI with imaging platforms to enable real-time diagnostics and the identification of novel predictive biomarkers for PACD. Ensuring AI algorithms are trained on diverse datasets will enhance their applicability across different populations and practice settings, fostering widespread adoption in PACD management.

Advanced risk stratification models

The development of advanced risk stratification models is central to enhancing PACD diagnostics. These models will likely utilize a combination of biometric data and machine learning algorithms to accurately predict disease progression and identify high-risk individuals. By incorporating patient-specific factors and high-resolution imaging data, these models can personalize monitoring and treatment plans. Future studies must validate these models' effectiveness using longitudinal data obtained in various clinical environments, ensuring they provide practical utility and integrate seamlessly into existing workflows.

Exploration of novel diagnostic biomarkers

Uncovering novel diagnostic biomarkers is essential for refining PACD diagnostics and facilitating early intervention. Integrating genomics, proteomics, and advanced imaging techniques can yield valuable insights into the molecular and biomechanical mechanisms driving PACD. The development of accessible, non-invasive tests for these biomarkers will enable clinicians to diagnose and monitor the disease more effectively. Multidisciplinary research collaborations will be key to identifying these biomarkers and translating findings into clinical practice.

Public health strategies for early detection

The impact of PACD cannot be overstated since it currently accounts for a significant portion of irreversible blindness worldwide. Developing robust public health strategies incorporating advanced diagnostics into primary care settings is crucial for reducing PACD's global impact, especially with earlier diagnosis leading to better visual outcomes. Emphasizing training healthcare personnel in using new diagnostic technologies and expanding telemedicine resources can extend specialized care to underserved areas. These strategies should be evaluated for cost-effectiveness and practical implementation to ensure they facilitate sustainable improvements in early detection and management of PACD globally.

Conclusion

The future of PACD diagnostics is bright, driven by technological advancements, novel analytical methods, and comprehensive public health strategies. By integrating these innovations into clinical practice, we can enhance early detection, personalize patient care, and reduce the global burden of PACD. Continued interdisciplinary collaboration and investment in these future directions will be imperative to achieving these goals and mitigating vision loss worldwide.

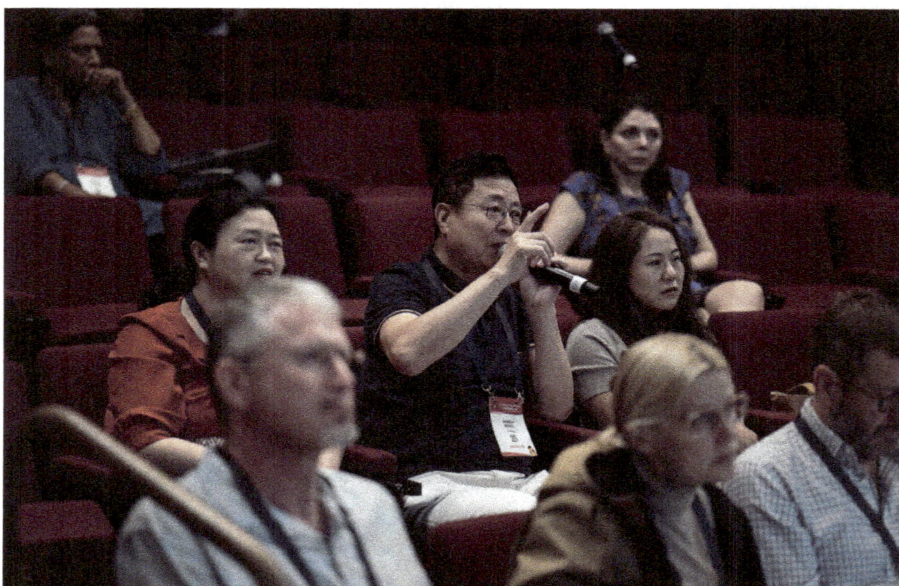

Ningli Wang

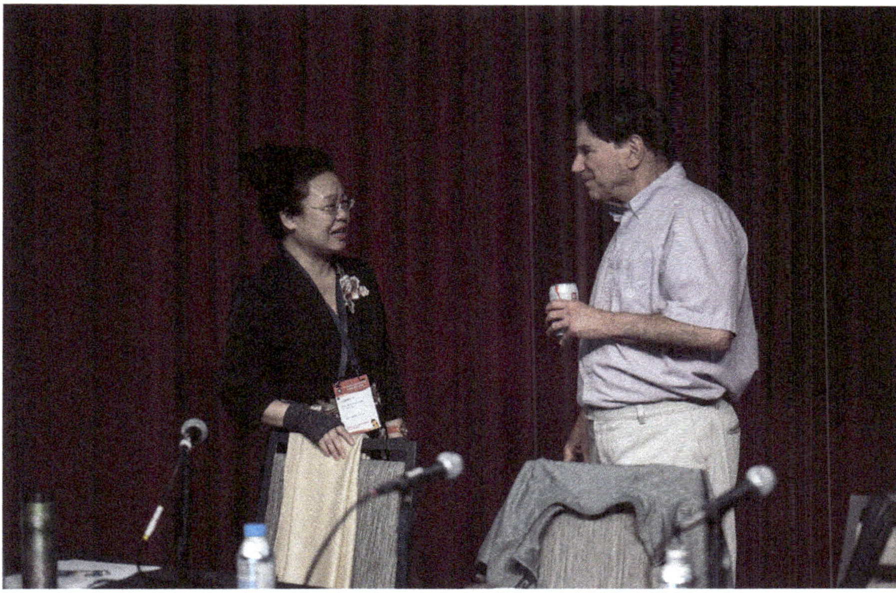

Xiulan Zhang and Robert N. Weinreb

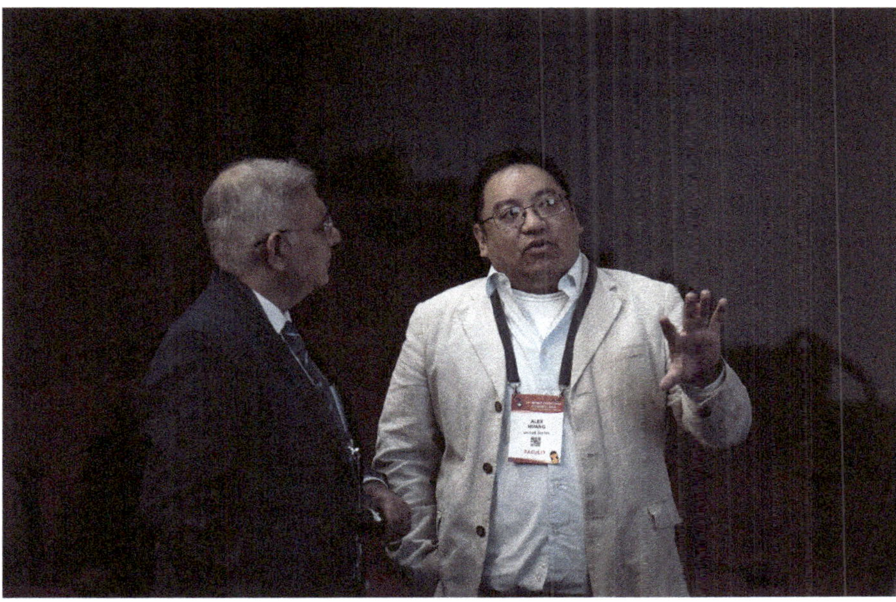

Tanuj Dada and Alex Huang

Section Leaders

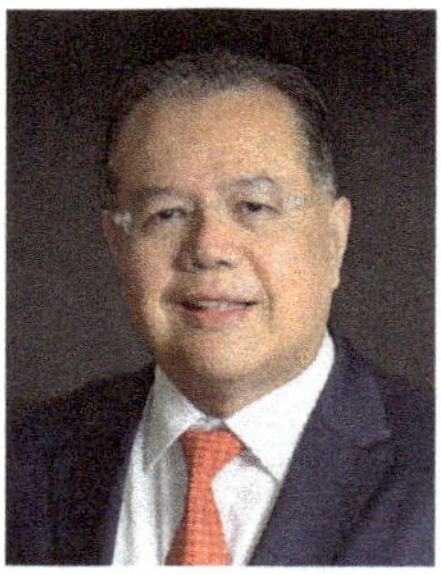

Ting Aung

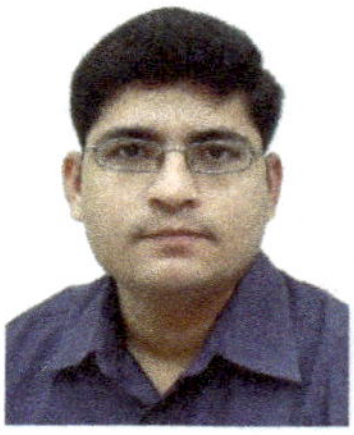

Mani Baskaran

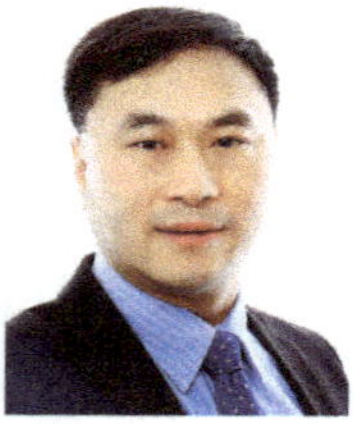

Shan Lin

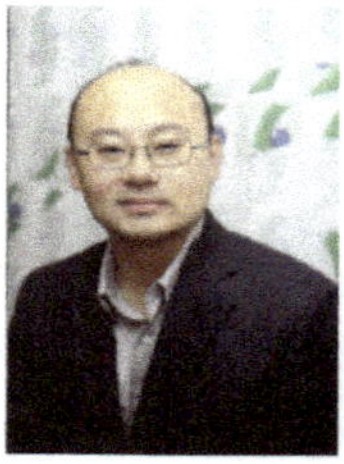

Lisandro Sakata

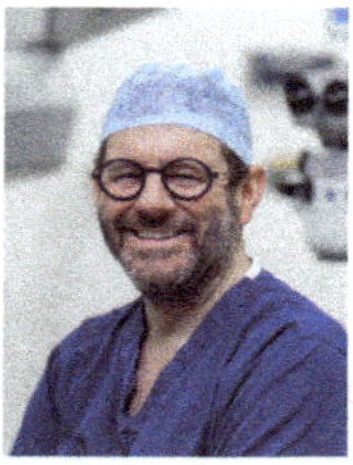

Gus Gazzard

4. MANAGEMENT: MEDICAL AND LASER

Tin Aung, Mani Baskaran, Shan Lin, Lisandro Sakata, Gus Gazzard

Abbreviations
AAC: acute angle closure
ACA: anterior chamber angle
ACD: anterior chamber depth
ACG: angle-closure glaucoma
ANA-LIS: Singapore Asymptomatic Narrow Angles Laser Iridotomy study
AOD: angle opening distance
ALPI: argon laser peripheral iridoplasty
APAC: acute primary angle closure
AS-OCT: anterior segment optical coherence tomography
CLE: clear lens extraction
EAGLE: Effectiveness of Early Lens Extraction for the Treatment of Primary Angle-Closure Glaucoma Trial
GRS: genetic risk score
IOP: intraocular pressure
ITC: iridotrabecular contact
LPI: laser peripheral iridotomy
PAC: primary angle closure
PACS: primary angle-closure suspect
PACD: primary angle-closure disease
PACG: primary angle closure-glaucoma
PAS: peripheral anterior synechiae
PIC: plateau iris configuration
POAG: primary open-angle glaucoma
SLT: selective laser trabeculoplasty
TM: trabecular meshwork
UBM: ultrasound biomicroscopy
ZAP: Zhongshan Angle-Closure Prevention Trial

Angle Closure and Angle-Closure Glaucoma, pp 1-19
Edited by Robert N. Weinreb, Benjamin Xu, Xiulan Zhang

Consensus statements

General approach

1. Gonioscopy is an indispensable part of the ophthalmic examination.
   - Gonioscopy should be performed with indentation to differentiate appositional from synechial closure.
   - The Van Herick test is not a substitute for gonioscopy.
   - Anterior segment imaging modalities can be used to augment the clinical examination but are not a substitute for gonioscopy, as features such as trabecular pigmentation, angle recession, and neovascularization cannot be reliably identified using AS-OCT or UBM.
2. Long-term follow-up with gonioscopy in phakic eyes is needed, as age-related lens thickening can further narrow the angle, increasing the risk of PACG.
3. Evaluation of the optic disc, visual field, and retinal nerve fiber layer is critical for detecting glaucomatous damage and progression.
4. An important goal of treatment in PACD is to alleviate ITC and prevent further impairment of aqueous drainage due to angle closure.
5. Even when the angle-closure process is controlled, further treatment may be necessary to avoid glaucoma progression.
   - Medications, lasers, and surgeries can recover or improve aqueous outflow in angle-closure eyes.

Medical treatment

6. In eyes with PACD, prostaglandin analogues are the most effective medical agent for IOP lowering regardless of the extent of synechial closure once pupillary block has been controlled.
7. Carbonic anhydrase inhibitors, beta blockers, and alpha-adrenergic agonists can be considered for second-line medical treatments.
   - Evidence on the IOP-lowering efficacy of Rho kinase inhibitors in angle closure is limited.
8. The role of miotics in PAC is unclear.
   - Miotics generally should not be used long-term as IOP-lowering agents in angle-closure eyes.
   - Miotics should be used in cases of APAC but may not be effective due to iris ischemia while the IOP is high.
   - Miotics may be considered for long-term use in plateau iris syndrome.
9. Cycloplegics should be considered in the setting of anterior chamber shallowing from secondary angle closure, such as aqueous misdirection.

Laser treatment

10. LPI is used to relieve relative pupillary block, which is the main mechanism in most patients with angle closure.
    - Angle closure persists in around a quarter of post-LPI eyes.
    - Angle assessment (gonioscopy or AS-OCT) should be performed post-LPI to assess the effect of LPI and identify other mechanisms, including plateau iris.
11. LPI is a safe procedure with very low risk of serious adverse events.
    - Sequential argon/Nd:YAG technique (argon first followed by Nd:YAG) requires less overall energy in patients with thick irides, specifically those of Asian and African descent or Hispanic ethnicity.
    - LPI location near the lid margins should be avoided to reduce risk of dysphotopsias.
    - LPI size should be a minimum of 200 μm in diameter
    - There is an increased risk of IOP spikes when performing LPI in eyes with elevated IOP and 2 or more quadrants of PAS.
12. LPI is not indicated in most PACS eyes (ZAP and ANA-LIS trials), although risk assessment for progression is suboptimal.
    - Factors to be considered for performing LPI include, for example, history of PACD in the fellow eye, older age, positive family history of PACG, need for frequent dilation (*e.g.*, in diabetics or glaucoma suspects), limited access to care, and need for hemodialysis.
    - Biometric features associated with greater risk for progression include higher IOP, smaller AOD500, smaller limbal ACD, and shallower ACD.
13. In APAC, LPI should be performed as soon as possible in the contralateral eye, which is at very high risk for a similar event.
14. Early lens extraction is an effective method of IOP lowering that is more cost-effective and results in better quality of life compared to LPI at certain stages of PACD (EAGLE trial).
    - Participants of the EAGLE Trial were aged 50 years or older and had PAC with IOP > 30 mmHg or PACG.
    - Patients who do not fulfill the EAGLE criteria may still benefit from early lens extraction, although these data are lacking
15. In APAC, laser peripheral iridoplasty or laser pupilloplasty may help to break the attack prior to definitive treatment.
    - LPIP widens the angle recess by contracting the iris away from the trabecular meshwork.

  - LPP contracts the iris tissue near the pupil, creating a peaked pupil and relieving pupillary block.
16. Iridoplasty can widen the angle in eyes with plateau iris syndrome that have persistent appositional angle closure after LPI.
  - Evidence does not support improved long-term IOP control.
  - Iridoplasty is not useful for synechial angle closure.
  - Iridoplasty may be associated with adverse effects, such as pupillary dilation, corneal endothelial damage, and progressive PAS formation.
17. SLT can be effective for IOP reduction in angle-closure eyes that have had LPI and/or lens extraction, allowing for visual access to the trabecular meshwork.

Future directions

- Additional data are needed on the efficacy of LPI treatment in diverse populations, especially with demographics differing from those of the ZAP and ANA-LIS trials.
- Further studies are needed to identify features of individuals who may be poorly responsive to LPI treatment and should be considered for alternative treatments, such as lens extraction, instead.

Clinical assessment of eyes with angle-closure disease

Poemen Chan

Anterior segment assessment

- Anterior chamber angle assessment should be a mandatory and integral part of ophthalmic assessment, especially for glaucoma patients.
- Identifying the presence and degree of ITC is crucial for glaucoma sub-classification (*i.e.*, open or closed angle), which influences the treatment algorithm.
- While gonioscopy is essential for assessing the anterior chamber – particularly, pigmentation of the TM, neovascularization of the angle, and differentiating appositional and synechial angle closure by indentation, UBM and AS-OCT may provide additional information about the angle status.
- Other slit-lamp illumination techniques may be considered to reasonably estimate the central or peripheral ACD (*i.e.*, the Van Herick and Redman-Smith tests), but should not be used to substitute for gonioscopy,

especially in cases where there is suspicion of narrow/closed angles. However, if the Van Herick test shows that the anterior chamber is at least half of the corneal thickness and the torchlight test is negative, there is a 98% chance that the angle is not closed.[1]

Comment: Gonioscopy is an essential part of the routine ophthalmic assessment. Anterior segmental imagining techniques can augment the assessment.

Gonioscopy

- Gonioscopy should be performed in a dark room, with a small and dim slit-lamp beam under high magnification and of a length that does not reach the pupillary area, so as to cause minimal closure of the pupillary area, and good topical anesthesia.
- A non-indentation goniolens (*e.g.*, Goldmann-style lens) with a larger diameter allows a magnified view to assess important anatomical landmarks and pathological signs in the angle, including pigmentation of the TM, neovascularization, and ITC. To visualize the angle over a convex iris, it may be necessary to alter the position of the mirror or gaze.[2-4]
- Differentiating appositional and synechial ITC requires an indentation goniolens (*i.e.*, Posner, Sussman, or Zeiss lenses) with a smaller diameter than the corneal diameter.

  Comment: Once ITC is identified, it is also essential to determine whether the ITC is appositional or synechial.
- Ideally, the position of iris insertion, angular width, peripheral iris configuration, and TM pigmentation observed under gonioscopy should be clearly documented (*e.g.*, the Spaeth method),[5] although the Schaffer method is more commonly used.

  Comment: The Spaeth classification provides a useful checklist of angle assessment.
- Gonioscopy assessment could be limited by patient discomfort, examiner subjectivity, and potential overestimation of the angle width. The latter could be due to unintentional corneal indentation and slit-lamp illumination causing pupil constriction.[6-8]

UBM

- UBM is a non-invasive contact imaging technique primarily used for evaluating the anterior segment, including pathologies of the angle, iris, lens, and ciliary body.

- There is a high agreement between UBM and gonioscopy in detecting irido-trabecular apposition.[3]
- The limitations of UBM include the requirement for direct contact of the transducer to the eye or through a water-bath immersion technique, which requires the patient to be in supine position and may falsely widen the anterior chamber. Its acquisition is patient- and operator-dependent.
- Image acquisition times are longer and there is a need for an experienced operator

  Comments: Despite its limitations, UBM is the only imaging technique that can consistently visualize the ciliary body and ciliary process.

AS-OCT

- High-speed, swept-source AS-OCT enables non-contact, quantitative, and repeatable 360° angle imaging. It can evaluate detailed iris configuration and various ACA dimensions, such as ACD, lens vault, and AOD.[9,10] It is sensitive in detecting angle closure, with a strong negative predictive value of over 95%.[11]
- Some AS-OCT devices can automatically identify the scleral spur using artificial intelligence. However, manual review may be beneficial to ensure measurement accuracy.

  Comment: Accurate identification of the scleral spur could affect the measurement of various ACA dimensions.
- AS-OCT has been extensively utilized in research studies and may be helpful in predicting outcomes. For instance, evaluation of untreated eyes of the ZAP trial participants[12] showed that AOD500 (the angle opening distance 500 μm anterior to the scleral spur to the anterior iris surface), horizontal iris curvature, and older age were significant risk factors for progression from PACS to PAC or AAC over a 6-year period.[13] However, the exact clinical role of AS-OCT remains undefined.
- The limitations of AS-OCT included upper and lower eyelid obscuration, a lack of indentation maneuver for angle status confirmation (appositional versus synechial closure), inability to observe TM pigmentation and neovascularization, and its inability to penetrate past the iris pigment epithelium. Therefore, assessment of the ciliary body and ciliary process relies on UBM.

  Comment: Although AS-OCT is a potentially superior clinical tool for anterior chamber assessment, it cannot entirely substitute the role of gonioscopy and UBM.

References

1. Van Herick W, Shaffer RN, Schwartz A. Estimation of width of angle of anterior chamber. Incidence and significance of the narrow angle. Am J Ophthalmol. Oct 1969;68(4):626-9. doi:10.1016/0002-9394(69)91241-0
2. European Glaucoma Society Terminology and Guidelines for Glaucoma, 5th Edition. Br J Ophthalmol. Jun 2021;105(Suppl 1):1-169. https://doi.org/10.1136/bjophthalmol-2021-egs-guidelines
3. Barkana Y, Dorairaj SK, Gerber Y, Liebmann JM, Ritch R. Agreement between gonioscopy and ultrasound biomicroscopy in detecting iridotrabecular apposition. Arch Ophthalmol. Oct 2007;125(10):1331-5. https://doi.org/10.1001/archopht.125.10.1331
4. Gedde SJ, Chen PP, Muir KW, et al. Primary Angle-Closure Disease Preferred Practice Pattern(R). Ophthalmology. Jan 2021;128(1):P30-P70. https://doi.org/10.1016/j.ophtha.2020.10.021
5. Spaeth GL. The normal development of the human anterior chamber angle: a new system of descriptive grading. Trans Ophthalmol Soc U K (1962). 1971;91:709-39.
6. Leung CK, Cheung CY, Li H, et al. Dynamic analysis of dark-light changes of the anterior chamber angle with anterior segment OCT. Invest Ophthalmol Vis Sci. Sep 2007;48(9):4116-22. https://doi.org/10.1167/iovs.07-0010
7. Porporato N, Baskaran M, Tun TA, et al. Understanding diagnostic disagreement in angle closure assessment between anterior segment optical coherence tomography and gonioscopy. Br J Ophthalmol. Jun 2020;104(6):795-799. https://doi.org/10.1136/bjophthalmol-2019-314672
8. Sakata LM, Lavanya R, Friedman DS, et al. Comparison of gonioscopy and anterior segment ocular coherence tomography in detecting angle closure in different quadrants of the anterior chamber angle. Ophthalmology. May 2008;115(5):769-74. https://doi.org/10.1016/j.ophtha.2007.06.030
9. Leung CK, Weinreb RN. Anterior chamber angle imaging with optical coherence tomography. Eye (Lond). Mar 2011;25(3):261-7. https://doi.org/10.1038/eye.2010.201
10. Chan PP, Lai G, Chiu V, Chong A, Yu M, Leung CK. Anterior chamber angle imaging with swept-source optical coherence tomography: comparison between CASIAII and ANTERION. Sci Rep. Oct 30 2020;10(1):18771. https://doi.org/10.1038/s41598-020-74813-3
11. Desmond T, Tran V, Maharaj M, Carnt N, White A. Diagnostic accuracy of AS-OCT vs gonioscopy for detecting angle closure: a systematic review and meta-analysis. Graefes Arch Clin Exp Ophthalmol. Jan 2022;260(1):1-23. https://doi.org/10.1007/s00417-021-05271-4
12. He M, Jiang Y, Huang S, et al. Laser peripheral iridotomy for the prevention of angle closure: a single-centre, randomised controlled trial. Lancet. Apr 20 2019;393(10181):1609-1618. https://doi.org/10.1016/S0140-6736(18)32607-2
13. Xu BY, Friedman DS, Foster PJ, et al. Ocular Biometric Risk Factors for Progression of Primary Angle Closure Disease: The Zhongshan Angle Closure Prevention Trial. Ophthalmology. Mar 2022;129(3):267-275. https://doi.org/10.1016/j.ophtha.2021.10.003

Posterior segment assessment
Jovina See

Posterior segment assessment consists of the evaluation of structure and function. With PACS and PAC, both structural and functional assessment remain normal as glaucomatous optic neuropathy is absent. In PACG, posterior segment assessment is performed to determine the extent of optic nerve damage. After laser or surgical treatment to open the angles, posterior segment analysis can be repeated to confirm stabilization of both structural and functional changes.

Treatment rationale or aims of treatment for angle-closure disease

George Kong, Roberto Vessani, John Thygensen

Angle closure
The primary aims of treatment for the angle-closure process include:

- Early detection of PACD.
- Prevent progression to PACG.
- Improve or prevent the worsening of narrow ACA configuration.
- Prevent development of PAS.
- Prevent the development of elevated IOP and treat if elevated IOP is present.
- Preserve optic nerve structure and visual function.
- Prevent APAC.

Early identification of patients with narrow ACAs should be part of the routine ophthalmic assessment, which includes gonioscopic assessment of the ACA or anterior segment imaging.

LPI is the cornerstone treatment for PACD by eliminating pupil block, improving angle configuration, and reducing further ITC. Thus, it should be considered in all eyes with PAC to prevent progression to PACG.[1,2] However, for PACS, current evidence does not support routine treatment with LPI in all cases and should be considered on a case-by-case basis. Cataract surgery should be considered to improve angle configuration if a visually significant cataract is present and for patients with PAC and high IOP or for patients with PACG.[3]

In eyes where residual appositional closure persists despite a patent PI, laser iridoplasty, or pilocarpine 1% twice daily can be considered in some cases, especially in eyes with plateau iris configuration. In cases of elevated IOP or fluctuating IOP despite patent PI, topical IOP-lowering medications should be considered to improve IOP control. SLT can be considered in selected cases of PAC if the narrow ACA structure is improved following LPI treatment and TM structures become visible on gonioscopy.[4]

When should LPI be considered for PACS?

Studies such as the ANA-LIS and ZAP trials showed that, while prophylactic LPI reduces the progression of PACS to PAC or PACG, the cumulative risk of progression is relatively low in a PACS population identified by screening.[5-7] In ANA-LIS, the number needed to treat to prevent a primary angle closure end point was 22 (95% CI, 12.8–57.5) at 5 years. Therefore, current evidence does not support the routine performance of LPI in all PACS cases, and such treatment should be performed in selected cases with a higher perceived risk.

The classification of PACS-plus, a subset of PACS individuals who carry additional risk factors for progression, helps clinicians identify patients who may benefit most from prophylactic LPI.[8] PACS-plus includes individuals with high-risk features such as a positive family history of angle-closure disease, hypermetropia, and those who require regular pupil dilation for ocular or medical reasons. These patients are more likely to have progression from PACS to PAC and PACG compared to PACS individuals without these features. In addition, LPI should also be considered for people living in remote locations (including people with occupations such as foreign aid workers, armed forces stationed overseas, oil rig workers, etc.) where regular ophthalmic examination and rapid access to emergency ophthalmic care is not possible.

Ongoing follow-up for PACS and PAC patients

Patients with PACS or PAC should undergo regular gonioscopic evaluations even after LPI to monitor for any changes in angle configuration and the formation of PAS. Patients should be made aware that even following LPI, there is still a risk of developing elevated IOP, intermittent IOP fluctuations, glaucomatous optic nerve damage, and vision loss.[6,7] Therefore, it is important to have routine assessments with their eye care professional. Regular assessment of optic nerve structure and function with slit-lamp examination, optic disc photography, OCT assessment of retinal nerve fiber layer, and standard automated perimetry should be considered even with IOP readings within normal limits and patent LPIs, as diurnal variations in IOP can still be a risk factor for progression.[9]

Advanced imaging techniques such as AS-OCT, Scheimpflug imaging, and UBM play a significant role in assessing angle structures, monitoring changes post-treatment, and excluding secondary causes of angle closure, such as ciliary body cysts.[10] These modalities enhance diagnostic accuracy and guide appropriate management strategies by providing detailed visualization of anterior segment anatomy. However, they should not be used in substitution of gonioscopy.

Educating patients and their caregivers about the nature of angle-closure disease, treatment options, and the importance of adherence to the management plan is vital for successful outcomes. Given that family history is a strong risk factor for the development of PACD,[11] patients should be encouraged to inform genetically related family members about their potential risk, promoting early screening and intervention.

References

1. Thomas R, Parikh R, Muliyil J, Kumar RS. Five-year risk of progression of primary angle closure to primary angle closure glaucoma: a population-based study. Acta Ophthalmol Scand. 2003 Oct;81(5):480-5. https://doi.org/10.1034/j.1600-0420.2003.00135.x
2. Nolan WP, Foster PJ, Devereux JG, Uranchimeg D, Johnson GJ, Baasanhu J. YAG laser iridotomy treatment for primary angle closure in east Asian eyes. Br J Ophthalmol. 2000 Nov;84(11):1255-9. https://doi.org/10.1136/bjo.84.11.1255
3. Azuara-Blanco A, Burr J, Ramsay C, et al. Effectiveness of early lens extraction for the treatment of primary angle-closure glaucoma (EAGLE): a randomised controlled trial. Lancet. 2016 Oct 1;388(10052):1389-1397.
4. Raj S, Thattaruthody F, Yadav D, et al. Long-Term Efficacy of Selective Laser Trabeculoplasty in Primary Angle-Closure Disease After Laser Peripheral Iridotomy. Semin Ophthalmol. 2024 Apr;39(3):235-241. https://doi.org/10.1080/08820538.2024.2312946
5. He M, Jiang Y, Huang S, et al. Laser peripheral iridotomy for the prevention of angle closure: a single-centre, randomised controlled trial. Lancet. 2019 Apr 20;393(10181):1609-1618. https://doi.org/10.1016/S0140-6736(18)32607-2
6. Yuan Y, Wang W, Xiong R, et al. Fourteen-Year Outcome of Angle-Closure Prevention with Laser Iridotomy in the Zhongshan Angle-Closure Prevention Study: Extended Follow-up of a Randomized Controlled Trial. Ophthalmology. 2023 Aug;130(8):786-794. https://doi.org/10.1016/j.ophtha.2023.03.024. Epub 2023 Apr 6. Erratum in: Ophthalmology. 2024 Jan;131(1):126. https://doi.org/10.1016/j.ophtha.2023.10.029
7. Baskaran M, Kumar RS, Friedman DS, et al. The Singapore Asymptomatic Narrow Angles Laser Iridotomy Study: Five-Year Results of a Randomized Controlled Trial. Ophthalmology. 2022 Feb;129(2):147-158. https://doi.org/10.1016/j.ophtha.2021.08.017

8. Foster PJ, Ng WS, Nolan WP, et al. Prevention of angle-closure glaucoma: balancing risk and benefit. Eye (Lond). 2022 Dec;36(12):2229-2231. https://doi.org/10.1038/s41433-021-01881-8
9. Srinivasan S, Choudhari NS, Baskaran M, George RJ, Shantha B, Vijaya L. Diurnal intraocular pressure fluctuation and its risk factors in angle-closure and open-angle glaucoma. Eye (Lond). 2016 Mar;30(3):362-8.
10. Xu BY, Pardeshi AA, Burkemper B, et al. Differences in Anterior Chamber Angle Assessments Between Gonioscopy, EyeCam, and Anterior Segment OCT: The Chinese American Eye Study. Transl Vis Sci Technol. 2019 Mar 26;8(2):5. https://doi.org/10.1167/tvst.8.2.5
11. Kong X, Chen Y, Chen X, Sun X. Influence of family history as a risk factor on primary angle closure and primary open angle glaucoma in a Chinese population. Ophthalmic Epidemiol. 2011 Oct;18(5):226-32. https://doi.org/10.3109/09286586.2011.595040

Primary angle-closure glaucoma

PACG is responsible for significant morbidity, especially in Asia.[1,2] PACG is likely more preventable than POAG due to its more IOP-dependent nature. PACG may result from acute emergencies, such as AAC, that requires urgent treatment, but it can be managed and controlled if the angle-closure process is diagnosed early.[3]

The aims of treatment of glaucomatous process in patients with PAC and PACG are:

- To prevent progression of the angle-closure process.
- To lower the IOP and prevent the development and worsening of glaucomatous optic neuropathy and visual field loss.

IOP measurement, dark-room dynamic gonioscopy, and optic disc and visual field evaluation are mandatory to assess the level of damage and for proper treatment planning. Focusing on the ACA is a principal management strategy for PAC and PACG. The choice of management is dependent on the type of presentation (AAC or chronic angle closure) and the stage of the disease.

Management of APAC

APAC requires emergent management that involves a rapid lowering of the IOP and resolution of relative pupil block – the most common mechanism of angle closure. Patients experiencing APAC should receive medical treatment (topical and systemic) to lower the IOP, and LPI should subsequently be performed in both eyes. A significant proportion of APAC patients do not respond adequately to medical treatment alone and other interventions might be considered.[3] ALPI is an alternative to conventional medical treatment that can mechanically open up the angle and reduce IOP in APAC.[4-6] In some cases where initial treatment fails to reduce IOP, additional treatments should be considered, including anterior chamber paracentesis under sterile conditions, surgical iridectomy, cyclodiode laser, or urgent phacoemulsification. Further details on the management of APAC are presented in Section 6.

Evidence on early lens extraction versus LPI for PACG: the EAGLE study

Recent evidence demonstrates that LPI and CLE can both be considered as a first-line therapy for patients aged 50 years or older with newly diagnosed PAC with IOP $\geq$ 30 mmHg or PACG and no advanced damage.[7] The EAGLE Trial demonstrated that significantly fewer participants who received CLE needed any further treatment to control IOP compared to patients subjected to LPI. Only 1 patient in the CLE group required further glaucoma surgery compared with 24 patients in the LPI group (difference of 10.9% in glaucoma surgery during the trial). Despite this, the need of additional medical therapy for long-term IOP control was significant in both treatment arms, with more than 30% for CLE and more than 80% for LPI with a follow-up of 36 months.[8]

It is important to understand which populations with PAC or PACG stand to benefit most from first-line therapy, whether LPI or CLE. Chinese ancestry, PAC without glaucoma, no glaucoma medications at baseline, better baseline visual field, and lower baseline IOP were factors associated with better long-term IOP control after either of these procedures.[8] However, if the angle is non-occludable after LPI, the benefit of CLE is reduced.

After LPI

Traditionally, the standard of care for PAC and PACG has been LPI to address pupillary block and open the drainage pathways and medical management with eye drops to reduce IOP.[9] Despite poor evidence of the IOP-lowering efficacy of ALPI for chronic PAC,[10] ALPI can effectively open the angle and may be considered in patients with persistent angle closure after LPI due to additional mechanisms such as plateau iris, nanophthalmos and iris and ciliary body cysts to improve angle anatomy and IOP control. After laser therapy, gonioscopy should be periodically repeated to confirm that the angle is open.

It is important to identify and manage patients with chronic IOP elevation that persists despite iridotomy or iridoplasty. A large proportion of these patients require medical therapy after laser intervention to achieve an adequate IOP level.[8] All the major classes of topical glaucoma medication can be used in angle closure patients.

SLT is an additional safe and effective method of reducing IOP in many eyes with PAC and PACG after a patent iridotomy in which there is a sufficient extent of visible trabecular meshwork.[11-13]

Other procedures such as lens extraction and/or incisional glaucoma surgery may be considered when IOP is not controlled by medication after laser therapy. The decision to add interventions depends on the IOP level as well as the degree and stability of glaucomatous damage and the extent of goniosynechiae. Patients with advanced PACG and elevated IOP often need a lower target IOP and have a higher risk of filtration surgery despite laser and medical therapy.

Recent available evidence suggests that cataract surgery in combination with MIGS can be safely and effectively performed in PACG and may be considered in the treatment rationale of this condition,[14] although it is considered an off-label use for most MIGS devices. One recent multicenter, randomized controlled trial investigated the effectiveness and safety of phacogoniotomy versus phacotrabeculectomy among Asian patients with advanced PACG and cataracts. After 12 months, phacogoniotomy demonstrated non-inferiority to phacotrabeculectomy in terms of IOP reduction.[15]

Long-term effect of iridotomy on glaucoma

There is still little evidence on the long-term benefit of iridotomy in the glaucomatous process. A recent meta-analysis that included 4 studies (1,543 participants) did not find sufficient evidence to draw any meaningful conclusions on the use of iridotomy for the purpose of slowing progression of visual field loss.[16] One recent study evaluated the contralateral eye of eyes with APAC 4 to 10 years after the attack. Most contralateral eyes treated with LPI had good vision and well-maintained IOP, and did not have glaucoma several years after presentation.[17] However, the evaluation of the angle after LPI is mandatory to assure that the angle is open.

Assessment of progression in PACG

Once IOP control has been achieved through the proposed therapy, patients with PAC or PACG should be monitored with structural (optic disc stereophotography, retinal nerve fiber layer thickness and macular ganglion cell layer/inner plexiform layer thickness measured by OCT) and functional exams (standardized automated perimetry) to assess control of glaucomatous damage. In addition to IOP and gonioscopy evaluation, the results of these exams will also indicate the need for additional interventions.

References

1. Foster PJ, Baasanhu J, Alsbirk PH, Munkhbayar D, Uranchimeg D, Johnson GJ. Glaucoma in Mongolia. A population-based survey in Hövsgöl province, northern Mongolia. Arch Ophthalmol. 1996 Oct;114(10):1235-41 https://doi.org/10.1001/archopht.1996.01100140435011
2. Foster PJ, Oen FT, Machin D, et al. The prevalence of glaucoma in Chinese residents of Singapore: a cross-sectional population survey of the Tanjong Pagar district. Arch Ophthalmol. 2000 Aug;118(8):1105-11. https://doi.org/10.1001/archopht.118.8.1105
3. Chan PP, Pang JC, Tham CC. Acute primary angle closure-treatment strategies, evidences and economical considerations. Eye. 2019;33 (1):110-119 https://doi.org/10.1038/s41433-018-0278-x
4. Ritch R. Argon laser treatment for medically unresponsive attacks of angle-closure glaucoma. Am J Ophthalmol. 1982;94:197-204. https://doi.org/10.1016/0002-9394(82)90075-7
5. Lai JS, Tham CC, Chua JK, Lam DS. Immediate diode laser peripheral iridoplasty as treatment of acute attack of primary angle closure glaucoma: a preliminary study. J Glaucoma. 2001; 10:89-94. https://doi.org/10.1097/00061198-200104000-00004
6. Lam DS, Lai JS, Tham CC, Chua JK, Poon AS. Argon laser peripheral iridoplasty versus conventional systemic medical therapy in treatment of acute primary angle-closure glaucoma: a prospective, randomized, controlled trial. Ophthalmology. 2002; 109:1591-6. https://doi.org/10.1016/S0161-6420(02)01158-2
7. Azuara-Blanco A, Burr J, Ramsay C, et al. Effectiveness of early lens extraction for the treatment of primary angle-closure glaucoma (EAGLE): a randomised controlled trial. Lancet. 2016 Oct 1;388(10052):1389-1397. https://doi.org/10.1016/S0140-6736(16)30956-4
8. Mitchell WG, Azuara-Blanco A, Foster PJ, et al. Predictors of long-term intraocular pressure control after lens extraction in primary angle closure glaucoma: results from the EAGLE trial. Br J Ophthalmol. 2023 Aug;107(8):1072-1078. https://doi.org/10.1136/bjophthalmol-2021-319765
9. American Academy of Ophthalmology Glaucoma Panel. Preferred practice pattern® guidelines. Primary angle closure. San Francisco, CA: American Academy of Ophthalmology, 2015.
10. Bayliss JM, Ng WS, Waugh N, Azuara-Blanco A. Laser peripheral iridoplasty for chronic angle closure. Cochrane Database Syst Rev. 2021 Mar 23;3(3):CD006746. https://doi.org/10.1002/14651858.CD006746.pub4
11. Ho CL, Lai JS, Aquino MV, et al. Selective laser trabeculoplasty for primary angle closure with persistently elevated intraocular pressure after iridotomy. J Glaucoma. 2009 Sep;18(7):563-6. https://doi.org/10.1097/IJG.0b013e318193c2d1
12. Narayanaswamy A, Leung CK, Istiantoro DV, et al. Efficacy of selective laser trabeculoplasty in primary angle-closure glaucoma: a randomized clinical trial. JAMA Ophthalmol. 2015 Feb;133(2):206-12. https://doi.org/10.1001/jamaophthalmol.2014.4893
13. Ali Aljasim L, Owaidhah O, Edward DP. Selective Laser Trabeculoplasty in Primary An-

gle-closure Glaucoma After Laser Peripheral Iridotomy: A Case-Control Study. J Glaucoma. 2016 Mar;25(3):e253-8. https://doi.org/10.1097/IJG.0000000000000282
14. Song Y, Zhang H, Zhang Y, et al. Minimally Invasive Glaucoma Surgery in Primary Angle-Closure Glaucoma. Asia Pac J Ophthalmol (Phila). 2022 Sep 1;11(5):460-469. https://doi.org/10.1097/APO.0000000000000561
15. Song Y, Lin F, Lv A, et al. Phacogoniotomy versus phacotrabeculectomy for advanced primary angle-closure glaucoma with cataract: A randomized non-inferiority trial. Asia Pac J Ophthalmol (Phila). 2024 Jan-Feb;13(1):100033. https://doi.org/10.1016/j.apjo.2024.100076
16. Rouse B, Le JT, Gazzard G. Iridotomy to slow progression of visual field loss in angle-closure glaucoma. Cochrane Database Syst Rev. 2023 Jan 9;1(1):CD012270. https://doi.org/10.1002/14651858.CD012270.pub3
17. Hamid S, Matarazzo F, Sun Z, Baboolal S, Muhundhakumar D, Foster PJ. Long-term outcomes after acute primary angle closure: case series from Moorfields Eye Hospital, UK. Br J Ophthalmol. 2024 May 13:bjo-2023-324748. https://doi.org/10.1136/bjo-2023-324748

Medical management

Sunee Chansangpetch, Remo Susanna, Shan Lin

The primary role of medications in angle closure is to reduce IOP. Patients with angle closure and elevated IOP often require IOP-lowering medications, either before or after angle-widening procedures. Medications are also used to prevent IOP elevation prophylactically after laser procedures, and to utilize the miotic effect for opening the angle in specific conditions.

IOP reduction

The initial management of angle closure focuses primarily on procedures designed to widen the ACA or prevent its further narrowing over time. These procedures are essential to address the underlying anatomical issue. Medications play a supportive role in this context, helping to lower IOP or to prevent it from rising, but they do not replace the need for definitive anatomical intervention.

Topical medications that reduce aqueous production or increase uveoscleral outflow—including beta-blockers, carbonic anhydrase inhibitors, alpha-2 adrenergic agonists, and prostaglandin analogs—work effectively in angle-closure glaucoma. Similar to the situation with open-angle glaucoma, prostaglandin analogs are the most effective medications for IOP control in angle-closure patients.[1] A meta-analysis reported that latanoprost reduced mean IOP by 7.9

mmHg (32.4%), peak IOP by 7.4 mmHg (29.8%), and trough IOP by 7.9 mmHg (32.5%) in PACG.[2] Another meta-analysis found that latanoprost was superior to timolol (mean difference 0.64) but slightly less effective than travoprost and bimatoprost (mean difference -0.19).[3] Prostaglandin analogs are effective in lowering IOP even in eyes with 360° of PAS.[4-6]

Cholinergic agonists, such as pilocarpine, induce miosis and pull the peripheral iris away from the trabecular meshwork, increasing angle space. Pilocarpine stimulates ciliary muscle contraction, increasing scleral spur tension, which enhances trabecular outflow and lowers IOP. Imaging studies have demonstrated that pilocarpine widens angle in narrow-angle patients.[7,8] However, it can paradoxically shallow the anterior chamber and increase the lens vault due to ciliary muscle contraction causing lens thickening and anterior movement of the lens-iris plane.[8] The IOP-lowering effect of pilocarpine is notably weaker than that of prostaglandins. A randomized trial in patients with PAC or PACG showed that 1% pilocarpine 4 times daily reduced IOP by 4.3 mmHg at 9 AM and 1.9 mmHg at 4 PM, compared to a consistent 7 mmHg reduction with travoprost.[9] Given its modest IOP-lowering effect and risks like posterior synechiae, long-term use of miotics for IOP reduction is generally not recommended.

More recent medications lower IOP through mechanisms involving increased trabecular outflow. Rho-kinase inhibitors, such as ripasudil and netarsudil, act on actin and myosin in the trabecular meshwork, increasing the permeability of Schlemm's canal endothelial cells. Latanoprostene bunod, a nitric oxide-donating prostaglandin, increases uveoscleral outflow via the latanoprost component and enhances aqueous outflow by relaxing the trabecular meshwork and Schlemm's canal through nitric oxide release. Omidenepag isopropyl (OMDI), a selective E-prostanoid subtype 2 (EP2) receptor agonist, stimulates EP2 receptors within the ciliary body and trabecular meshwork, promoting aqueous humor outflow through both pathways.

Limited evidence exists on the efficacy of drugs promoting trabecular outflow in angle-closure eyes. A post-marketing surveillance study of ripasudil reported a significant IOP reduction in PACG eyes, with a mean decrease of 3.9 ± 5.3 mmHg (14.4%). In comparison, a mean IOP reduction of 2.9 ± 4.2 mmHg (13.4%) was observed in open-angle glaucoma eyes in the same report.[10] Another study found that adding netarsudil to existing glaucoma treatments reduced IOP equally in both open-angle glaucoma and PAC.[11] Real-world data from Japan demonstrated a significant IOP reduction of 1.7 ± 2.8 mmHg in naïve PACG patients treated with OMDI monotherapy.[12] While this reduction appears smaller than the 2.7 ± 2.6 mmHg observed in open-angle glaucoma patients, no statistical comparison between the groups was conducted. Although the PACG sample size was smaller, the data suggest that narrow angles may not significantly limit IOP-lowering efficacy of drugs enhancing trabecular outflow. However, these studies lacked details on factors such as synechiae and the extent of angle closure, which may influence drug efficacy.

Drugs delivered via intracameral implants, such as the bimatoprost and travoprost implants, require sufficient angle space, particularly in the inferior angle. Clinical trials for these implants have been conducted exclusively in open-angle glaucoma or ocular hypertension eyes with angles graded ≥ 3 by the Shaffer system and peripheral anterior chamber depths ≥ 0.5 corneal thickness by Van Herick examination, limiting their use in angle closure.[13,14] Angle closure eyes that have undergone angle-widening procedures may be eligible for treatment with these implants. However, no data are currently available on the safety profile of these devices in eyes with PACD.

Systemic medications

In acute angle-closure crisis, rapid IOP reduction and symptom relief are priorities. Systemic and topical antiglaucoma medications should be promptly administered if there are no contraindications, with systemic drugs providing rapid, potent IOP reduction. Stabilized IOP allows for further interventions based on the underlying mechanisms, such as LPI in APAC with pupillary block. Systemic options include oral/intravenous acetazolamide and osmotic agents (oral glycerin or intravenous mannitol), with intravenous forms suitable for patients unable to take oral medications or experiencing severe vomiting. However, intravenous medications can cause systemic side effects and should be used with caution in elderly or at-risk patients.

Although miotics may help break an early acute pupillary block, they are ineffective in conditions of markedly high IOP leading to ischemia in the iris. Additionally, they may worsen angle closure by increasing the lens's anterior-posterior diameter and causing forward displacement of lens-iris diaphragm. For this reason, miotics should be avoided in lens-induced secondary angle closure, such as phacomorphic glaucoma or anterior lens subluxation.

Cycloplegic agents can stabilize the anterior chamber by increasing zonular tension, flattening the lens. This effect also pulls the lens-iris diaphragm posteriorly, counteracting the forward force of the vitreous. Cycloplegics are included as part of initial medical management for malignant glaucoma or medication-induced ciliary effusion. Due to their opposing effect to cycloplegics, miotics are contraindicated in these conditions.

Preoperative medications for laser

Topical miotics are used preoperatively for laser procedures in angle closure to constrict the pupil. Stretching the iris stroma aids LPI, while flattening the peripheral iris facilitates laser peripheral iridoplasty. Alpha-adrenergic agonists, including brimonidine and apraclonidine, have a fast onset of action and are frequently used prophylactically to prevent transient IOP elevation following laser procedures. These agents reduce the frequency and magnitude of IOP spikes. Randomized controlled trials have shown that a single preoperative drop of brimonidine or apraclonidine have comparable efficacy in preventing IOP elevations after anterior segment laser surgeries, including LPI and ALPI.[15-17] Brimonidine may additionally have a stronger miotic effect than apraclonidine.[16]

References

1. Cheng JW, Cai JP, Li Y, Wei RL. A meta-analysis of topical prostaglandin analogs in the treatment of chronic angle-closure glaucoma. J Glaucoma. Dec 2009;18(9):652-7. https://doi.org/10.1097/IJG.0b013e31819c49d4
2. Chen R, Yang K, Zheng Z, Ong ML, Wang NL, Zhan SY. Meta-analysis of the Efficacy and Safety of Latanoprost Monotherapy in Patients With Angle-closure Glaucoma. J Glaucoma. Mar 2016;25(3):e134-44. https://doi.org/10.1097/IJG.0000000000000158
3. Li J, Lin X, Yu M. Meta-analysis of randomized controlled trials comparing latanoprost with other glaucoma medications in chronic angle-closure glaucoma. Eur J Ophthalmol. Jan-Feb 2015;25(1):18-26. https://doi.org/10.5301/ejo.5000506
4. Aung T, Chan YH, Chew PT, Group ES. Degree of angle closure and the intraocular pressure-lowering effect of latanoprost in subjects with chronic angle-closure glaucoma. Ophthalmology. Feb 2005;112(2):267-71. https://doi.org/10.1016/j.ophtha.2004.08.024
5. Kook MS, Cho HS, Yang SJ, Kim S, Chung J. Efficacy of latanoprost in patients with chronic angle-closure glaucoma and no visible ciliary-body face: a preliminary study. J Ocul Pharmacol Ther. Feb 2005;21(1):75-84. https://doi.org/10.1089/jop.2005.21.75
6. Vyas P, Naik U, Gangaiah JB. Efficacy of bimatoprost 0.03% in reducing intraocular pressure in patients with 360 degrees synechial angle-closure glaucoma: a preliminary study. Indian J Ophthalmol. Jan-Feb 2011;59(1):13-6. https://doi.org/10.4103/0301-4738.73708
7. Kobayashi H, Kobayashi K, Kiryu J, Kondo T. Pilocarpine induces an increase in the anterior chamber angular width in eyes with narrow angles. Br J Ophthalmol. May 1999;83(5):553-8. https://doi.org/10.1136/bjo.83.5.553
8. Mogil RS, Khezri N, Ren R, et al. Changes in Iridocorneal Angle and Anterior Chamber Structure in Eyes With Anatomically Narrow Angles: Laser Iridotomy Versus Pilocarpine. J Glaucoma. Dec 2018;27(12):1073-1078. https://doi.org/10.1097/IJG.0000000000001097
9. Wu LL, Huang P, Gao YX, Wang ZX, Li B. A 12-week, double-masked, parallel-group study

of the safety and efficacy of travoprost 0.004% compared with pilocarpine 1% in Chinese patients with primary angle-closure and primary angle-closure glaucoma. J Glaucoma. Aug 2011;20(6):388-91. https://doi.org/10.1097/IJG.0b013e3181efb358

10. Tanihara H, Kakuda T, Sano T, et al. Safety and Efficacy of Ripasudil in Japanese Patients with Glaucoma or Ocular Hypertension: 3-month Interim Analysis of ROCK-J, a Post-Marketing Surveillance Study. Adv Ther. Feb 2019;36(2):333-343. https://doi.org/10.1007/s12325-018-0863-1
11. Pham AT, Bradley C, Casey C, Jampel HD, Ramulu PY, Yohannan J. Effectiveness of Netarsudil versus Brimonidine in Eyes already Being Treated with Glaucoma Medications at a Single Academic Tertiary Care Practice: A Comparative Study. Curr Ther Res Clin Exp. 2023;98:100689. https://doi.org/10.1016/j.curtheres.2022.100689
12. Miki A, Miyamoto E, Ishida N, Shii D, Hori K, Group LR. Efficacy and Safety of Omidenepag Isopropyl 0.002% Ophthalmic Solution: A Retrospective Analysis of Real-World Data in Japan. Adv Ther. May 2022;39(5):2085-2095. https://doi.org/10.1007/s12325-022-02069-6
13. Bacharach J, Tatham A, Ferguson G, et al. Phase 3, Randomized, 20-Month Study of the Efficacy and Safety of Bimatoprost Implant in Patients with Open-Angle Glaucoma and Ocular Hypertension (ARTEMIS 2). Drugs. Nov 2021;81(17):2017-2033. https://doi.org/10.1007/s40265-021-01624-9
14. Sarkisian SR, Jr., Ang RE, Lee AM, et al. Phase 3 Randomized Clinical Trial of the Safety and Efficacy of Travoprost Intraocular Implant in Patients with Open-Angle Glaucoma or Ocular Hypertension. Ophthalmology. Sep 2024;131(9):1021-1032. https://doi.org/10.1016/j.ophtha.2024.02.022
15. Chen TC, Ang RT, Grosskreutz CL, Pasquale LR, Fan JT. Brimonidine 0.2% versus apraclonidine 0.5% for prevention of intraocular pressure elevations after anterior segment laser surgery. Ophthalmology. Jun 2001;108(6):1033-8. https://doi.org/10.1016/s0161-6420(01)00545-0
16. Yuen NS, Cheung P, Hui SP. Comparing brimonidine 0.2% to apraclonidine 1.0% in the prevention of intraocular pressure elevation and their pupillary effects following laser peripheral iridotomy. Jpn J Ophthalmol. Mar-Apr 2005;49(2):89-92. https://doi.org/10.1007/s10384-004-0149-9
17. Chen TC. Brimonidine 0.15% versus apraclonidine 0.5% for prevention of intraocular pressure elevation after anterior segment laser surgery. J Cataract Refract Surg. Sep 2005;31(9):1707-12. https://doi.org/10.1016/j.jcrs.2005.02.035

Laser therapy

Lisandro Sakata

LPI

Chungkwon Yoo, Rodolfo Grossman, Theodoros Filippopoulos

Aims of treatment

- Prevention of AAC: LPI has been shown to be effective in preventing subsequent episodes of angle closure in the fellow eyes of patients with AAC crisis. If untreated, there is a 50% risk of an AAC attack within 5 years for these eyes.[1,2] Fellow phakic eyes of those affected by PAC/PACG should undergo LPI treatment to mitigate these risks.
- Long-term IOP control: In patients with PAC/PACG who have elevated IOP, LPI treatment aims to achieve target IOP levels by addressing the reversible component of the disease: appositional angle closure. However, PAC/PACG patients treated with LPI are likely to require additional long-term medical or surgical treatment, and LPI is less effective than cataract extraction for long-term IOP control.[3]
- Prevention of PAS formation and progressive glaucomatous optic nerve damage: This is achieved by eliminating appositional closure caused by pupillary block, thereby removing the primary mechanism responsible for PAS development. By doing so, it results in either lowering of the coexisting elevated IOP and/or preventing future IOP rises that contribute to the development or progression of glaucomatous optic neuropathy.

Mechanisms of action

Laser iridotomy relieves pupillary block by providing an alternate pathway for aqueous humor to bypass the pupil. This eliminates the pressure differential between the anterior and posterior chambers, allowing the iris to lose its convex configuration and to move away from the trabecular meshwork, thereby widening the angle.[4]

Techniques for performing LPI

An adequate view of the iris and cooperation of the patient are mandatory. Patients presenting with newly diagnosed PAC or PACG with markedly elevated IOP can be treated with topical and systemic medications to achieve a safe IOP level (< 30 mmHg) prior to undergoing LPI. Pretreatment with pilocarpine is helpful to stretch and thin the iris, and allows the laser to penetrate the iris more easily iris. Pretreatment with apraclonidine or brimonidine may help mitigate IOP spikes. Topical anesthesia is used. An Abraham iridotomy lens is used with methylcellulose gel. Pretreatment of the iris with a green argon laser is useful in patients with a high risk of bleeding (*e.g.*, anticoagulant use).

Optimal size and location of LPI

The LPI is often recommended to be placed in the peripheral third of the iris, between 11 and 1 o'clock, to reduce visual symptoms. However, some prefer the 3 and 9 o'clock positions to minimize LPI-related dysphotopsias. Sites with iris crypts, where the iris is thinner, are ideal if they are suitably located.

Fleck determined that an iridotomy should have a minimum size of 15 μm to effectively prevent pupillary block, but he recommended aiming for a size between 150 μm and 200 μm. One of the factors considered in his model was the thickness of the iris. Brown Asian irides, thicker and more substantial than blue ones, may require a larger iridotomy.

LPI methods

<u>Thermal (green) LPI</u>

Argon or green laser proved effective but required melanin for energy absorption, making it harder to penetrate light blue irides.

<u>Nd:YAG LPI</u>

In the late 1980s, the Nd:YAG laser replaced thermal laser as the primary tool for performing LPI. Using Q-switched mode, it creates high energy ionic plasma to photodisrupt tissues. This laser does not need melanin pigment for iris absorption and uses less energy than argon lasers.

- Suggested settings:
    - Check that the defocus is set to zero. Surgeons may use low power (1–3 mJ) to thin the iris or higher power (4–5 mJ) to quickly penetrate it. Pigment release from the posterior chamber signals iridotomy patency. Transillumination is useful to locate the iridotomy and confirm patency. Once a hole is made, enlarge it horizontally to an adequate size, ideally with lower energy.

<u>Sequential green/Nd:YAG LPI</u>

In patients with darker irides, large amounts of energy may be required to achieve a patent PI when using the Nd:YAG laser. Thermal green laser pre-treatment to thin the iris results in the need for less energy with the Nd:YAG laser, which is then used to penetrate the iris and create an iridotomy.[5,6] The coagulative effect of the green laser reduces the risk of bleeding from the iridotomy site.

- Green laser settings:
  - Stage 1 (optional): Use a 50-µm spot size, 100 mW power, and 0.05-second duration. Apply 30 shots in a rosette pattern to thin the iris and prevent large bubbles with higher power.
  - Stage 2: Increase the power to 800 mW and set the duration to 0.1 seconds for 10–15 shots (or more if not employing Stage 1) to create a deep central crater.
- Nd:YAG laser settings:
  - Set power to 1–3 mJ and increase to the power required to penetrate iris in the green argon laser pre-treated area. Enlarge as for Nd:YAG PI.

Post-laser treatment

The IOP needs to be checked 45–60 minutes after LPI. Administer topical steroids to reduce inflammation and taper according to the clinical response. An alpha-agonist or oral acetazolamide should be prescribed in cases where there is concern of post-laser IOP spike, *e.g.*, in cases with raised IOP or advanced PACG.

Complications of LPI

Bleeding

Nd:YAG laser can cause bleeding when it hits iris vessels, but pressure on the globe with the laser lens typically stops it.

Cornea

Previous reports have indicated that using high-energy green laser for creating iridotomies could cause direct injury to the corneal epithelium or endothelium.[7] A study utilizing specular microscopy to examine the corneal endothelium after Nd:YAG laser procedures, including iridotomies, found dark areas in the endothelium corresponding to the amount of Nd:YAG energy used. However, 6 months post-iridotomy, there was no statistically significant loss of corneal endothelial cells.[8]

Anterior lens capsule

Avoid this rare LPI complication by placing the iridotomy in the peripheral iris away from the lens and setting laser defocus to zero before treatment.

IOP elevation

The incidence of acute IOP increase following LPI is low, primarily due to the routine pretreatment with topical alpha-agonists.[9] However, patients with advanced PACG and extensive PAS are more likely to experience an IOP spike. The limited trabecular meshwork not occluded by PAS may have compromised outflow function and can become obstructed by iris pigment and tissue from the PI, resulting in an acute increase in IOP. For patients with advanced PACG undergoing LPI, a course of oral acetazolamide initiated immediately after the procedure and continued for 2 to 3 days may be considered.

Patients may experience sustained IOP increases after LPI, requiring close monitoring and treatment with IOP-lowering medications. Topical steroids might cause prolonged IOP elevation post-LPI; thus, non-steroidal anti-inflammatory agents are a suitable alternative. Excessive anterior chamber inflammation post-laser is more likely in individuals with thick, dark irides, such as Asians.

Dysphotopsia

Dysphotopsias (lines, ghost images, glare, or halos) may occur and are presumed to be associated with proximity of the iridotomy to the tear meniscus at the lid-cornea interface, which directs the light rays upward acting as a base-up prism. Some studies recommend horizontal placement of the iridotomy at a distance from the tear meniscus. However, other recent studies do not support the notion that the iridotomy location influences the likelihood of dysphotopsias.[10-12]

Posterior synechiae

The development of posterior synechiae after LPI can lead to a permanently miotic pupil. Possible factors that may contribute to the formation of posterior synechiae include increased contact between the posterior iris and the anterior lens surface following LPI, the use of miotic agents, and inflammation of the anterior chamber.

Accelerated cataract formation

LPI might cause or worsen cataracts. A prior study noted progression of posterior subcapsular lens opacities in eyes treated with LPI, but without a control group, and other factors, such as underlying PAC or medication use, may influence these results.[13] This is more concerning for asymptomatic ITC patients considering prophylactic LPI. However, LPI benefits outweigh the cataract risk for those with established PAC and PACG.

References

1. Lowe RF. Acute angle-closure glaucoma. The second eye: an analysis of 200 cases. Br J Ophthalmol 1962;46:641-650. https://doi.org/10.1136/bjo.46.11.641
2. Snow JT. Value of prophylactic iridectomy on the second eye in angle-closure glaucoma. Trans Ophthalmol Soc UK 1997;97:189-191.
3. Radhakrishnan S, Chen PP, Junk AK, et al. Ophthalmic Technology Assessment: Laser peripheral iridotomy in primary angle closure: a report by the American Academy of Ophthalmology. Ophthalmology. 2018;125:1110-1120. https://doi.org/10.1016/j.ophtha.2018.01.015
4. Jin JC, Anderson DR. The effect of iridotomy on iris contour. Am J Ophthalmol 1990;110:260-263. https://doi.org/10.1016/S0002-9394(14)76341-X
5. Lim L, Seah SKL, Lim ASL. Comparison of argon laser iridotomy and sequential argon and YAG laser iridotomy in dark irides. Ophthal Surg Lasers 1996;27:285-288. https://doi.org/10.3928/1542-8877-19960401-08
6. Ho T, Fan R. Sequential argon-YAG laser iridotomies in dark irides. Br J Ophthalmol 1992;76:329-331. https://doi.org/10.1136/bjo.76.6.329
7. Pollack IP. Use of Argon laser energy to produce iridotomies. Ophthalmic Surg 1980;11:506-515
8. Kozobolis VP, Detorakis ET, Vlachonikolis IG, Pallikaris IG. Endothelial corneal damage after neodymium:YAG laser treatment: Pupillary membranectomies, iridotomies, capsulotomies. Ophthal Surg Lasers 1998;29:793-802. https://doi.org/10.3928/1542-8877-19981001-03
9. Lewis R, Perkins TW, Gangnon R, et al. The rarity of clinically significant rise in intraocular pressure after laser peripheral iridotomy with apraclonidine. Ophthalmology 1998;105: 2256-2259. https://doi.org/10.1016/S0161-6420(98)91225-8
10. Vera V, Naqi A, Belovay GW, Varma DK, Ahmed IIK. Dysphotopsia after temporal versus superior laser peripheral iridotomy: a prospective randomized paired eye trial. Am J Ophthalmol. 2014157:929-935. https://doi.org/10.1016/j.ajo.2014.02.010
11. Srinivasan K, Zebardast N, Krishnamurthy P, et al. Comparison of new visual disturbances after superior versus nasal/ temporal laser peripheral iridotomy: a prospective randomized trial. Ophthalmology. 2018;125:345-351. https://doi.org/10.1016/j.ophtha.2017.09.015
12. Balas M, Mathew DJ. Dysphotopsia and location of laser iridotomy: a systematic review. Eye. 2024;38:1240-1245. https://doi.org/10.1038/s41433-023-02913-1
13. Lim LS, Husain R, Gazzard G, et al. Cataract progression after prophylactic laser peripheral iridotomy: potential implications for the prevention of glaucoma blindness. Ophthalmology 2005;112:1355-1359. https://doi.org/10.1016/j.ophtha.2005.02.026

Risk-assessment recommendations for LPI

Evan M. Chen, Ying Han

PACS definition

PACS is defined as 180° or more of ITC without elevated IOP, PAS, or evidence of related optic nerve damage.[1] In contrast to management recommendations for PAC and PACG, there has been less consensus on the use of LPI for PACS.

ZAP study

Two landmark studies have provided important insight on the efficacy of LPI for PACS. The ZAP study was a prospective randomized contralateral eye study that 889 patients with PACS managed with LPI in 1 eye vs observation in the other.[2] The primary outcome of the study was progression to PAC (defined as an increase in IOP greater than 25 mmHg or subsequent development of PAS) or PACG. In 6 years of follow-up, eyes that received LPI progressed to PAC at nearly half the rate (2.1% vs 4.1%) compared to eyes that were observed. Of note, most patients who progressed were categorized as such due to the development of PAS rather than an elevation in IOP. This difference was statistically significant. The rate of PACG was 0.1% vs 0.6% for LPI vs observation eyes. In secondary analysis, the ZAP study also found that different definitions of PACS, including 3 or 4 quadrants of angle closure, did not result in significantly different results. The findings from this study led the authors to conclude that due to the low rate of progression overall, which were largely attributed to visually insignificant anatomic changes, widespread utilization of LPI for PACS was not recommended.

ANA-LIS

A second landmark clinical trial, ANA-LIS was published shortly after the ZAP study.[3] This study examined 480 eyes with PACS over 5 years of follow-up with 1 eye randomized to prophylactic LPI and the other to observation. The rate of progression to PAC was slightly higher than in the ZAP study but showed that LPI reduced the rate of progression by approximately half (5.5% vs 10.2%). Similar to the ZAP study, development of PAS was the most common endpoint. In both studies, there were very few adverse events associated with LPI treatment.

Limitations of existing studies

These studies are the largest and most robust to date examining the utility of LPI for PACS, although several important limitations should be considered. First, these studies included homogeneous Chinese and Singaporean participants for ZAP and

ANA-LIS, respectively, limiting generalizability. Furthermore, high-risk PACS patients and those with visually significant cataracts were excluded; in ANA-LIS, patients with retinal conditions who had previously experienced symptoms of potential angle closure during dilation were also excluded. Strict exclusion criteria likely result in an underestimation of progression rates. Of note, prior studies have identified higher rates of progression from PAC to PACG.[4] Second, the studies have limited follow-up periods. Differences between treatment and observation in these studies increased with longer follow-up, so it is possible that differences in progression rates may further increase over time. This is an important consideration given PACS is a chronic condition that can be present for decades. Indeed, a 14-year follow-up of the ZAP study found that the difference in rate of progression had widened (6.6% vs 20.9%), with a relative decreased rate of progression of 69% among the LPI group compared to 47% among the control eyes at 6 years.[5] Third, these studies take place in single health systems with idealized follow-up schedules.

While these studies demonstrated a limited utility of LPI for PACS, the decision to proceed with LPI must still be considered on a patient-by-patient basis. The ANA-LIS study found higher rates of progression in individuals with older age, elevated IOP after dilation, and diabetes mellitus.[3] Other reports have suggested racial and gender differences in progression risk as well as anatomic factors.[6,7] Systems-level factors—including lack of access to routine and emergent ophthalmic care, including cataract surgery—should also be considered when considering deferring prophylactic LPI.[8]

Racial/ethnic considerations

Racial/ethnic differences in PACG prevalence and conversion from PACS to PACG

Studies examining the global prevalence of PACG globally have identified differences in rates of disease by race with Asian countries having the greatest prevalence of PACG.[9] However, many prior international studies have examined racially and ethnically homogeneous populations. Studies in the United States with diverse populations have found low PACG rates among elderly Black and White patients.[10] They have also not identified a significant difference in the rate of conversion from anatomical narrow angles to PACG based on race/ethnicity.[11]

Racial/ethnic differences in impact of PACG disease

While the prevalence of PACG and risk of conversion to PACG may not be significantly greater in specific racial groups, the impact of disease can be greater. In a recent study of patients in the United States from the Intelligent Research in Sight (IRIS) Registry, Black and Hispanic patients with PACG were found to have significantly higher odds of blindness compared to non-Hispanic White patients even after accounting for IOP and other ocular comorbidities.[12] This may in part be due to lower rates of detection of anatomical narrow angles in these racial groups which, in turn, may be related to differences in access to care or provider biases.[13]

Racial/ethnic differences in response to LPI

It is also noted that racial differences in adverse events following prophylactic LPI have been reported. In a study of 2,407 eyes, IOP elevation and iritis were significantly more common in patients who had self-identified as Black.[14] Differences in adverse event prevalence is postulated to be attributed to differences in pigmentation and iris thickness.[15]

In summary, few large studies have examined racial/ethnic differences in PACG prevalence, risk of progression from PACS to PAC/PACG and response to LPI. A clinical trial with a racially/ethnically diverse patient population emulating the ZAP and ANA-LIS studies could provide critical insight to the utility of LPI in specific racial groups. Elucidation of these differences is particularly important given the higher risk of blindness from PACG and lower rates of detection of ANA among minority populations.

References

1. Gedde SJ, Chen PP, Muir KW, et al. Primary Angle-Closure Disease Preferred Practice Pattern®. Ophthalmology. 2021;128(1):P30-P70. https://doi.org/10.1016/j.ophtha.2020.10.021
2. He M, Jiang Y, Huang S, et al. Laser peripheral iridotomy for the prevention of angle closure: a single-centre, randomised controlled trial. Lancet Lond Engl. 2019;393(10181):1609-1618. https://doi.org/10.1016/S0140-6736(18)32607-2
3. Baskaran M, Kumar RS, Friedman DS, et al. The Singapore Asymptomatic Narrow Angles Laser Iridotomy Study: Five-Year Results of a Randomized Controlled Trial. Ophthalmology. 2022;129(2):147-158. https://doi.org/10.1016/j.ophtha.2021.08.017
4. Thomas R, George R, Parikh R, Muliyil J, Jacob A. Five year risk of progression of primary angle closure suspects to primary angle closure: a population based study. Br J Ophthalmol. 2003;87(4):450-454. https://doi.org/10.1136/bjo.87.4.450

5. Yuan Y, Wang W, Xiong R, et al. Fourteen-Year Outcome of Angle-Closure Prevention with Laser Iridotomy in the Zhongshan Angle-Closure Prevention Study: Extended Follow-up of a Randomized Controlled Trial. Ophthalmology. 2023;130(8):786-794. https://doi.org/10.1016/j.ophtha.2023.03.024
6. Lavanya R, Wong TY, Friedman DS, et al. Determinants of angle closure in older Singaporeans. Arch Ophthalmol Chic Ill 1960. 2008;126(5):686-691. https://doi.org/10.1001/archopht.126.5.686
7. Zhang Y, Thomas R, Zhang Q, Li SZ, Wang NL. Progression of Primary Angle Closure Suspect to Primary Angle Closure and Associated Risk Factors: The Handan Eye Study. Invest Ophthalmol Vis Sci. 2021;62(7):2. https://doi.org/10.1167/iovs.62.7.2
8. Apolo G, Bohner A, Pardeshi A, et al. Racial and Sociodemographic Disparities in the Detection of Narrow Angles Prior to Primary Angle Closure Glaucoma in the United States. Ophthalmol Glaucoma. 2022;5(4):388-395. https://doi.org/10.1016/j.ogla.2022.01.001
9. Zhang N, Wang J, Chen B, Li Y, Jiang B. Prevalence of Primary Angle Closure Glaucoma in the Last 20 Years: A Meta-Analysis and Systematic Review. Front Med. 2020;7:624179. https://doi.org/10.3389/fmed.2020.624179
10. Friedman DS, Jampel HD, Muñoz B, West SK. The Prevalence of Open-angle Glaucoma Among Blacks and Whites 73 Years and Older: The Salisbury Eye Evaluation Glaucoma Study. Arch Ophthalmol. 2006;124(11):1625-1630. https://doi.org/10.1001/archopht.124.11.1625
11. Yoo K, Apolo G, Zhou S, et al. Rates and Patterns of Diagnostic Conversion from Anatomical Narrow Angle to Primary Angle-Closure Glaucoma in the United States. Ophthalmol Glaucoma. 2023;6(2):169-176. https://doi.org/10.1016/j.ogla.2022.08.016
12. Shah SN, Zhou S, Sanvicente C, et al. Prevalence and Risk Factors of Blindness Among Primary Angle Closure Glaucoma Patients in the United States: An IRIS Registry Analysis. Am J Ophthalmol. 2024;259:131-140. https://doi.org/10.1016/j.ajo.2023.11.007
13. Apolo G, Bohner A, Pardeshi A, et al. Racial and Sociodemographic Disparities in the Detection of Narrow Angles Prior to Primary Angle Closure Glaucoma in the United States. Ophthalmol Glaucoma. 2022;5(4):388-395. https://doi.org/10.1016/j.ogla.2022.01.001
14. Adetunji MO, Meer E, Whitehead G, et al. Self-identified Black Race as a Risk Factor for Intraocular Pressure Elevation and Iritis Following Prophylactic Laser Peripheral Iridotomy. J Glaucoma. 2022;31(4):218. https://doi.org/10.1097/IJG.0000000000001995
15. Waisbourd M, Shafa A, Delvadia R, et al. Bilateral Same-day Laser Peripheral Iridotomy in the Philadelphia Glaucoma Detection and Treatment Project. J Glaucoma. 2016;25(10):e821-e825. https://doi.org/10.1097/IJG.0000000000000409

Clinical assessment after LPI

LPI is effective in relieving the pupillary block mechanism, but it is not equally effective in the context of other mechanisms, such as thick peripheral iris, anterior iris insertion, plateau iris configuration (PIC), progressive lens thickening, or a combination of these factors.[1,2] In a Chinese population, one study estimated that one-third of PACS cases are due to PIC. UBM also demonstrated that 60% of PACS eyes in this study group still present ITC in at least 1 quadrant after LPI.[2]

Regular ACA assessment is still mandatory, even after prophylactic LPI. Despite the development of different imaging devices to evaluate the ACA, there is a lack of evidence to determine which devices or biometric parameters should be used for PACS follow-up. Indeed, dynamic gonioscopy (*i.e.*, gonioscopy with and without indentation) remains the gold-standard technique for angle evaluation, and it is the only method that allows differentiation between appositional and permanent angle closure.[3] Patients should also be monitored regularly for IOP elevation.

Further evaluation is required when there is no change in ACA profile after LPI or in case of progression (development of PAS and/or IOP rise) It is estimated that PIC is detected in up to one-third of Asian eyes after LPI.[2,4] The forward rotation of the ciliary processes present in PIC eyes can be visualized by UBM, the only imaging technique capable of assessing the ciliary body and processes.

Progressive lens thickening associated with aging also contributes to angle narrowing,[5] which may partially explain the role of aging as a significant risk factor for progression from PACS. This reinforces the need for continuous and systematic follow-up over time. Of note, in both the ZAP and ANA-LIS trials,[6,7] participants were around 6 decades of age (59.3 ± 5.0 and 62.8 ± 6.9 years, respectively). The relatively younger age, combined with good visual acuity profile (visual acuity worse than 20/40 was an exclusion criteria), prevented significant cataract cases from being included in both trials, possibly contributing to the low rate of progression in these trials. Cataract may affect ACD, and ACD was identified as a risk factor for angle closure.[8-10] ACD can be measured by AS-OCT, Scheimpflug imaging, or ultrasound, but measurements obtained with different techniques are not interchangeable.

Recommendations on how to follow untreated PACS individuals

The same regular follow-up after LPI applies to untreated PACS individuals. However, it is worth noting that progressive angle narrowing may continue as a result of lens thickening associated with aging. Untreated eyes tend to present a more rapid angle width decrease in comparison to LPI-treated eyes,[11] raising the level of attention and risk for untreated eyes.

In parallel to monitoring for the occurrence of further narrowing and/or synechiae development, patients must be thoroughly educated about the severity of the angle-closure process. They should also be informed about symptoms of acute or intermittent PAC. It is critical to consider that severe complications of AAC attack, as well as the severity of PACG, both serious vision-threatening conditions, could be effectively avoided by a successful well-timed LPI.

References

1. Ramakrishnan R, Mitra A, Abdul Kader M, Das S. To Study the Efficacy of Laser Peripheral Iridoplasty in the Treatment of Eyes With Primary Angle Closure and Plateau Iris Syndrome, Unresponsive to Laser Peripheral Iridotomy, Using Anterior-Segment OCT as a Tool. J Glaucoma. 2016 May;25(5):440-6. https://doi.org/10.1097/IJG.0000000000000307
2. He M, Friedman DS, Ge J, et al. Laser peripheral iridotomy in primary angle-closure suspects: biometric and gonioscopic outcomes: the Liwan Eye Study. Ophthalmology. 2007 Mar;114(3):494-500. https://doi.org/10.1016/j.ophtha.2006.06.053
3. Riva I, Micheletti E, Oddone F, et al. Anterior Chamber Angle Assessment Techniques: A Review. J Clin Med. 2020 Nov 25;9(12):3814. https://doi.org/10.3390/jcm9123814
4. Kumar RS, Baskaran M, Chew PT, et al. Prevalence of plateau iris in primary angle closure suspects an ultrasound biomicroscopy study. Ophthalmology. 2008 Mar;115(3):430-4. https://doi.org/10.1016/j.ophtha.2007.07.026
5. Klein BE, Klein R, Moss SE. Correlates of lens thickness: the Beaver Dam Eye Study. Invest Ophthalmol Vis Sci. 1998 Jul;39(8):1507-10.
6. He M, Jiang Y, Huang S, et al. Laser peripheral iridotomy for the prevention of angle closure: a single-centre, randomised controlled trial. Lancet. 2019;393(10181):1609-1618. https://doi.org/10.1016/S0140-6736(18)32607-2
7. Baskaran M, Kumar RS, Friedman DS, et al. The Singapore Asymptomatic Narrow Angles Laser Iridotomy Study: Five-Year Results of a Randomized Controlled Trial. Ophthalmology. 2022;129(2):147-158. https://doi.org/10.1016/j.ophtha.2021.08.017
8. Leung CK, Palmiero PM, Weinreb RN, et al. Comparisons of anterior segment biometry between Chinese and Caucasians using anterior segment optical coherence tomography. Br J Ophthalmol. 2010 Sep;94(9):1184-9. https://doi.org/10.1136/bjo.2009.167296
9. Zhang Y, Zhang Q, Thomas R, Li SZ, Wang NL. Development of angle closure and associated risk factors: The Handan eye study. Acta Ophthalmol. 2022 Feb;100(1):e253-e261. https://doi.org/10.1111/aos.14887

10. Zhang Y, Thomas R, Zhang Q, Li SZ, Wang NL. Progression of Primary Angle Closure Suspect to Primary Angle Closure and Associated Risk Factors: The Handan Eye Study. Invest Ophthalmol Vis Sci. 2021 Jun 1;62(7):2 https://doi.org/10.1167/iovs.62.7.2
11. Jiang Y, Chang DS, Zhu H, et al. Longitudinal changes of angle configuration in primary angle-closure suspects: the Zhongshan Angle-Closure Prevention Trial. Ophthalmology. 2014 Sep;121(9):1699-1705. https://doi.org/10.1016/j.ophtha.2014.03.039

LPI in the management of PAC and PACG

Winnie Nolan

Mechanism of action of LPI

An adequately sized iridotomy creates a hole in the iris which eliminates pupillary block by allowing aqueous humor a shortcut from the posterior to anterior chamber bypassing the pupil. In doing so, the iris loses convexity and, depending on the degree of pupillary block, the iris will flatten and fall away from the trabecular meshwork, which results in partial or complete opening of the angle.

Indications for LPI in PAC

- Fellow eye of affected eye in AAC crisis. Initial studies on surgical iridectomy found that LPI protects the fellow eye from developing AAC. Untreated, the fellow eye has a 50% risk of developing AAC over 5 years.[1,2]
- PAC with elevated IOP (> 21 mmHg), evidence of PAS, or symptoms suggestive of angle closure.
- PAC eyes with IOP > 30 mmHg are eligible for CLE following publication of the EAGLE trial, which found CLE to be more effective than LPI in controlling IOP.[3] However, LPI is still indicated or should be offered to certain groups of patients who do not fulfil the criteria for inclusion in the EAGLE trial due to higher risk of complications or potential adverse outcomes of surgery:
    - o Eyes with very short axial lengths (< 21 mm) that are at risk of poor refractive outcomes or aqueous misdirection.
    - o Young patients (< 50 years old) who may be more at risk of retinal detachment and will develop early onset presbyopia with CLE.
    - o Patients who do not wish to have CLE surgery as first-line treatment.

Indications for LPI in PACG

- PACG eyes with IOP >21 mmHg should be offered clear lens extraction due to better outcomes in the EAGLE trial. As with PAC, LPI can be offered instead of CLE in patients with PACG who may be at higher risk of complications of surgery or poorer outcomes as described in the previous section.

LPI techniques

<u>Positioning of LPI</u>

The iridotomy can be positioned superiorly or temporally and should be placed as peripheral as possible in the iris to avoid lens damage from the laser. There is conflicting evidence from small randomized controlled trials on whether positioning the iridotomy superiorly or temporally affects the rate of dysphotopsia.[4,5] However, the occasional patient can develop prolonged and distressing symptoms of photopsia, which is thought to be due to the prismatic effect of the tear film when the eyelid transects the iridotomy. Therefore, it may be advisable to position the iridotomy at or close to the 12 o'clock position superiorly (completely covered by the upper lid) or at the 3 or 9 o'clock position temporally (completely uncovered). In thick irides it may be easier to position the iridotomy in a crypt, where the iris is thinner.

<u>Nd:YAG LPI</u>

The Nd:YAG laser in Q-switched mode causes photodisruption of the iris tissue and is the commonly used method for performing LPI.

- If patients have significantly elevated IOP, medical treatment should be prescribed to reduce IOP before the laser procedure.
- Pre-treat the eye with pilocarpine 2% or 4% to constrict the pupil and stretch the iris, and a topical alpha-agonist (apraclonidine 1% or brimonidine) to reduce bleeding and post-laser IOP spikes.[7]
- Instill topical anesthesia into the eye to be treated.
- Use a coupling fluid with an iridotomy lens such as the Abraham lens and place the
- lens on the eye.
- Set the defocus to zero.
- Ask the patient to either look down or slightly horizontally (depending on whether aiming for superior, nasal or temporal iridotomy) so that the laser beam will be perpendicular to the iris.
- Start with a lower power setting (1–3mJ).

- Deliver single shots to the iris until a gush of pigment demonstrates penetration of the iris
- Enlarge the iridotomy once patent.

Sequential argon/Nd:YAG LPI

In patients with thick brown irides, argon laser can be used prior to Nd:YAG laser to prepare the iris by contracting and thinning the tissues, so that less energy is required for the Nd:YAG laser to penetrate. Additionally, the coagulation of the iris by the argon laser reduces the chances of hemorrhage. Sequential argon/ Nd:YAG laser is the preferred technique for iridotomies in patients with dark brown irides, *e.g.*, patients of Asian or African descent.[6]

- Argon laser pre-treatment:
  - Prepare the eye as above applying drops and laser lens.
  - Initial stage (optional): Deliver 5–30 low power shots (50-μm spot size, 100 mW power, 0.01 seconds). This may help avoid bubbles.
  - Second stage: Deliver 10–15 higher power shots (50 μm, 400m W, 0.1 seconds) to form a deep central crater in the iris without penetration.
- Nd:YAG laser: Once the argon laser pre-treatment is complete, proceed with Nd:YAG laser as described in above to penetrate the iris and form the iridotomy.

Post-laser management

- Instill a further drop of alpha-agonist following the treatment.
- Check the IOP 30–60 minutes after treatment.
- Topical steroids should be prescribed for a week after laser to reduce inflammation.
- Consider a short course of oral acetazolamide post-laser in patients with advanced glaucomatous optic neuropathy or very high IOP prior to laser.
- The patient should be examined a week after treatment to check that the iridotomy is patent and large enough. Gonioscopy or anterior segment imaging can be repeated to check if the angle is more open and the pupillary block has been eliminated.

Complications of LPI

Immediate

- Iris hemorrhage: This is often self-limiting but if persistent then pressure on the globe with the laser lens can be used to stop the bleeding. If the blood is obscuring the view, it is best to stop and continue later or on another day when the blood has cleared.

- Corneal or lens damage from the laser: This is rare and minimized by setting the defocus to zero and ensuring the iridotomy is peripheral, and therefore beyond the edge of the lens.
- Inability to complete the iridotomy: This may be due to a thick iris, poor view due to corneal opacity or bleeding, or poor tolerance of the procedure by patient. The options are to attempt to complete the iridotomy at another sitting or to switch to another procedure instead, *e.g.*, surgical iridectomy or lens extraction.

Intermediate

- Iridotomy too small or non-patent: Top up laser at second sitting.
- Intraocular inflammation or posterior synechiae: This can be prevented by using intensive topical steroids hourly (daytime) for the first 24 hours after laser and then 4 times a day for a week.
- IOP spike: Patients at higher risk of IOP spikes include those with advanced glaucoma, poorly controlled IOP prior to laser, and cases with high cumulative laser energy. Some patients can also develop a steroid response, which can be minimized by pre- and post-laser topical alpha-agonists and a course of acetazolamide in patients at higher risk.

Effectiveness of laser iridotomy in PAC and PACG

The multicenter EAGLE trial in 2016 randomized patients with PAC (with IOP ≥ 30 mmHg) or PACG to LPI or CLE. At 3 years of follow-up, 60% of patients treated with iridotomy required medication to control the IOP compared with 20% of the CLE group. Only 1 patient in the CLE group required further glaucoma surgery compared with 24 patients in the LPI group (difference of 10.9% in glaucoma surgery during the trial). CLE was superior to LPI in terms of IOP control, patient-reported outcomes, and cost-effectiveness.[3]

The effectiveness of LPI may vary depending on the severity of disease. Older retrospective studies show that LPI is less likely to control IOP without medications in eyes with extensive PAS or optic disc damage compared with those without these features.[8,9]

References

1. Lowe RF. Acute angle-closure glaucoma: the second eye: an analysis of 200 cases. Br J Ophthalmol. 1962;46(11):641-50. https://doi.org/10.1136/bjo.46.11.641

2. Salmon JT. Value of prophylactic peripheral iridectomy on the second eye in angle-closure glaucoma. Trans Ophthalmol Soc U K. 1977;97:322-5.
3. Azuara-Blanco A, Burr J, Ramsay C, et al. Effectiveness of early lens extraction for the treatment of primary angle-closure glaucoma (EAGLE): a randomised controlled trial. Lancet. 2016;388(10052):1389-97. https://doi.org/10.1016/S0140-6736(16)30956-4
4. Vera V, Naqi A, Belovay GW, Varma DK, Ahmed II. Dysphotopsia after temporal versus superior laser peripheral iridotomy: a prospective randomized pair-eye trial. Am J Ophthalmol. 2014;157(5):929-35. https://doi.org/10.1016/j.ajo.2014.02.010
5. Wang D, Lin S. New developments in anterior segment optical coherence tomography for glaucoma. Curr Opin Ophthalmol. 2016;27(2):111-7. https://doi.org/10.1097/ICU.0000000000000243
6. De Silva DJ, Gazzard G, Foster P. Laser iridotomy in dark irides. Br J Ophthalmol. 2007;91(2):222-5. https://doi.org/10.1136/bjo.2006.104315
7. Rosenberg LF, Krupin T, Ruderman J, et al. Apraclonidine and anterior segment laser surgery: comparison of 0.5% versus 1.0% apraclonidine for prevention of postoperative intraocular pressure rise. Ophthalmology. 1995;102(9):1312-8. https://doi.org/10.1016/S0161-6420(95)30869-X
8. Salmon JF. Long-term intraocular pressure control after Nd-YAG laser iridotomy in chronic angle-closure glaucoma. J Glaucoma. 1993;2(4):291-6. https://doi.org/10.1097/00061198-199300240-00012
9. Nolan WP, Foster PJ, Devereux JG, Uranchimeg D, Johnson GJ, Baasanhu J. YAG laser iridotomy treatment for primary angle closure in east Asian eyes. Br J Ophthalmol. 2000;84(11):1255-9. https://doi.org/10.1136/bjo.84.11.1255

Iridoplasty

Seng Kheong Fang, Niklas Telinius, Gus Gazzard

ALPI was first proposed by Ritch[1] in 1982 to treat unresponsive APAC. The technique was then adapted by Ritch and colleagues to include plateau iris syndrome.[2] The aim of ALPI is to widen the angle and reduce ITC. The mechanisms by which ALPI acts is to induce contraction of the iris stroma peripheral to the burn site, thereby physically pulling the angle open,[2] as well as by thinning out the iris stroma at the burn site.[3] ALPI does not eliminate pupillary block and is thus not a definitive treatment for PACD but is rather a potential secondary procedure. In 10%–80% of PACS, the ACA remains appositionally closed after an iridotomy and the question whether additional interventions are needed to reestablish a normal chamber anatomy is highly relevant.[4,5] In the following section, the evidence in favor of using ALPI in different scenarios of the PACD spectrum will be reviewed with focus on randomized clinical trials (RCTs).

Indications

From PACS to PACG

A recent Cochrane review reviewed the evidence for ALPI in chronic angle closure. Four RCTs were identified, but all studies showed elements of high risk of bias. Three different clinical scenarios were tested.

- Iridoplasty versus no treatment: A single RCT[6] evaluated the use of ALPI as a secondary procedure compared to no further treatment in 22 PACS or PAC subjects over 3 months. There was some effect on diurnal IOP measurements, with a mean reduction of -1.81 mmHg (95% CI: -3.11 to -0.51) of maximum IOP. There was no effect on minimum IOP. Angle anatomy was assessed with AS-OCT, which demonstrated an increase in all measured parameters. Of note, no AS-OCT data were reported for the control group.
- Iridoplasty versus medication: One RCT compared ALPI to travoprost 0.004% as a secondary procedure after iridotomy in 80 subjects with PAC or PACG (1:1 randomization) over 12 months.[7] The primary endpoint of the study revealed a higher success rate (IOP < 21 mmHg without additional medications) of 85% for the travoprost group compared to 35% for the ALPI group. The Kaplan-Meier curve showed that the ALPI failures primarily started to occur at approximately 6 months. Laser treatment resulted in widening of the angle. Despite this, there was a significant increase in PAS formation in the ALPI group (from 1.7 to 2.6 clock hours) but interestingly not in the travoprost group (1.8 to 1.6 clock hours). There were no serious adverse events reported, with mild complications limited to 2 cases of post-laser IOP spike in the ALPI group, with 1 requiring glaucoma surgery.
- Iridoplasty plus iridotomy versus iridotomy alone: Two RCTs[8,9] evaluated the use of ALPI in combination with peripheral iridotomy compared to peripheral iridotomy alone as a primary intervention for either PACS[8] or PAC/PACG.[9] The 2 studies included 174 subjects in total. The main finding was that there was no significant effect of adding ALPI as measured by several important clinical outcome measures. The final mean IOP was similar and not significant different between groups, with a mean difference of 0.39 mmHg (95% CI: -1.07 to 1.85) at 3 and 12 months.[10] The mean difference in glaucoma medications was also non-significant at 0.10 drops (95% CI: -0.34 to 0.54) at 12 months. Anterior chamber anatomy was assessed with Scheimpflug imaging in 1 study, which demonstrated minor additional deepening of the chamber in the

ALPI group.[8] In the other study, the angle was assessed with gonioscopy and the extent of PAS reported.[9] Interestingly the iridotomy group had a reduction in PAS formation (1 clock hour); however, the iridotomy plus ALPI group had a significantly higher reduction in PAS formation (2 clock hours). Complications were mild and uncommon across groups, and ALPI did not result in additional complications. The only severe complication reported was 1 case of malignant glaucoma in the ALPI group in the study by Sun *et al.*[9]

Plateau iris

Plateau iris is a condition in which an enlarged or anteriorly positioned ciliary body maintains the iris root near the trabecular meshwork, leading to angle closure. The ALPI mechanism of action is to induce thinning of the superficial iris tissue and thus to reduce ITC. However, this procedure has no effect on the ciliary body anteposition. The underlying cause is therefore not treated. Any element of pupillary block should be eliminated with an iridotomy or lens removal before ALPI is considered. A systematic review by Bourdon *et al.*[11] from 2019 identified 1 prospective and 7 retrospective studies with at least 1 month of follow-up on ALPI for plateau iris syndrome. No RCT has been conducted. In general, most studies include the whole primary angle closure as one group and does not distinguish between the plateau iris phenotype and other phenotypes and there is a lack of high-quality studies that allow conclusions to be drawn.

The effect on the angle anatomy has primarily been evaluated with gonioscopy. Success in widening the angle varies between studies, from 46%[12] to 100%.[13] Gain of 1 Shaffer or Spaeth grade in 2 quadrants can be an expected outcome. Re-treatment has been reported to be necessary in 10%–18% of cases because of gradual narrowing of the angle with time.[13] Less data is available on the anatomical effects of ALPI using more objective measures, such as AS-OCT. Ramakrishnan *et al.* used AS-OCT and found that the angle-opening distance at 500 μm from the scleral spur (AOD500) increased from 0.132 ± 0.016 mm at baseline to 0.179 ± 0.062 mm ($p < 0.001$) after 1 year.[12] The most important factor to assess the efficacy of ALPI in plateau iris syndrome is the reduction in IOP. In the systematic review by Bourdon,[11] the weighted mean IOP decreased from 19.6 mmHg at baseline to 15.6 mmHg after 1 year of follow-up, equivalent to a reduction of 4.0 mmHg or 20%. In studies with a 6-year follow-up, the weighted mean IOP was 18.7 mmHg at baseline and 18.5 mmHg at the last visit, indicating a minimal decrease of 0.2 mm Hg or 1%.

ALPI seems to lower IOP and widen the iridocorneal angle in the short run but there is no data to support any long-term efficacy of ALPI for plateau iris syndrome. As ALPI does not abolish accommodation, ALPI may be considered in young patients in need of additional treatment in place of lens removal. In conclusion, there is a lack of evidence to define a clear role for ALPI in plateau iris syndrome.

APAC

ALPI can be used to break an episode of APAC, either as initial treatment, when iridotomy is not feasible due to corneal edema or for episodes not responding to conventional treatment (medications and iridotomy). The procedure does not eliminate pupillary block, which still needs to be addressed after the attack has been broken. The procedure can be performed in the entire 360° or to a lesser extent, *e.g.*, 1 or 2 quadrants. The concept of using ALPI as primary treatment instead of systemic medications was first tested in a prospective trial by Lam *et al.*,[14] where 8 out of 10 patients had an IOP below 21 mmHg after 1 hour and all patients after 2 hours.

The role of ALPI in different APAC scenarios has subsequently been tested in 3 RCTs.[15–17] Two studies have tested ALPI versus medications and 1 study has tested ALPI in combination with surgical iridectomy versus trabeculectomy.

In the study by Lam *et al.*,[15] ALPI was tested after initial pilocarpine (4%) and timolol (0.5%) against intravenous acetazolamide (and mannitol if IOP was over 60 mmHg) in cases where iridotomy was not possible. Laser produced favorable outcomes in terms of greater IOP reduction during the first 2 hours, after which there was no significant difference between the groups. All patients received iridotomy at a later time point as definitive treatment. There was no difference in IOP or glaucoma medications between the groups after 6 months. The effect on angle anatomy was investigated in the study by Sng *et al.*[17] where ALPI resulted in a larger increase in angle width measurements (AOD750 and TISA750) compared with medical treatment. Appositional contact in an inflamed eye may lead to PAS formation. It appears logical that ALPI treatment can reduce PAS formation since it reduces the time needed to break the attack and increases the angle width. This was addressed in the study by Lai *et al.*[18] and the proportion of eyes with of PAS $\geq 90°$ in the ALPI group was indeed lower compared to the medical arm (22% vs 44.7%, respectively).

In the RCT by Nguyen *et al.*,[16] ALPI was tested in a different setting, in combination with surgical iridectomy and compared with trabeculectomy. Sixty-seven patients with unresponsive APAC were randomized to one of the procedures. Both groups achieved high success rates (IOP < 21 mmHg without medications) of 97.3% and 93.3% in the ALPI-iridectomy and trabeculectomy groups, respectively. Complications were more frequent in the ALPI-iridectomy group.

Despite the close proximity between iris and cornea during APAC, there are no reports that suggest corneal safety issues in this setting. Endothelial cell loss was not different between ALPI-treated eyes and medication only.[18]

In summary, ALPI can effectively break APAC, including cases where corneal edema precludes successful iridotomy. The benefit of ALPI in terms of greater IOP reduction during APAC appears to disappear after 2 hours. ALPI may result in better anatomical outcomes but data that demonstrate that this translates to better clinical outcomes in terms of IOP is lacking. The role of ALPI as primary treatment for all cases is thus debatable, but ALPI has a role in unresponsive cases. Lastly, ALPI does not replace iridotomy or lens removal to eliminate pupillary block for definitive treatment.

Iridoplasty techniques

Pre-treatment

Pupil constriction is essential to stretch the iris and is achieved with pilocarpine (2%–4%). IOP-lowering medications may be used to prevent or blunt a post-laser IOP spikes. If corneal edema is present, glycerin or glucose can be applied to draw water out of the stroma via osmosis, which can facilitate the procedure.

Laser treatment

The whole procedure typically involves 20 to 24 burns across 360°, while maintaining a separation of approximately 2 spot-diameters between each burn and avoiding prominent radial vessels.[19] Overlapping applications may result in iris necrosis and should be avoided.

The argon laser is configured to deliver contraction burns using a 150–500 μm spot size (often closer to 500 μm), a duration of 0.4 to 0.7 seconds, and an initial power setting of 100–200 mW (depending on spot size).[11,19] Using an Abraham lens, the laser beam is directed at the most peripheral portion of the iris. Care must be taken to place the application as peripherally as possible, and it is an option to let the aiming beam minimally overlap onto the adjacent sclera. Any arcus senilis should be ignored and does not constitute a problem. With each laser application, visible contraction of the iris must be observed. If not, the power should be increased. Successful contraction burns are often accompanied by a noticeable deepening of the peripheral anterior chamber at the burn sites and discomfort from the patient. If bubble formation or pigment release occurs, power should be reduced. As the procedure progresses, laser burns may be applied to more peripheral areas than initially accessible. This is a result of prior contraction burns retracting the iris stroma, thereby exposing more peripheral parts of the angle.

Post-laser treatment

IOP-lowering medications (brimonidine is commonly referenced in the literature) may be used to prevent or blunt a post-laser IOP spikes. A short course of topical steroids is recommended and could be dexamethasone 0.1% or prednisolone acetate 1%, 4 to 6 times daily for up to 1 week.

Complications

Complications are predominantly transient and mild, whereas severe and persistent complications are rare.[10] The most common complication is a low-grade inflammation that is responsive to topical steroids. Isolated cases of persistent uveitis lasting beyond 2 weeks and iris hemorrhage have been documented, both resolving with conservative management. Symptomatic persistent mydriasis unresponsive to pilocarpine after uneventful ALPI have been reported.[20] However, all cases resolved within 1 year. Corneal burns may occur, although they typically resolve within a few days. Loss of endothelial cells has not been reported in the studies that investigated this.[7,9,18] Iris necrosis due to application of confluent spots has been observed.[2]

Summary

A recent Cochrane review based on 4 RCTs concluded that ALPI does not appear to be an effective IOP-lowering option and does not have a major role in chronic primary angle closure. Although ALPI may have a positive effect on angle anatomy, this observation does not appear to translate into long-term IOP reduction, and the clinical impact of this intervention is thus minimal. Plateau iris syndrome has been a traditional indication for ALPI but the data that support its use do not derive from RCTs. The increasing availability of phacoemulsification and the EAGLE study[21] supporting lens removal in PAC and PACG also diminishes the role of ALPI in the treatment of PACD. In young patients, ALPI has the obvious advantage over lens removal that it does not result in loss of accommodation. The one setting where ALPI does have a clear role is in medically unresponsive APAC, where ALPI has been shown to be successful in lowering IOP more rapidly.

References

1. Ritch R. Argon laser treatment for medically unresponsive attacks of angle-closure glaucoma. Am J Ophthalmol. 1982;94:197-204. https://doi.org/10.1016/0002-9394(82)90075-7
2. Ritch R, Tham CCY, Lam DSC. Argon laser peripheral iridoplasty (ALPI): an update. Surv Ophthalmol. 2007;52:279-288. https://doi.org/10.1016/j.survophthal.2007.02.006
3. Liu J, Lamba T, Belyea DA. Peripheral laser iridoplasty opens angle in plateau iris by thinning the cross-sectional tissues. Clin Ophthalmol. 2013;7:1895-1897. https://doi.org/10.2147/OPTH.S47297
4. Baskaran M, Yang E, Trikha S, Kumar RS, et al. Residual angle closure one year after laser peripheral iridotomy in primary angle closure suspects. Am J Ophthalmol. 2017;183:111-117. https://doi.org/10.1016/j.ajo.2017.08.016
5. Gupta B, Angmo D, Yadav S, Dada T, Gupta V, Sihota R. Quantification of iridotrabecular contact in primary angle-closure disease. J Glaucoma. 2020;29:681-688. https://doi.org/10.1097/IJG.0000000000001572
6. Bourne RRA, Zhekov I, Pardhan S. Temporal ocular coherence tomography-measured changes in anterior chamber angle and diurnal intraocular pressure after laser iridoplasty: IMPACT study. Br J Ophthalmol. 2017;101:886-891. https://doi.org/10.1136/bjophthalmol-2016-308720
7. Narayanaswamy A, Sakata LM, He M, et al. Argon laser peripheral iridoplasty for primary angle-closure glaucoma. Ophthalmology. 2016;123:514-521. https://doi.org/10.1016/j.ophtha.2015.11.002
8. Lee JR, Choi JY, Kim YD, Choi J. Laser peripheral iridotomy with iridoplasty in primary angle closure suspect: anterior chamber analysis by Pentacam. Korean J Ophthalmol. 2011;25:252-256. https://doi.org/10.3341/kjo.2011.25.4.252
9. Sun X, Liang YB, Wang NL, et al. Laser peripheral iridotomy with and without iridoplasty for primary angle-closure glaucoma: 1-year results of a randomized pilot study. Am J Ophthalmol. 2010;150:68-73. https://doi.org/10.1016/j.ajo.2010.02.004
10. Bayliss JM, Ng WS, Waugh N, Azuara-Blanco A. Laser peripheral iridoplasty for chronic angle closure. Cochrane Database Syst Rev. 2021;(3):CD012722. https://doi.org/10.1002/14651858.CD006746.pub4
11. Bourdon H, Aragno V, Baudouin C, Labbé A. Iridoplasty for plateau iris syndrome: a systematic review. BMJ Open Ophthalmol. 2019;4:e000273. https://doi.org/10.1136/bmjophth-2019-000340
12. Ramakrishnan R, Mitra A, Abdul Kader M, Das S. To study the efficacy of laser peripheral iridoplasty in the treatment of eyes with primary angle closure and plateau iris syndrome, unresponsive to laser peripheral iridotomy, using anterior-segment OCT as a tool. J Glaucoma. 2016;25:440-446. https://doi.org/10.1097/IJG.0000000000000207
13. Romito N, Bluwol E, Graber M, Le Pape C, Lachkar Y. Argon laser iridoplasty for plateau iris syndrome: long-term outcomes of 48 eyes. J Glaucoma. 2019;28:767-771. https://doi.

org/10.1097/IJG.0000000000001313
14. Lam DSC, Lai JSM, Tham CCY. Immediate argon laser peripheral iridoplasty as treatment for acute attack of primary angle-closure glaucoma: a preliminary study. Ophthalmology. 1998;105:2231-2236. https://doi.org/10.1016/S0161-6420(98)92237-0
15. Lam D. Argon laser peripheral iridoplasty versus conventional systemic medical therapy in treatment of acute primary angle-closure glaucoma: a prospective, randomized, controlled trial. Ophthalmology. 2002;109:1591-1596. https://doi.org/10.1016/S0161-6420(02)01158-2
16. Nguyen HX, Nguyen ND, Nguyen HT, et al. Comparing combined laser iridoplasty and surgical iridectomy with trabeculectomy in treatment of refractory acute primary angle closure without significant cataract: a randomized controlled trial. Eye (Lond). 2023;37:2139-2144. https://doi.org/10.1038/s41433-022-02311-z
17. Sng CC, Aquino MC, Liao J, Zheng C, Ang M, Chew PT. Anterior segment morphology after acute primary angle closure treatment: a randomised study comparing iridoplasty and medical therapy. Br J Ophthalmol. 2016;100:542-548. https://doi.org/10.1136/bjophthalmol-2015-307087
18. Lai JS, Tham CC, Chua JK, et al. To compare argon laser peripheral iridoplasty (ALPI) against systemic medications in treatment of acute primary angle-closure: mid-term results. Eye (Lond). 2006;20:309-314. https://doi.org/10.1038/sj.eye.6701867
19. Wong MOM, Chow CWY, Ritch R, Tham CCY. Laser peripheral iridoplasty: procedures and pitfalls. Expert Rev Ophthalmol. 2024;19:333-339. https://doi.org/10.1080/17469899.2024.2368806
20. Espana EM, Ioannidis A, Tello C, Liebmann JM, Foster P, Ritch R. Urrets-Zavalia syndrome as a complication of argon laser peripheral iridoplasty. Br J Ophthalmol. 2007;91:427-429. https://doi.org/10.1136/bjo.2006.105098
21. Azuara-Blanco A, Burr J, Ramsay C, et al. Effectiveness of early lens extraction for the treatment of primary angle-closure glaucoma (EAGLE): a randomised controlled trial. Lancet. 2016;388:1389-1397. https://doi.org/10.1016/S0140-6736(16)30956-4

Laser pupilloplasty

Sophia Wang, Rajesh Sasikumar, Gus Gazzard

Mechanism and aims

Laser pupilloplasty is a procedure performed to assist in breaking an AAC attack.[1,2] Unlike laser iridoplasty, which targets the peripheral iris to contract the iris stroma and open the angle, pupilloplasty targets the pupillary sphincter to relieve pupillary block when the pupillary sphincter is cramped (Fig. 1). The laser procedure contracts the pupillary sphincter in a small area, creating a peaked pupil which pulls away from the lens surface, thus establishing a connection from the posterior to anterior chamber that allows aqueous flow (Fig. 2).

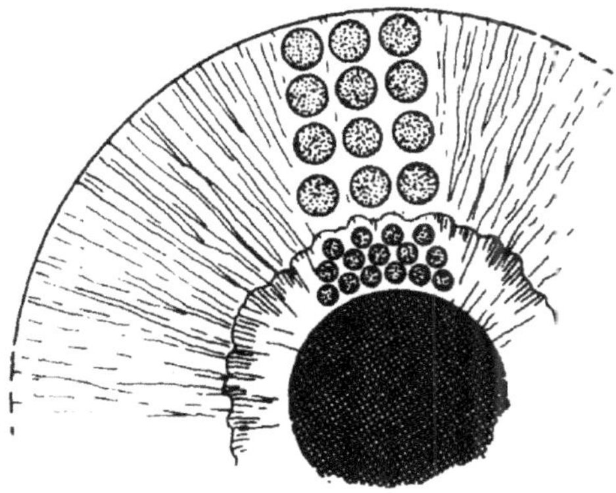

Fig. 1. Pupilloplasty combined with iridoplasty. Smaller burns (200 μm) are used on the sphincter. Image and caption reproduced from Ritch.1

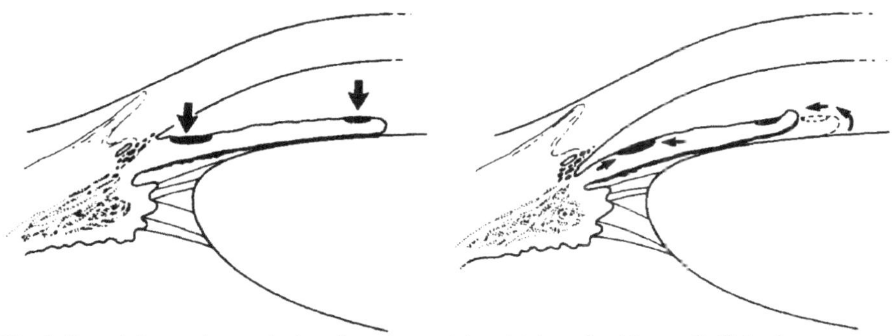

Fig. 2. Stretch burns (arrows) placed on the peripheral iris and sphincter (left) lead to construction of peripheral iris stroma and opening of the angle (right) and contraction and elevation of the sphincter (arrows). The peripheral burns break the mechanical block caused by apposition of the iris to trabecular meshwork, while the burns on the sphincter break the relative pupillary block. Image and caption reproduced from Ritch.[1]

Indications

Laser pupilloplasty is typically performed in conjunction with laser iridoplasty. These procedures can be helpful as a temporizing measure if LPI is unable to immediately be performed. In conditions of prolonged high IOP, the pupil experiences ischemia and is poorly responsive to miotics; without the pupil stretch provided by effective miosis, it may be more challenging to successfully perform LPI through thick iris stroma.[1] In addition, in cases where corneal edema precludes LPI, iridoplasty and pupilloplasty may still be feasible as these procedures do not require as much visibility. In a case series of 27 eyes of 23 patients that evaluated combined iridoplasty and pupilloplasty in patients with medically unresponsive acute angle-closure glaucoma, combined laser iridoplasty and pupilloplasty was successful in 20 eyes at lowering IOP within 6 hours.[2] Overall, the IOP was lowered from approximately 52 mmHg to 38 mmHg at 1 hour, 28 mmHg at 2 hours, and 20 mmHg at 6 hours.[2]

Technique

There have been different argon laser settings described to perform laser pupilloplasty. A topical numbing agent such as proparacaine 0.5% is used, and a laser contact lens (*e.g.*, Abraham lens) is applied. Ritch recommended 200-μm spot size, 0.5 seconds duration, and 200 mW power.[1] Zhou *et al.* described laser settings of 280–380-μm spot size, 0.2–0.25 seconds duration, and 260–320 mW power.[2] Laser is applied near the margin of the pupil to target the pupillary sphincter muscle. A smaller spot size is desirable because larger diameter laser burns might encompass some of the pupillary aperture. A higher power than that used for iridoplasty was also described as desirable as the iris is thicker at the sphincter than in the periphery.[1] Not all patients require extensive treatment to get the desired peaked pupil; Zhou *et al.* proposed 4–6 spots being placed in one area to achieve pupil peaking,[2] while Ritch illustrated 15 spots.[1] In addition to the pupil peaking and pulling away from the lens surface at the area of treatment, aqueous humor flow can be directly observed as well. Over time, the iris configuration may become flatter.

Complications

Additional sequelae of treatment include deformation of the pupil, pupillary thinning, and poor response to light, although some of these may be due to simultaneous iridoplasty.[2] Corneal epithelial and endothelial injuries may also occur.[2] In some cases, the procedure may fail to lower the IOP if aqueous humor flow from the posterior towards the anterior chamber cannot be established. This can occur in cases with high lens vault, where the lens and iris have a larger area of contact. Pupilloplasty may not be sufficient under those circumstances to bring the iris fully out of contact from the underlying lens to establish the aqueous pathway necessary to break the pupillary block.[2]

References

1. Ritch R. Argon laser treatment for medically unresponsive attacks of angle-closure glaucoma. Am J Ophthalmol. 1982 Aug 1;94(2):197–204. https://doi.org/10.1016/0002-9394(82)90075-7
2. Zhou W, Zhao F, Shi D, Qadri M, Jiang L, Ma L. Argon laser peripheral iridoplasty and argon laser pupilloplasty: Alternative management for medically unresponsive acute primary angle closure. J Ophthalmol. 2019 Aug 14;2019:1876912. https://doi.org/10.1155/2019/1876912

SLT: mechanisms, indications, and complications

Gus Gazzard, Augusto Azuara Blanco, Austin Nakatsuka

SLT is a laser-based intervention utilized for the management of IOP in patients with open-angle glaucoma or ocular hypertension. As a non-invasive procedure, SLT offers an effective alternative or adjunct to pharmacological therapies, with the potential to reduce dependency on long-term medications.[1]

Mechanism of action

SLT employs a frequency-doubled Q-switched Nd:YAG laser (wavelength 532 nm) that selectively targets pigmented trabecular meshwork cells through the principle of selective photothermolysis.[2] The energy delivered is absorbed by melanocytes in the TM, sparing adjacent non-pigmented cells and minimizing collateral thermal damage. This process triggers the activation of macrophages and cytokines, leading to remodeling of the extracellular matrix and enhancement of aqueous humor outflow.[3] It is theorized that less histopathological destruction is seen with SLT than argon laser trabeculoplasty due to its ability to selectively photolyse pigmented TM cells without causing collateral damage due to photocoagulation. This is thought to be due to its shorter pulse duration (3 nsec) than the thermal relaxation time of melanin (1 msec).[4,5]

There are a few theorized mechanisms of structural remodeling in SLT, since minimal structural damage directly to the TM and adjacent stuctures occurs. A rabbit model demonstrated transient increase in aqueous lipid peroxide, suggesting that SLT leads to liberation of free oxygen radicals which induce this peroxidation process.[6] Another study showed disassembly of tight junctions in Schlemm's canal cells exposed to media conditioned by lasered TM cells.[7] Other studies have demonstrated proliferative responses in inflammatory cells such as monocytes and other chemokines that lead to release of TNFα which are postulated to alter TM permeability.[8]

Indications

SLT is indicated for a variety of glaucomatous conditions. SLT is frequently recommended as a first-line therapy for POAG or ocular hypertension, particularly for patients unable or unwilling to adhere to long-term pharmacologic treatment.[9] A number of peer-reviewed studies have demonstrated the IOP-lowering efficacy of SLT in a range from 20% to 30%.[10-12] Other secondary OAG, such as pseudoexfoliative or pigmentary glaucoma, have been demonstrated to respond even better to SLT than POAG, due to greater numbers of melanocytic cells in the TM.[13] However, it should be noted that in heavily pigmented eyes, there can be a paradoxical and persistent rise in IOP.

In regard to angle-closure glaucoma, SLT is typically not considered a first-line treatment as the pathophysiology of the disease runs directly opposed to the anatomical considerations in OAG. In angle closure, the iris or parts of the iris are blocking the aqueous humor from accessing the TM. SLT requires direct application of laser energy to the TM in order to be efficacious. However, it sometimes becomes possible to apply SLT to the TM after angle-closure treatments such as LPI or surgical methods such as CLE. Some studies have shown efficacy of adjunct SLT being effective in further lowering IOP after these procedures.[14-16] In fact, some studies have shown an IOP reduction of up to 30%.[16-17] Kurysheva *et al.* postulated, based on the work of Sihota *et al.* showing similar histological changes in the TM in both chronic PACG and POAG using electron microscopy, that SLT should be an equally effective treatment in either of these diseases.[17-18]

Chang and authors compared the outcome of SLT between POAG and pseudophakic PACG patients receiving maximal medical therapy and found the 1-year efficacy of SLT was equivalent. In fact, SLT was found to be more effective in eyes with PACG than eyes with POAG when focusing on those with a lower baseline IOP.[19] Another study looked at the efficacy of SLT in PAC and PACG eyes with previous LPI compared to POAG eyes and also found equivalent safety and efficacy.[20]

Techniques/methods

SLT is typically performed in an outpatient setting and requires minimal preparation and recovery time.

- <u>Pre-procedure preparation</u>: Patients are administered topical anesthesia and pre-procedural IOP-lowering medications (*e.g.*, apraclonidine or brimonidine) to reduce the risk of post-procedural IOP spikes.
- <u>Laser delivery</u>: A goniolens is used to visualize the TM. The laser is applied at 50–100 evenly spaced non-overlapping locations along 180° or 360° of the TM. Each pulse delivers approximately 0.4–1.2 mJ of energy. Clinically, the energy level used for SLT is titrated according to the appearance of microbubbles in the angle. There is evidence to support cell death occurring at the energy threshold needed for microbubble formation.[2]
- <u>Post-procedure care</u>: Anti-inflammatory medications, typically corticosteroids or nonsteroidal anti-inflammatory drugs, are prescribed to manage mild anterior chamber inflammation. Follow-up visits are scheduled to monitor IOP response and potential complications.[2]

Complications

Although SLT is associated with a favorable safety profile, certain complications may arise, necessitating careful patient monitoring and management. One of the most common of these is a transient IOP elevation. A temporary rise in IOP occurs in up to 20% of cases, usually within the first 1–2 hours post-treatment. This is attributed to the release of pigment and debris into the aqueous humor. IOP-lowering medications can mitigate this risk.[21-23] Mild anterior uveitis is another common complication, characterized by trace to 1+ cells and flare. This typically resolves within a few days to weeks with topical anti-inflammatory therapy.[7] Rarely, corneal edema may develop due to energy dispersion or pre-existing endothelial dysfunction. This complication is usually self-limiting.[24] Minimal bleeding (hyphema) in the anterior chamber is an infrequent occurrence and typically resolves spontaneously without intervention.[25-26]

SLT efficacy diminishes over time in some patients, necessitating repeat treatments. While repeat SLT is generally safe, the success rate may decline after multiple sessions. Other rare complications can include visual disturbances, such as transient blurring or halos, and rarely, systemic side effects from preoperative medications.

Conclusion

While SLT is not typically considered as a first-line treatment for chronic angle-closure glaucoma, several studies have demonstrated efficacy after initial treatment such as LPI or lens extraction. SLT may be a safe and effective adjunct treatment in the algorithm for angle closure and angle-closure glaucoma patients. However, the authors recommend that SLT should not be utilized in angle-closure glaucoma unless the trabecular meshwork structures are visible to allow safe performance of the procedure.

References

1. Kennedy JB, SooHoo JR, Kahook MY, Seibold LK. Selective Laser Trabeculoplasty: An Update. Asia Pac J Ophthalmol (Phila). 2016 Jan-Feb;5(1):63-9. https://doi.org/10.1097/APO.0000000000000175
2. Latina M.A., Sibayan S.A., Shin D.H., Noecker R.J., Marcellino G. Q-switched 532-nm Nd:YAG laser trabeculoplasty (selective laser trabeculoplasty): A multicenter, pilot, clinical study11Dr. Mark A. Latina has financial interest in this technology. Ophthalmology. 1998;105:2082-2090. https://doi.org/10.1016/S0161-6420(98)91129-0
3. Melamed S, Kottler H, Epstein DL. Selective laser trabeculoplasty: A clinical trial. Arch Ophthalmol. 2003;121(7):957-960. https://doi.org/10.1001/archopht.121.7.957

4. van Buskirk EM, Pond V, Rosenquist RC. Argon laser trabeculoplasty. Studies of mechanism of action. Ophthalmology. 1984;91:1005-1010. https://doi.org/10.1016/S0161-6420(84)34197-5
5. van Buskirk EM. Pathophysiology of laser trabeculoplasty. Surv Ophthlamol. 1989;33:264-272. https://doi.org/10.1016/0039-6257(82)90152-7
6. Guzey M, Vural H, Satici A, Karadede S, Dogan Z. Increase of free oxygen radicals in aqueous humour induced by selective Nd:YAG laser trabeculoplasty in the rabbit. Eur J Ophthalmol. 2001;11(1):47-52. https://doi.org/10.1177/112067210101100109
7. Leahy K, Sarris M, Di Girolamo N, Watson SL, et al. Investigation of corneal endothelial changes post selective laser trabeculoplasty. Invest Ophthalmol Vis Sci. 2014;55(13):6162. https://doi.org/10.1111/ceo.13172
8. Bradley JM, Anderssohn AM, Colvis CM, et al. Mediation of laser trabeculoplasty-induced matrix metalloproteinase expression by IL-1beta and TNFalpha. Invest Ophthalmol Vis Sci. 2000;41(2):422-430.
9. Gazzard G, Konstantakopoulou E, Garway-Heath D, et al. Selective Laser Trabeculoplasty versus Eye Drops for First-Line Treatment of Ocular Hypertension and Glaucoma (LiGHT): a Multicentre Randomised Controlled Trial. Lancet. 2019;393:1505-16. https://doi.org/10.1016/S0140-6736(18)32213-X
10. Gracner T. Intraocular pressure response of capsular glaucoma and primary open-angle glaucoma to selective Nd:YAG laser trabeculoplasty: a prospective, comparative clinical trial. Eur J Ophthalmol. 2002;12:287-92. https://doi.org/10.1177/112067210201200406
11. Lai JS, Chua JK, Tham CC, Lam DS. Five-year follow up of selective laser trabeculoplasty in Chinese eyes. Clin Exp Ophthalmol. 2004;91:361-5. https://doi.org/10.1111/j.1442-9071.2004.00839.x
12. Kano K, Kuwayama Y, Mizoue S, et al. Clinical results of selective laser trabeculoplasty. Nippon Ganka Gakkai Zasshi. 1999;103:612-6.
13. Ayala M, Chen E. Comparison of selective laser trabeculoplasty (SLT) in primary open angle glaucoma and pseudoexfoliation glaucoma. Clin Ophthalmol. 2011;5:1469-1473. https://doi.org/10.2147/OPTH.S25636
14. Wongwuticomjon T, Chansangpetch S, Inobhas A, Tantisevi V. Efficacy of Selective Laser Trabeculoplasty in Primary Angle-closure Glaucoma after Peripheral Iridotomy. J Curr Glaucoma Pract. 2022 May-Aug;16(2):124-127. https://doi.org/10.5005/jp-journals-10078-1377
15. Ho CL, Lai JS, Aquino MV, et al. Selective laser trabeculoplasty for primary angle closure with persistently elevated intraocular pressure after iridotomy. J Glaucoma. 2009 Sep;18(7):563-6. https://doi.org/10.1097/IJG.0b013e318193c2d1
16. Narayanaswamy A, Leung CK, Istiantoro DV, et al. Efficacy of Selective Laser Trabeculoplasty in Primary Angle-Closure Glaucoma: A Randomized Clinical Trial. JAMA Ophthalmol. 2015;133(2):206-212. https://doi.org/10.1001/jamaophthalmol.2014.4893
17. Kurysheva NI, Lepeshkina LV. Selective Laser Trabeculoplasty Protects Glaucoma Progres-

sion in the Initial Primary Open-Angle Glaucoma and Angle-Closure Glaucoma after Laser Peripheral Iridotomy in the Long Term. Biomed Res Int. 2019 Dec 21;2019:4519412. https://doi.org/10.1155/2019/4519412

18. Sihota R, Goyal A, Gupta V, Kaur J, Nag T. Scanning electron microscopy of the trabecular meshwork: understanding the pathogenesis of primary angle closure glaucoma. Indian J Ophthalmol. 2012;60(3):183-188. https://doi.org/10.4103/0301-4738.95868
19. Chang PY, Wang JY, Wang JK, Huang TL, Hsu YR. Comparison of Treatment Outcomes of Selective Laser Trabeculoplasty for Primary Open-Angle Glaucoma and Pseudophakic Primary Angle-Closure Glaucoma Receiving Maximal Medical Therapy. J Clin Med. 2021 Jun 28;10(13):2853. https://doi.org/10.3390/jcm10132853
20. Ali Aljasim L, Owaidhah O, Edward DP. Selective Laser Trabeculoplasty in Primary Angle-closure Glaucoma After Laser Peripheral Iridotomy: A Case-Control Study. J Glaucoma. 2016 Mar;25(3):e253-8. https://doi.org/10.1097/IJG.0000000000000282
21. Latina MA, de Leon JM. Selective laser trabeculoplasty. Ophthalmol Clin North Am. 2005;18(3):409-419. https://doi.org/10.1016/j.ohc.2005.05.005
22. Francis BA, Hong B, Winarko J, Kawji S. Repeatability of selective laser trabeculoplasty for open-angle glaucoma. Ophthalmology. 2005;112(12):2047-2053.
23. Barkana Y, Belkin M. Selective Laser Trabeculoplasty. Surv Ophthalmol. 2007;52:634-654. https://doi.org/10.1016/j.survophthal.2007.08.014
24. Moubayed SP, Hamid M, Choremis J, Li G. An unusual finding of corneal edema complicating selective laser trabeculoplasty. Can J Ophthalmol. 2009;44:337-38 https://doi.org/10.3129/i09-025
25. Rhee DJ, Krad O, Pasquale LR. Hyphema following selective laser trabeculoplasty. Ophtalmic Surg Lasers Imaging. 2009;40:493-4. https://doi.org/10.3928/15428877-20090901-09
26. Shihadeh WA, Ritch R, Liebmann JM. Hyphema occurring during selective laser trabeculoplasty. Ophthalmic Surg Lasers Imaging. 2006;37(5):432-3. https://doi.org/10.3928/15428877-20060901-14

Future directions

Jeff Liebmann, Mineo Ozaki, Miriam Kolko

The future of angle-closure glaucoma management is evolving, driven by a range of pivotal studies that explore various treatment strategies and offer valuable insights into personalized care for patients with this condition.[1]

Precision care of angle-closure disease

The EAGLE study, published in 2016, clearly demonstrated that lens extraction outperforms LPI in reducing IOP and enhancing quality of life for PACG patients above 50 years of age, establishing lens extraction as a viable or even preferred treatment for early-stage PACG. However, as we look ahead, the role of lens extraction in combination with other treatments for more advanced stages of the disease remains an area for further exploration.[2,3] The 2023 study *Predictors of Long-term Intraocular Pressure Control After Lens Extraction in Primary Angle-Closure Glaucoma* offers additional insights, revealing that patients who undergo CLE are significantly more likely to maintain stable, drop-free IOP control compared to those receiving LPI. This highlights CLE as a promising treatment, especially for those in the early stages of PACG. However, factors such as non-Chinese ethnicity, higher baseline IOP, and prior glaucoma medication use were found to be predictors of less favorable long-term IOP outcomes, emphasizing the importance of personalized treatment strategies moving forward.[4] Finally, the *Ten-Year Clinical Outcomes of Acute Primary Angle-Closure* study, published in 2021, offered a critical perspective on APAC cases. This research demonstrated that early phacoemulsification significantly outperformed initial LPI, yielding better clinical outcomes, such as reduced reliance on medication, fewer PAS, and a lower incidence of blindness.[5] These findings reinforce lens extraction as the preferred intervention for acute angle-closure scenarios, addressing both the immediate and long-term challenges associated with APAC.

Looking ahead, lens extraction continues to establish its importance in managing angle-closure glaucoma, yet its role in advanced cases remains less clear, particularly when combined with other surgical interventions, such as trabeculectomy. Further studies are needed to delineate these scenarios. In addition, as research deepens, understanding how factors such as ethnicity, baseline IOP, and treatment history impact long-term outcomes will be essential for tailoring strategies to improve patient care comprehensively.

While the shift towards CLE has gained significant momentum, more studies have investigated the clinical benefits of LPI. In this context, ANA-LIS, published in 2022, followed asymptomatic narrow-angle patients for 5 years and found that while LPI reduced the incidence of angle-closure events, the overall rate of progression was low.[6] This highlights the need for a more selective, targeted approach to prophylactic treatment, suggesting that LPI should be reserved for higher-risk patients who are more likely to develop ACG.

Similarly, the ZAP study and its extended follow-up, published in 2019,[7] as well as the *Laser Peripheral Iridotomy for the Prevention of Angle Closure* trial,[8] provide novel insights on the role of prophylactic LPI in managing PACS. The ZAP study's 14-year follow-up highlights that while LPI significantly reduces the incidence of PAC by two-thirds, the overall risk of progression in a community-based PACS population remains relatively low. This suggests that while LPI is effective in lowering risk, its universal application in all PACS cases may not be necessary, particularly in populations with a low baseline risk of progression. The study also underscores the need to identify additional risk factors beyond IOP and anterior chamber parameters, such as IOP elevation after dark room prone provocative testing, to enhance the precision of predicting PAC development and guiding intervention.[7] The *Laser Peripheral Iridotomy for the Prevention of Angle Closure* trial similarly cautions against widespread prophylactic use of LPI. The findings indicate that LPI does not offer significant advantages in reducing angle-closure progression for asymptomatic individuals with no elevated IOP or related symptoms. This further emphasizes the importance of a more targeted approach, reserving LPI for individuals at higher risk of PAC or PACG development.[8]

One potential advantage of LPI is its minimal effect on cataract progression. A study by Chang *et al.*, published in 2023, on cataract progression after LPI found no significant increase in cataract formation in PACS eyes after LPI, suggesting that the procedure might not significantly exacerbate cataract progression, unlike other surgical interventions. This could make LPI an appealing option for certain patients with PACS who do not yet have advanced cataracts.[9]

Overall, these recent landmark studies underline the importance of tailoring treatment strategies to the individual patient, carefully weighing the risks and benefits of each intervention based on factors such as baseline IOP, symptom severity, and progression risk. Although CLE is increasingly favored for its long-term effectiveness, LPI, however, still holds value, but its application must be selective and evidence-driven. In this context, The *Anatomic Changes and Predictors of Angle Widening after Laser Peripheral Iridotomy* study, published in 2021, sheds light on the significance of laser technique, showing that superior LPI is more effective than temporal LPI in widening the angle. This finding highlights that, when considering LPI as a treatment option, the location of the procedure should be carefully considered to optimize outcomes.[10]

In terms of diagnostic approaches, the *Darkroom Prone Provocative Testing* study, published in 2019, demonstrated that this test could not reliably differentiate the risk of angle-closure between PACS and individuals with open angles.

This suggests that while provocative testing can be useful in certain clinical situations, it is not sufficient as a standalone test for determining the risk of angle closure, and clinicians should rely on a more comprehensive diagnostic approach.[11] Therefore, further work establishing clinical tests that help identify high-risk cases of angle closure is needed.

Novel treatments for angle closure-disease

In the past decade, no significant new studies have emerged regarding eye drop treatments for angle-closure glaucoma. As a result, prostaglandin analogs remain the first-line choice for pharmacologic management.[12] However, as we look to the future, it will be essential to explore innovative alternatives and refine our understanding of adjunct therapies that could optimize outcomes. With evolving treatment landscapes, ongoing research could reveal more personalized options, particularly as we better understand the long-term effects and response variations across diverse patient populations.

In contrast to the lack of recent studies on eye drops, newer treatments such as SLT and MIGS are gaining traction in the management of angle-closure glaucoma. The 2024 study by Raj *et al.* highlighted SLT's long-term efficacy in controlling IOP post-LPI, reinforcing its potential in managing PACG.[13] Similarly, Wongwuticomjon *et al.* found SLT effective in reducing IOP after LPI in a study published in 2022,[14] and Kurysheva and Lepeshkina published a study in 2019 reporting that SLT protected against glaucoma progression in patients with PACG.[15] Finally, Aljasim *et al.* published a study in 2016, in which they concluded that SLT could benefit PACG patients post-LPI.[16]

The use of MIGS in PACG is still largely experimental, with limited published data and no official approval for this specific indication. Studies such as those by Chansangpetch *et al.*, published in 2018,[17] and Hernstadt *et al.*, published in 2019,[18] have explored the combination of cataract surgery with trabecular microbypass stents such as the iStent in angle-closure glaucoma patients, showing promising results in terms of IOP reduction and medication reduction. These approaches have particularly benefited patients who have undergone laser iridotomy but still face elevated IOP.

Despite these encouraging findings, challenges remain due to the anatomy of ACG, where the iris may obstruct the TM, complicating the effectiveness of MIGS devices like trabecular microbypass stents or other surgical options aimed at improving drainage. Surgeons should therefore take special care to ensure that stent outlets are not obstructed by the iris, a potential complication that could hinder long-term IOP control.

Overall, while MIGS techniques show potential for angle-closure glaucoma, further research is needed to establish their efficacy and safety in this specific patient population. The procedure is not yet standardized for angle closure and remains experimental.

Drug-induced angle closure

In addition to the aforementioned advancements in ACG management, there is growing recognition of drug-induced ACG as an important factor in both diagnosis and treatment. A recent study, *Blind Spots in Therapy: Unveiling Drug-Induced Angle-Closure Glaucoma Through a National Analysis*, published in 2024, highlighted how commonly prescribed medications, such as topiramate, along with lesser-known drugs such as olanzapine, phentermine, and ranibizumab, can induce ACG.[19] This underlines the necessity for clinicians to be vigilant in recognizing and managing potential drug-induced cases of ACG. Awareness of the effects of these drugs is critical in ensuring appropriate treatment and preventing exacerbation of angle-closure conditions. As the understanding of drug-induced glaucoma continues to evolve, clinicians will need to factor this into their treatment plans, particularly in patients with a history of ACG or those at risk.

Novel risk-stratification strategies

GRS are increasingly being recognized as valuable tools in the management of PACG. Incorporating genetic information into clinical decision-making could help identify patients who are at a higher genetic risk for developing more severe forms of PACG, enabling more tailored and proactive interventions. For example, a study by Liu *et al.*, published in 2021, identified significant genetic susceptibility loci associated with severe PACG, particularly the *EPDR1* gene, which was found to predispose individuals to more aggressive disease development. Their findings suggest that individuals with a higher GRS may be at greater risk of experiencing severe PACG, potentially guiding clinicians to monitor these patients more closely or initiate earlier, more aggressive treatments to prevent progression.[20] In a study published in 2022, Sekimitsu *et al.* demonstrated the utility of GRS in identifying individuals at higher risk for PACG, with their study also exploring how the interaction between genetic factors and environmental influences, such as the use of psychotropic medications, may impact PACG diagnosis. This highlights the potential of GRS not only in risk assessment but also in understanding how external factors may modify disease risk in genetically predisposed individuals.[21]

However, integrating genetic data into clinical practice remains a work in progress. A study by Nongpiur *et al.* published in 2019 showed that while genetic data is significant on its own, its inclusion alongside biometric data, such as ACD, provides only marginal improvement in PACG detection.[22] As research continues to refine genetic markers and their predictive power, it is likely that GRS will become an integral part of decision-making, helping to personalize treatment strategies and improve patient outcomes in ACG management.

Conclusion

In conclusion, the management of ACG is set for transformative progress, underpinned by continuous research and the development of personalized treatment approaches. While lens extraction remains integral in early-stage ACG, combining it with additional interventions, particularly for advanced cases, is an area ripe for further exploration. The incorporation of GRS into clinical practice holds promise for refining risk assessments and enabling earlier interventions tailored to individual patient profiles.

Despite the decline in the use of LPI, its safety profile suggests it may still have a role in certain situations, while newer treatments like SLT and MIGS are emerging but require more rigorous validation for their specific use in angle closure. Moving forward, the focus must be on refining personalized treatment strategies that consider ethnic and genetic diversity, ensuring that approaches are both effective and safe for each patient.

To fully harness these advancements, future research must bridge gaps in ethnic representation, with more studies needed across non-Asian populations. Such efforts will help move the field from a generalized model of care to one that addresses the unique characteristics of each individual, ensuring optimal outcomes for ACG patients globally.

References

1. Jayaram H, Kolko M, Friedman DS, Gazzard G. Glaucoma: now and beyond. Lancet. 2023 Nov 11;402(10414):1788-1801. https://doi.org/10.1016/S0140-6736(23)01289-8
2. Azuara-Blanco A, Burr J, Ramsay C, et al. Effectiveness of early lens extraction for the treatment of primary angle-closure glaucoma (EAGLE): a randomised controlled trial. Lancet. 2016 Oct 1;388(10052):1389-1397. https://doi.org/10.1016/S0140-6736(16)30956-4
3. Tanner L, Gazzard G, Nolan WP, Foster PJ. Has the EAGLE landed for the use of clear lens extraction in angle-closure glaucoma? And how should primary angle-closure suspects be treated? Eye (Lond). 2020 Jan;34(1):40-50. https://doi.org/10.1038/s41433-019-0634-5
4. Mitchell WG, Azuara-Blanco A, Foster PJ, Halawa O, Burr J, Ramsay CR, Cooper D, Cochran C, Norrie J, Friedman D, Chang D. Predictors of long-term intraocular pressure control after

lens extraction in primary angle closure glaucoma: results from the EAGLE trial. Br J Ophthalmol. 2023 Aug;107(8):1072-1078. https://doi.org/10.1136/bjophthalmol-2021-319765

5. Chan PP, Tang FY, Leung DY, Lam TC, Baig N, Tham CC. Ten-Year Clinical Outcomes of Acute Primary Angle Closure Randomized to Receive Early Phacoemulsification Versus Laser Peripheral Iridotomy. J Glaucoma. 2021 Apr 1;30(4):332-339. https://doi.org/10.1097/IJG.0000000000001799
6. Baskaran M, Kumar RS, Friedman DS, et al. The Singapore Asymptomatic Narrow Angles Laser Iridotomy Study: Five-Year Results of a Randomized Controlled Trial. Ophthalmology. 2022 Feb;129(2):147-158. https://doi.org/10.1016/j.ophtha.2021.08.017
7. Yuan Y, Wang W, Xiong R, et al. Fourteen-Year Outcome of Angle-Closure Prevention with Laser Iridotomy in the Zhongshan Angle-Closure Prevention Study: Extended Follow-up of a Randomized Controlled Trial. Ophthalmology. 2023 Aug;130(8):786-794. https://doi.org/10.1016/j.ophtha.2023.03.024. Epub 2023 Apr 6. Erratum in: Ophthalmology. 2024 Jan;131(1):126. https://doi.org/10.1016/j.ophtha.2023.10.029
8. He M, Jiang Y, Huang S, Chang DS, Munoz B, Aung T, Foster PJ, Friedman DS. Laser peripheral iridotomy for the prevention of angle closure: a single-centre, randomised controlled trial. Lancet. 2019 Apr 20;393(10181):1609-1618. https://doi.org/10.1016/S0140-6736(18)32607-2
9. Chang DS, Jiang Y, Kim JA, Huang S, Munoz B, Aung T, He M, Foster PJ, Friedman D. Cataract progression after Nd:YAG laser iridotomy in primary angle-closure suspect eyes. Br J Ophthalmol. 2023 Sep;107(9):1264-1268. https://doi.org/10.1136/bjophthalmol-2021-320929
10. Xu BY, Friedman DS, Foster PJ, et al. Anatomic Changes and Predictors of Angle Widening after Laser Peripheral Iridotomy: The Zhongshan Angle Closure Prevention Trial. Ophthalmology. 2021 Aug;128(8):1161-1168. https://doi.org/10.1016/j.ophtha.2021.01.021
11. Friedman DS, Chang DS, Jiang Y, Huang S, Kong X, Munoz B, Aung T, Foster PJ, He M. Darkroom prone provocative testing in primary angle closure suspects and those with open angles. Br J Ophthalmol. 2019 Dec;103(12):1834-1839. https://doi.org/10.1136/bjophthalmol-2018-313362
12. Aung T, Wong HT, Yip CC, Leong JY, Chan YH, Chew PT. Comparison of the intraocular pressure-lowering effect of latanoprost and timolol in patients with chronic angle closure glaucoma: a preliminary study. Ophthalmology. 2000 Jun;107(6):1178-83. https://doi.org/10.1016/s0161-6420(00)00073-7
13. Raj S, Thattaruthody F, Yadav D, et al. Long-Term Efficacy of Selective Laser Trabeculoplasty in Primary Angle-Closure Disease After Laser Peripheral Iridotomy. Semin Ophthalmol. 2024 Apr;39(3):235-241. https://doi.org/10.1080/08820538.2024.2312946
14. Wongwuticomjon T, Chansangpetch S, Inobhas A, Tantisevi V. Efficacy of Selective Laser Trabeculoplasty in Primary Angle-closure Glaucoma after Peripheral Iridotomy. J Curr Glaucoma Pract. 2022 May-Aug;16(2):124-127. https://doi.org/10.5005/jp-journals-10078-1377
15. Kurysheva NI, Lepeshkina LV. Selective Laser Trabeculoplasty Protects Glaucoma Progres-

sion in the Initial Primary Open-Angle Glaucoma and Angle-Closure Glaucoma after Laser Peripheral Iridotomy in the Long Term. Biomed Res Int. 2019;2019:4519412.

16. Ali Aljasim L, Owaidhah O, Edward DP. Selective Laser Trabeculoplasty in Primary Angle-closure Glaucoma After Laser Peripheral Iridotomy: A Case-Control Study. J Glaucoma. 2016 Mar;25(3):e253-8. https://doi.org/10.1097/IJG.0000000000000282
17. Chansangpetch S, Lau K, Perez CI, Nguyen N, Porco TC, Lin SC. Efficacy of Cataract Surgery With Trabecular Microbypass Stent Implantation in Combined-Mechanism Angle Closure Glaucoma Patients. Am J Ophthalmol. 2018 Nov;195:191-198. https://doi.org/10.1016/j.ajo.2018.08.003
18. Hernstadt DJ, Cheng J, Htoon HM, Sangtam T, Thomas A, Sng CCA. Case Series of Combined iStent Implantation and Phacoemulsification in Eyes with Primary Angle Closure Disease: One-Year Outcomes. Adv Ther. 2019 Apr;36(4):976-986. https://doi.org/10.1007/s12325-019-00899-5
19. Aftab OM, Khan H, Khouri AS. Blind Spots in Therapy: Unveiling Drug-Induced Angle-Closure Glaucoma Through a National Analysis. Ophthalmol Glaucoma. 2024 Sep-Oct;7(5):485-490. https://doi.org/10.1016/j.ogla.2024.04.006. Epub 2024 Apr 27. Erratum in: Ophthalmol Glaucoma. 2025 May-Jun;8(3):326. https://doi.org/10.1016/j.ogla.2025.01.003
20. Liu C, Nongpiur ME, Cheng CY, Khor CC, Yu M, Husain R, Ho CL, Wong TT, Boey PY, Perera S, Wong TY, Vithana EN, Aung T. Evaluation of Primary Angle-Closure Glaucoma Susceptibility Loci for Estimating Angle Closure Disease Severity. Ophthalmology. 2021 Mar;128(3):403-409. https://doi.org/10.1016/j.ophtha.2020.07.027
21. Sekimitsu S, Wang J, Elze T, Segrè AV, Wiggs JL, Zebardast N. Interaction of background genetic risk, psychotropic medications, and primary angle closure glaucoma in the UK Biobank. PLoS One. 2022 Jun 28;17(6):e0270530. https://doi.org/10.1371/journal.pone.0270530
22. Nongpiur ME, Khor CC, Cheng CY, et al. Integration of Genetic and Biometric Risk Factors for Detection of Primary Angle Closure Glaucoma. Am J Ophthalmol. 2019 Dec;208:160-165. https://doi.org/10.1016/j.ajo.2019.07.022

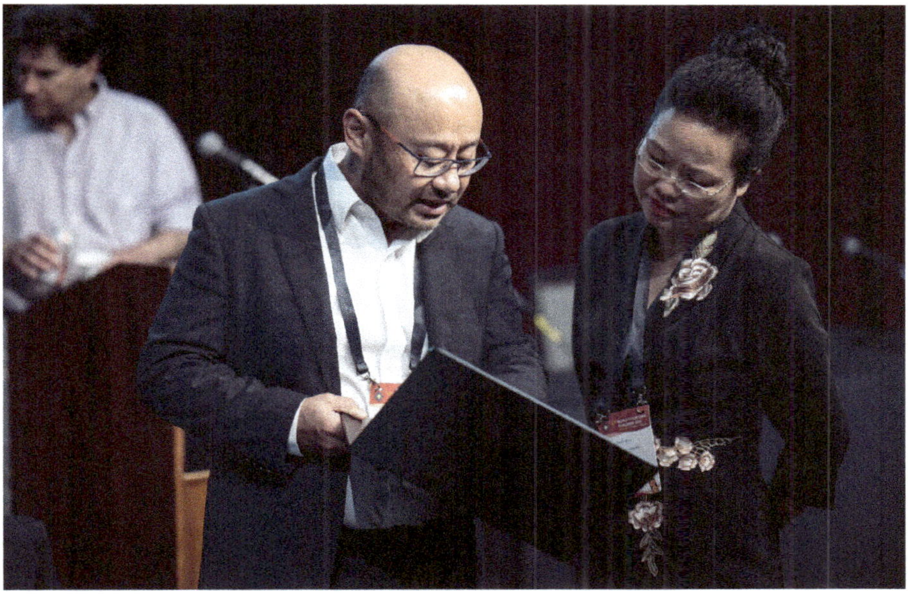

Lisandro Sakata and Xiulan Zhang

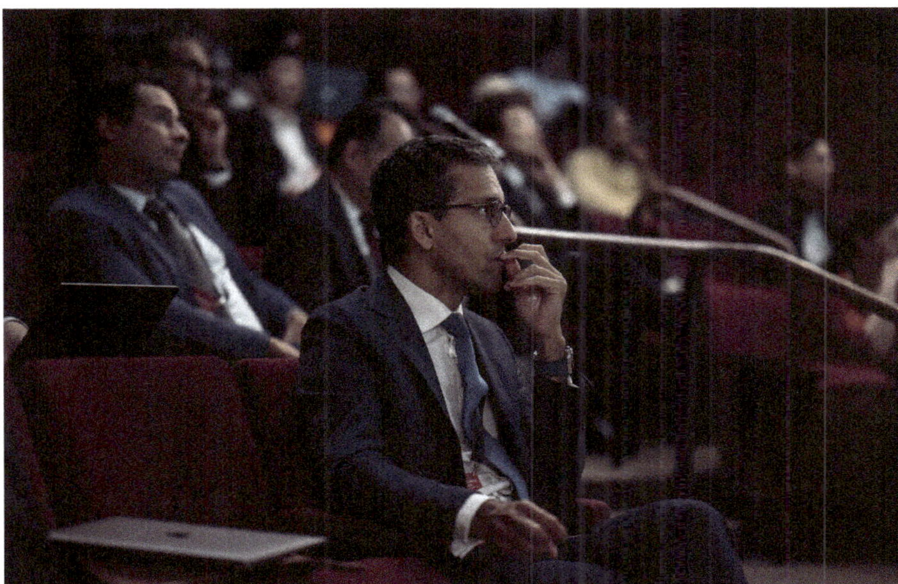

Kaweh Mansouri

Section Leaders

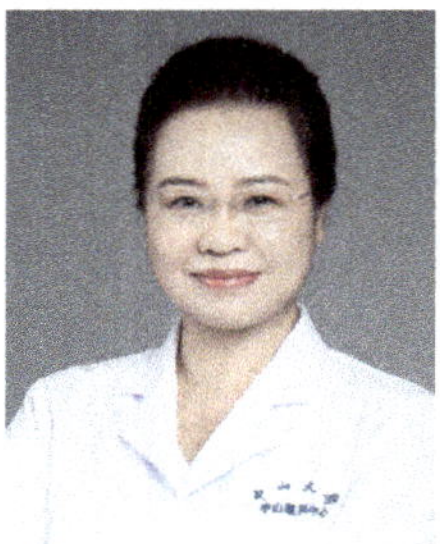

Xiuan Zhang

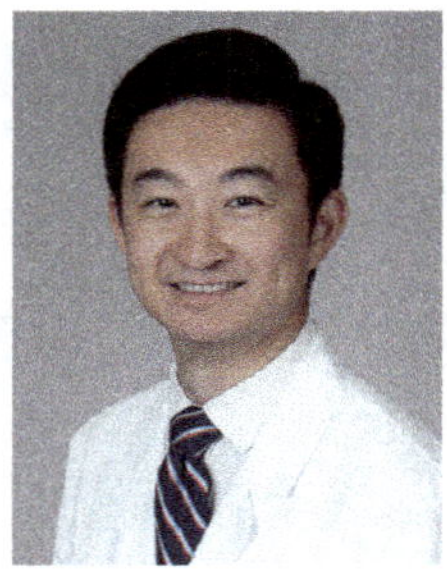

Benjamikn Xu

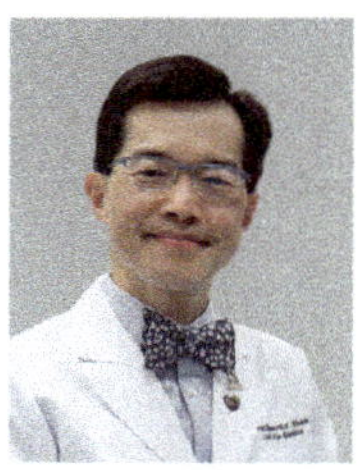

Clement Tham

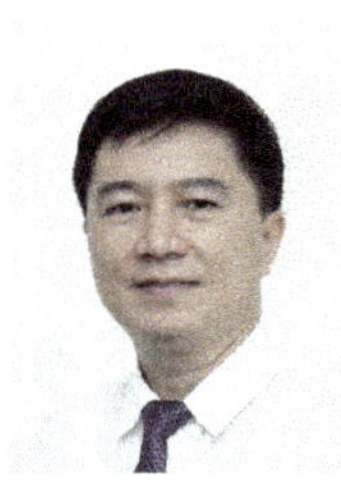

Do Tan

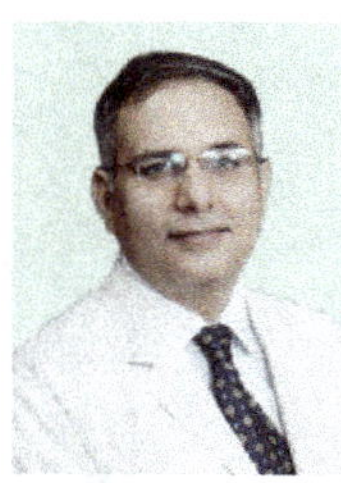

Tanuj Dada

5. SURGICAL MANAGEMENT

Xiulan Zhang, Benjamin Xu, Clement Tham, Tanuj Dada, Do Tan

Abbreviations

AC: anterior chamber
ACG: angle-closure glaucoma
ACD: angle-closure disease
APAC: acute primary angle closure
CB: ciliary body
CLE: clear lens extraction
EAGLE: Effectiveness of Early Lens Extraction for the Treatment of Primary Angle-Closure Glaucoma Trial
ECP: endoscopic cyclophotocoagulation
FDA: Food and Drug Administration
GDD: glaucoma drainage device
GSL: goniosynechiolysis
GT: goniotomy
IOL: intraocular lens
IOP: intraocular pressure
ITC: iridotrabecular contact
LPI: laser peripheral iridotomy
MIGS: minimally invasive glaucoma surgery
MMC mitomycin C
MP-TLT: micropulse laser trans-scleral laser therapy
OAG: open-angle glaucoma
OCT: optical coherence tomography
OVD: ophthalmic viscosurgical devices
PAC: primary angle closure
PACD: primary angle-closure disease
PACG: primary angle-closure glaucoma
PAS: peripheral anterior synechiae
Phaco: phacoemulsification
RCT: randomized controlled trial

Angle Closure and Angle-Closure Glaucoma, pp 1-19
Edited by Robert N. Weinreb, Benjamin Xu, Xiulan Zhang

SC: Schlemm's canal
SPI: surgical peripheral iridectomy
TM: trabecular meshwork
UCP: ultrasound cycloplasty

Consensus statements

1. Lens extraction can lead to significant reduction in IOP and medication burden in PACD.
    - Lens extraction can effectively lower IOP regardless of whether the glaucoma is controlled or uncontrolled preoperatively.
    - Lens extraction alone may not achieve target IOP or medication-free control in those with poorly controlled PACG and advanced disease.
    - Glaucoma surgery (*e.g.*, trabeculectomy, MIGS) at the time of lens extraction may be indicated to achieve IOP control, particularly when the glaucoma is moderate to severe.
    - Lens extraction can alter visual field and OCT results, necessitating a new baseline for subsequent glaucoma monitoring.
2. Lens extraction is an option as a first-line treatment for PACG and PAC with raised IOP (EAGLE trial).
    - Lens extraction demonstrated superior effectiveness in lowering IOP, medication needs, the rate of subsequent glaucoma surgeries, and was associated with better quality of life score compared to standard care with LPI and topical medications.
    - Phaco with IOL placement in the capsular bag is the recommended method of lens extraction.
    - If Phaco is not available, the benefits and risks of the available surgical techniques must be carefully evaluated.
3. There are inconclusive data on the benefit of Phaco + GSL for better IOP lowering as compared to Phaco alone in patients with PACG, cataract, and PAS.
    - Evidence is inconclusive that Phaco + GSL is superior to Phaco alone in terms of IOP control, reduction of PAS, and the need for medications.
4. Combining Phaco with GSL and MIGS, including goniotomy, may be more effective than Phaco alone in reducing IOP in patients with PACG.
    - Data are limited on the types of MIGS and the specific stages of PACD appropriate for this treatment.

- Some MIGS devices are off-label for use in PACD.
- GSL may need to be performed to access the TM.
- Phaco with GSL and goniotomy (phacogoniotomy) can be a viable option for IOP reduction in patients with PACG and cataract.
- One RCT reported similar cumulative rates of surgical success between phacogoniotomy and phacotrabeculectomy in advanced PACG eyes.

5. Trabeculectomy alone can provide effective IOP lowering in PACG eyes, particularly in the pseudophakic eye.
   - In the phakic eye, trabeculectomy promotes cataract progression and there is an increased risk of shallow AC and iris incarceration in the sclerectomy.
   - Subsequent cataract surgery can increase the risk of bleb scarring.
6. Combining Phaco with trabeculectomy (phacotrabeculectomy).
   - Phacotrabeculectomy is a viable option for PACG eyes.
   - Phacotrabeculectomy addresses the underlying issue of a crowded AC or a bulky lens and reduces the risk of further shallowing of the AC.
7. GDD implantation is typically reserved for PACG eyes at higher risk for failure and/or complications than with other interventions or for those patients who have unsuccessful outcomes with other IOP-lowering surgeries.
   - Combined Phaco and GDD implantation can be considered in eyes with significant cataract or very shallow AC due to a thick crystalline lens.
8. Cycloablation is an alternative treatment for the management of PACG.
   - Results are variable and treatment often needs to be repeated.
   - It may be particularly useful when the patient wishes to avoid the risks of incisional surgery or is not systemically fit for or unable to access the operating room.
   - Large prospective RCTs on the use of cycloablation for PACG are needed.
   - ECP combined with Phaco may provide greater IOP lowering than Phaco alone.

Surgical management

Xiulan Zhang, Tanuj Dada

In addition to medication and laser treatment, surgical intervention is a primary method for managing PAC/PACG. Historically, trabeculectomy has been a mainstay in the treatment of PACG. However, it carries an increased risk of potential complications, especially in phakic PACG eyes and is currently not preferred as the initial surgical option in many cases. In the last 2 decades, the popularization of Phaco with early lens extraction marked a paradigm shift in the surgical treatment of PACG. Currently, with the advancement of MIGS techniques, the combination of Phaco, GSL, and MIGS after holds great promise in the treatment of PACG. There is a paucity of long-term studies on Phaco-MIGS and this approach in PACG is not yet fully explored and adopted across the globe. However, there is no doubt that the landscape of surgical treatment of PACG is changing with the introduction of surgical innovations.

Lens extraction in the surgical management of primary angle-closure glaucoma

Noel Chan, Jolly Tsui, Clement Tham

Lens extraction has become safer with the popularization of Phaco,[1] and it is effective in reducing IOP and the need for IOP-lowering medications, especially in eyes with PACD. Depending on disease severity and control, Phaco with or without concomitant glaucoma surgeries may be indicated. This section reviews the current evidence on the indications, mechanisms, and efficacy of lens extraction in PACG. Complications and postoperative management are also explored.

Indications for lens extraction in PACG

Visual function and lens status

Extraction of visually significant cataract can improve visual function and vision-related quality of life even in those with advanced glaucoma.[2-5] Clearing of the visual axis may also improve the accuracy of visual field assessment and optic nerve monitoring. Even for PACG without visually significant cataract, studies have found that lens extraction can help maintain good visual acuity and function by correcting of hypermetropia and lowering IOP,[6] medications, and need for subsequent glaucoma interventions.[7]

Persistence or progression of angle closure and PAS

Aging-related increases in ITC and angle crowding from progressive lenticular enlargement irrespective of lens status exacerbate both pupillary block and appositional angle closure.[8,9] Even though LPI has long been the first-line treatment for PACG, angles in up to 58% of eyes with patent iridotomies remained closed due to unaddressed non-pupillary block mechanisms.[10,11] As lens extraction targets a different pathophysiology in PACG by eliminating lens-related mechanisms and further widening the AC angle, eyes with persistent or progression in angle closure may benefit from the procedure.[12,13]

Poorly controlled disease or poor intolerance/compliance to medications

In eyes that fail to meet target IOP and show recent glaucomatous progression despite maximally tolerated medical treatment, surgical intervention should be considered. Based on disease status and patient preference, Phaco alone or combined with other glaucoma surgeries may be considered to achieve complete or qualified success.

In preparation for other intraocular glaucoma surgeries

Development of opacities will accelerate after initial glaucoma procedures secondary to the combination of aging, surgical manipulation, and postoperative steroid use. Performing lens extraction prior to other intraocular glaucoma surgeries eliminates the risk of subsequent cataract progression and therefore prevents progressive angle crowding and the need for future lens extraction, which can potentially further jeopardize the drainage function established previously.[14]

Mechanism of action of lens extraction in PACG

PACG is a glaucomatous optic neuropathy with an untreated IOP of > 21 mmHg due to occlusion of the TM by the peripheral iris, defined as the presence of ≥ 180° ITC on gonioscopy.[15] Apart from pupillary block, non-pupillary block mechanisms of angle closure are also important in PACG and these include angle crowding from plateau iris, thick peripheral iris rolls, or innately abnormally thick and anteriorly positioned lenses that grow with age.[7,16]

Multiple studies have found that lens extraction may potentially reverse the underlying pathophysiology in PACG by deepening the AC, reopening the appositionally closed parts of the angle, and modifying iris configuration.[12,17] These anatomical alterations may prevent pupillary block and lead to enhanced aqueous drainage through the TM, thereby improving postoperative IOP control. However, IOP lowering can be observed in eyes with different types of glaucoma, and not all PACG eyes can achieve satisfactory IOP reduction after lens extraction alone.[18-20] The exact underlying mechanism for its IOP-lowering effect in PACG remains unclear. Apart from the anatomical changes in angle configuration, other possible hypotheses include tissue meshwork extracellular matrix remodeling and reduction of TM pigment.[21,22]

Prospective longitudinal studies that systematically investigate factors affecting the degree and duration of IOP reduction after lens extraction are still lacking but potential prognostic factors include higher preoperative IOP,[19,23-26] shallower central AC, greater lens vault,[23,27-29] and longer ITC length.[26]

Efficacy of lens extraction in PACG

Among the different types of glaucoma, lens extraction provides the most significant IOP-lowering effect in eyes affected by PACG.[8,9,12,18,25,29-32] Regardless of the level of preoperative medical control, PACG eyes with visually significant cataract may benefit from Phaco alone, which is associated with reductions in IOP and medication burden.[33-35] Studies have also shown reduced IOP fluctuations after lens extraction.[3,36] A recent meta-analysis summarizing the efficacy of Phaco for PACG with optically significant cataract identified a reduction of postoperative IOP by ≥ 3 mmHg and ≥ 5 mmHg in 19% and 1% of those with medically controlled disease, respectively,[20,25] while in medically uncontrolled disease, the percentages increased to 65% and 53%, respectively.[25] However, for patients with moderate to severe glaucoma who need greater IOP and medication reduction or drop-free control, combined cataract surgery with trabeculectomy, cyclophotocoagulation or MIGS may be considered, balancing against the increased risks of operative complications and cost-effectiveness.[20,34,37-50] Phaco alone may not be sufficient to effectively control IOP, especially when there are PAS after lens extraction, as demonstrated by the significant IOP reduction achieved by gonioscopy-assisted GSL and goniotomy procedures following Phaco in advanced PACG cases.[37-45] Details will be covered in other sections.

Despite improved safety with the evolution of lens extraction, removal of optically clear lenses as a treatment for PACG was not widely accepted until recently. The first RCT that investigated the efficacy and safety of CLE versus trabeculectomy was conducted by Tham *et al.*[51] Although trabeculectomy was associated with lower medication requirements at postoperative 24 months, CLE alone resulted in a similar reduction of IOP with significantly fewer complications. The superiority of CLE over conventional treatment was further delineated in the pivotal EAGLE trial published in 2016.[7] This multicenter international RCT involved 419 patients with either PACG or newly diagnosed PAC with IOP > 30 mmHg. In comparison to standard treatment with LPI and topical medications, eyes randomized to receive CLE had lower mean IOP (1.18 mmHg lower), glaucoma medication burden, and rate of subsequent trabeculectomy

(0.5% vs 2.8%). At postoperative 36 months, 61% and 21% of the patients attained medication-free control in the CLE and standard care groups, respectively, an outcome that was 10 times more likely with initial CLE.[52] Chinese ethnicity and initial drop-free status were predictors for optimal IOP response to CLE over the postoperative 36 months. Differences in the rate of visual field progression were however, not found. In terms of visual function, visual acuity, and vision-related quality of life scores were better in those who received CLE compared to standard care, likely due to the reduced need of glaucoma medications and surgery, improved visual quality, and the correction of refractive error, allowing the patients to be spectacle-free postoperatively. A separate analysis on the CLE group in the EAGLE cohort confirmed the significantly reduced refractive error but reported suboptimal refractive predictability, with 59% and 85% of the eyes within ± 0.5 D and ± 1.0 D of target refraction, respectively.[53] No serious adverse events were reported in both groups of treatment. Based on a subgroup of 179 patients recruited from United Kingdom centers, economic analysis favored CLE, which was again demonstrated in another secondary analysis showing higher quality-adjusted life years with CLE, even though the initial service costs were higher.[54] In the setting of their healthcare system, CLE would be cost-effective by 3 years and cost-saving by 10 years after the procedure.

While lens extraction was previously mainly performed for visual rehabilitation, these studies provided strong evidence for its cost-effectiveness and IOP lowering. Therefore, lens extraction has been recently advocated as a first-line treatment in PACG and should be considered earlier even in the absence of visually significant cataract. However, it is important to note that the EAGLE trial included a specific cohort of patients aged 50 years or older (to lessen the effect of loss of accommodation from CLE with mild to moderate PACG), hence limiting generalizability of the study results. The benefit of CLE in advanced and medically controlled PACG with patent LPI or good accommodative function will need to be confirmed in long-term prospective clinical trials.

Phaco with IOL implantation in the capsular bag is the recommended method of lens extraction. If Phaco is not available, the risks and benefits of the available surgical techniques must be carefully evaluated before implementation in these eyes.

Complications of Phaco in PACG

Even though lens extraction has been shown to be effective in treating PACG, the procedure can be technically challenging in PACG eyes. It should be performed by experienced surgeons to minimize inherent risks, such as posterior capsular rupture, zonular dehiscence, and malignant glaucoma, to justify this management choice, especially for those with advanced disease or otherwise good vision in the absence of cataract.

Small or atonic pupils can complicate lens extraction and are often encountered in PACG eyes that require miotic agents for control or with a history of acute angle-closure attack. Preoperatively, it is crucial to withhold any miotic agents and ensure adequate pharmacological pupil dilatation. Intraoperatively, posterior synechiae should be lysed with OVD and further pupil enlargement may be achieved by intracameral injection of dilating agents or mechanical stretching with hooks or expansion devices. Postoperatively, anti-inflammatory agents should be prescribed to control any ocular inflammation from iris manipulation to prevent intense ocular inflammation and cystoid macular oedema.

One of the most common complications even after uneventful lens extraction is an IOP spike, which is more frequently observed in glaucomatous eyes and has been reported in 1%–5% of those with PACG.[7,19,23,55-57] Those with advanced disease are particularly at risk of the wipe-out phenomenon from intra- and post-operative IOP spikes. Extra care should therefore be taken to optimize preoperative IOP control, minimize intraoperative AC fluctuations, maintain minimal bottle height, avoid retention of OVD, and control the immediate postoperative IOP with prophylactic topical and/or systemic glaucoma medications.[55,58 59]

Although loss of corneal endothelial cells is common after Phaco even in normal eyes,[60-62] it is likely exacerbated in PACG due to the closer proximity between the Phaco probe and the endothelium in eyes with shallow AC.[63] Incidence of corneal edema after lens extraction in PACG ranged from 0.5% to 9.5% in different studies.[7,57,64] To avoid corneal decompensation, endothelial cell count can be evaluated preoperatively for risk stratification, especially in those with history of acute angle closure,[65] and the endothelium should be protected with OVD while applying minimal Phaco energy and minimizing intraocular manipulations. Other complications include prolonged AC inflammation, which was observed in 2% to 16% of PACG eyes that underwent Phaco.[7,24,30,57] Refractive surprise is another complication that can significantly affect the patients' daily activities, particularly in those with preoperative 20/20 vision who undergo CLE.[66]

Management of PACG after lens extraction

Depending on disease severity and postoperative IOP response, clinicians should re-titrate glaucoma medications against target IOP after lens extraction with the aim to reduce medication burden. Apart from IOP-lowering effects, numerous studies have revealed significant changes in visual field,[2,4,67,68] OCT, and scanning laser polarimetry results of the retinal nerve fiber layer and the ganglion cell complex after extraction of optically significant cataract.[69-72] Therefore, new baseline examinations after lens extraction are recommended to allow accurate monitoring of any PACG progression.

Comments

While lens extraction is associated with significant reduction in IOP and medication needs in PACG with or without cataract, concomitant glaucoma surgeries should be considered in those with advanced or poorly controlled disease. Currently, there is limited evidence for CLE in advanced PACG, medically controlled PACG with patent LPI, and patients with good accommodative function. Predictive factors for IOP reduction after lens extraction also need to be further studied.

References

1. Davis G. The Evolution of Cataract Surgery. Mo Med 2016;113(1):58-62.
2. Bhandari S, Pandyal I, Khanal SP, Thapa SS. Effect of phacoemulsification surgery on various parameters in patients with glaucoma. Nepal J Ophthalmol. 2014;6(11):46-55. https://doi.org/10.3126/nepjoph.v6i1.10772
3. Özyol P, Özyol E, Sül S, et al. Intra-ocular pressure fluctuation after cataract surgery in primary angle-closure glaucoma eyes medically controlled after laser iridotomy. Acta Ophthalmol. 2016;94(7):e528-e33. https://doi.org/10.1111/aos.13023
4. Musch DC, Gillespie BW, et al. Cataract extraction in the collaborative initial glaucoma treatment study: incidence, risk factors, and the effect of cataract progression and extraction on clinical and quality-of-life outcomes. Arch Ophthalmol. 2006;124(12):1694-700. https://doi.org/10.1001/archopht.124.12.1694
5. Xu X, Sun Q, Ma YY, Zou HD. Vision-related Quality of Life Outcomes of Cataract Surgery in Advanced Glaucoma Patients. J Glaucoma. 2016;25(1):e5-11. https://doi.org/10.1097/IJG.0000000000000299
6. Shen L, Melles RB, Metlapally R, et al. The Association of Refractive Error with Glaucoma in a Multiethnic Population. Ophthalmology. 2016;123(1):92-101. https://doi.org/10.1016/j.ophtha.2015.07.002
7. Azuara-Blanco A, Burr J, Ramsay C, et al. Effectiveness of early lens extraction for the treatment of primary angle-closure glaucoma (EAGLE): a randomised controlled trial. Lancet. 2016;388(10052):1389-97. https://doi.org/10.1016/S0140-6736(16)30956-4
8. Brown RH, Zhong L, Lynch MG. Lens-based glaucoma surgery: using cataract surgery to reduce intraocular pressure. J Cataract Refract Surg. 2014;40(8):1255-62. https://doi.org/10.1016/j.jcrs.2014.06.001
9. Razeghinejad MR, Myers JS. Contemporary approach to the diagnosis and management of

primary angle-closure disease. Surv Ophthalmol. 2018;63(6):754-68. https://doi.org/10.1016/j.survophthal.2018.05.001

10. Costa VP, Leung CKS, Kook MS, Lin SC. Clear lens extraction in eyes with primary angle closure and primary angle-closure glaucoma. Surv Ophthalmol. 2020;65(6):662-74. https://doi.org/10.1016/j.survophthal.2020.04.003
11. Yeung BY, Ng PW, Chiu TY, et al. Prevalence and mechanism of appositional angle closure in acute primary angle closure after iridotomy. Clin Exp Ophthalmol. 2005;33(5):478-82. https://doi.org/10.1111/j.1442-9071.2005.01065.x
12. Hayashi K, Hayashi H, Nakao F, Hayashi F. Changes in anterior chamber angle width and depth after intraocular lens implantation in eyes with glaucoma. Ophthalmology. 2000;107(4):698-703. https://doi.org/10.1016/S0161-6420(00)00007-5
13. Ong AY, Ng SM, Vedula SS, Friedman DS. Lens extraction for chronic angle-closure glaucoma. Cochrane Database Syst Rev. 2021;3(3):Cd005555. https://doi.org/10.1002/14651858.CD005555.pub3
14. Gedde SJ, Heuer DK, Parrish RK, 2nd. Review of results from the Tube Versus Trabeculectomy Study. Curr Opin Ophthalmol. 2010;21(2):123-8. https://doi.org/10.1097/ICU.0b013e3283360b68
15. European Glaucoma Society Terminology and Guidelines for Glaucoma, 5th Edition. Br J Ophthalmol. 2021;105(Suppl 1):1-169. https://doi.org/10.1136/bjophthalmol-2021-egsguidelines
16. Weinreb RN, Aung T, Medeiros FA. The pathophysiology and treatment of glaucoma: a review. JAMA. 2014;311(18):1901-11. https://doi.org/10.1001/jama.2014.3192
17. Tham CC, Leung DY, Kwong YY, et al. Effects of phacoemulsification versus combined phaco-trabeculectomy on drainage angle status in primary angle closure glaucoma (PACG). J Glaucoma. 2010;19(2):119-23. https://doi.org/10.1097/IJG.0b013e31819d5d0c
18. Pasquali A, Varano L, Ungaro N, et al. Does Cataract Extraction Significantly Affect Intraocular Pressure of Glaucomatous/Hypertensive Eyes? Meta-Analysis of Literature. J Clin Med. 2024;13(2). https://doi.org/10.3390/jcm13020508
19. Chen PP, Lin SC, Junk AK, et al. The Effect of Phacoemulsification on Intraocular Pressure in Glaucoma Patients: A Report by the American Academy of Ophthalmology. Ophthalmology. 2015;122(7):1294-307. https://doi.org/10.1016/j.ophtha.2015.03.021
20. Fang Z, Song Y, Jin L, et al. Phacoemulsification combined with trabecular meshwork-Schlemm canal-based minimally invasive glaucoma surgery in primary angle-closure glaucoma: a systematic review and meta-analysis. BMC Ophthalmol. 2025;25(1):168. https://doi.org/10.1186/s12886-025-04005-y
21. Wang N, Chintala SK, Fini ME, Schuman JS. Ultrasound activates the TM ELAM-1/IL-1/NF-kappaB response: a potential mechanism for intraocular pressure reduction after phacoemulsification. Invest Ophthalmol Vis Sci. 2003;44(5):1977-81. https://doi.org/10.1167/iovs.02-0631

22. Damji KF, Konstas AG, Liebmann JM, et al. Intraocular pressure following phacoemulsification in patients with and without exfoliation syndrome: a 2-year prospective study. Br J Ophthalmol. 2006;90(8):1014-8. https://doi.org/10.1136/bjo.2006.091447
23. Liu CJ, Cheng CY, Ko YC, Lau LI. Determinants of long-term intraocular pressure after phacoemulsification in primary angle-closure glaucoma. J Glaucoma. 2011;20(9):566-70. https://doi.org/10.1097/IJG.0b013e3181efe1e9
24. Shams PN, Foster PJ. Clinical outcomes after lens extraction for visually significant cataract in eyes with primary angle closure. J Glaucoma. 2012;21(8):545-50. https://doi.org/10.1097/IJG.0b013e31821db1db
25. Masis M, Mineault PJ, Phan E, Lin SC. The role of phacoemulsification in glaucoma therapy: A systematic review and meta-analysis. Surv Ophthalmol. 2018;63(5):700-10. https://doi.org/10.1016/j.survophthal.2017.08.006
26. Selvan H, Angmo D, Tomar AS, et al. Changes in Intraocular Pressure and Angle Status After Phacoemulsification in Primary Angle Closure Hypertension. J Glaucoma. 2019;28(2):105-10. https://doi.org/10.1097/IJG.0000000000001137
27. Perez CI, Chansangpetch S, Nguyen A, et al. How to Predict Intraocular Pressure Reduction after Cataract Surgery? A Prospective Study. Curr Eye Res. 2019;44(6):623-31. https://doi.org/10.1080/02713683.2019.1580375
28. Shin HC, Subrayan V, Tajunisah I. Changes in anterior chamber depth and intraocular pressure after phacoemulsification in eyes with occludable angles. J Cataract Refract Surg. 2010;36(8):1289-95. https://doi.org/10.1016/j.jcrs.2010.02.024
29. Huang G, Gonzalez E, Lee R, et al. Association of biometric factors with anterior chamber angle widening and intraocular pressure reduction after uneventful phacoemulsification for cataract. J Cataract Refract Surg. 2012;38(1):108-16. https://doi.org/10.1016/j.jcrs.2011.06.037
30. Lam DS, Leung DY, Tham CC, et al. Randomized trial of early phacoemulsification versus peripheral iridotomy to prevent intraocular pressure rise after acute primary angle closure. Ophthalmology. 2008;115(7):1134-40. https://doi.org/10.1016/j.ophtha.2007.10.033
31. Moghimi S, Hashemian H, Chen R, et al. Early phacoemulsification in patients with acute primary angle closure. J Curr Ophthalmol. 2015;27(3-4):70-5. https://doi.org/10.1016/j.joco.2015.12.001
32. Brown RH, Zhong L, Whitman AL, et al. Reduced intraocular pressure after cataract surgery in patients with narrow angles and chronic angle-closure glaucoma. J Cataract Refract Surg. 2014;40(10):1610-4. https://doi.org/10.1016/j.jcrs.2014.01.038
33. Tham CC, Kwong YY, Leung DY, et al. Phacoemulsification versus combined phacotrabeculectomy in medically controlled chronic angle closure glaucoma with cataract. Ophthalmology. 2008;115(12):2167-73.e2. https://doi.org/10.1016/j.ophtha.2008.06.016
34. Tham CC, Kwong YY, Leung DY, et al. Phacoemulsification versus combined phacotrabeculectomy in medically uncontrolled chronic angle closure glaucoma with cataracts. Ophthal-

mology. 2009;116(4):725-31, 31.e1-3. https://doi.org/10.1016/j.ophtha.2008.12.054

35. Baig N, Kam KW, Tham CC. Managing Primary Angle Closure Glaucoma - The Role of Lens Extraction in this Era. Open Ophthalmol J. 2016;10:86-93. https://doi.org/10.2174/1874364101610010086
36. Tojo N, Otsuka M, Miyakoshi A, et al. Improvement of fluctuations of intraocular pressure after cataract surgery in primary angle closure glaucoma patients. Graefes Arch Clin Exp Ophthalmol. 2014;252(9):1463-8. https://doi.org/10.1007/s00417-014-2666-7
37. Song Y, Xie L, Zhu X, et al. Two-year outcome of phacogoniotomy for advanced primary angle-closure glaucoma with cataracts: a multicentre study. Br J Ophthalmol. 2025;109(7):770-4. https://doi.org/10.1136/bjo-2024-325375
38. Song Y, Zhang Y, Li F, et al. One-Year Results of a Multicenter Study: Intraocular Pressure-Lowering Effect of Combined Phacoemulsification, Goniosynechialysis, and Goniotomy for Cases of Advanced Primary Angle-Closure Glaucoma With Cataract. Asia Pac J Ophthalmol (Phila). 2022;11(6):529-35. https://doi.org/10.1097/APO.0000000000000579
39. Song Y, Fan S, Tang L, et al. Two-Year Outcomes of Phacogoniotomy vs Phacotrabeculectomy for Advanced Primary Angle-Closure Glaucoma With Cataract: A Noninferiority Randomized Clinical Trial. JAMA Ophthalmol. 2025;143(6):462-9. https://doi.org/10.1001/jamaophthalmol.2025.0685
40. Song Y, Lin F, Lv A, et al. Phacogoniotomy versus phacotrabeculectomy for advanced primary angle-closure glaucoma with cataract: A randomized non-inferiority trial. Asia Pac J Ophthalmol (Phila). 2024;13(1):100033. https://doi.org/10.1016/j.apjo.2023.100033
41. Lin F, Zhang Y, Zhu X, et al. Impact of Peripheral Anterior Synechiae on the Outcome of Combined Phacoemulsification, Goniosynechialysis, and Goniotomy for Primary Angle Closure Glaucoma and Cataract: A Multicenter Observational Study. J Glaucoma. 2024;33(8):587-93. https://doi.org/10.1097/IJG.0000000000002435
42. Dorairaj S, Tam MD, Balasubramani GK. Two-Year Clinical Outcomes of Combined Phacoemulsification, Goniosynechialysis, and Excisional Goniotomy For Angle-Closure Glaucoma. Asia Pac J Ophthalmol (Phila). 2020;10(2):183-7. https://doi.org/10.1097/APO.0000000000000321
43. Gupta S, Sethi A, Yadav S, et al. Safety and efficacy of incisional goniotomy as an adjunct with phacoemulsification in primary angle-closure glaucoma. J Cataract Refract Surg. 2021;47(4):504-11. https://doi.org/10.1097/j.jcrs.0000000000000481
44. Tanito M, Sugihara K, Tsutsui A, et al. Midterm Results of Microhook ab Interno Trabeculotomy in Initial 560 Eyes with Glaucoma. J Clin Med. 2021;10(4). https://doi.org/10.3390/jcm10040814
45. Song Y, Zhang H, Zhang Y, et al. Minimally Invasive Glaucoma Surgery in Primary Angle-Closure Glaucoma. Asia Pac J Ophthalmol (Phila). 2022;11(5):460-9. https://doi.org/10.1097/APO.0000000000000561
46. El Sayed YM, Elhusseiny AM, Albalkini AS, et al. Mitomycin C-augmented Phacotrabeculec-

tomy Versus Phacoemulsification in Primary Angle-closure Glaucoma: A Randomized Controlled Study. J Glaucoma. 2019;28(10):911-5. https://doi.org/10.1097/IJG.0000000000001345

47. Tham CC, Leung DY, Kwong YY, et al. Factors correlating with failure to control intraocular pressure in primary angle-closure glaucoma eyes with coexisting cataract treated by phacoemulsification or combined phacotrabeculectomy. Asia Pac J Ophthalmol (Phila). 2015;4(1):56-9. https://doi.org/10.1097/APO.0000000000000091
48. Lai ISW, Chan NCY, Ling A, et al. Combined Phacoemulsification-Endoscopic Cyclophotocoagulation versus Phacoemulsification Alone in Primary Angle-Closure Glaucoma: A Pilot Randomized Controlled Trial. Ophthalmol Glaucoma. 2021;4(6):589-96. https://doi.org/10.1016/j.ogla.2021.03.007
49. Hansapinyo L, Choy BNK, Lai JSM, Tham CC. Phacoemulsification Versus Phacotrabeculectomy in Primary Angle-closure Glaucoma With Cataract: Long-Term Clinical Outcomes. J Glaucoma. 2020;29(1):15-23. https://doi.org/10.1097/IJG.0000000000001397
50. Chan PP, Li EY, Tsoi KKF, et al. Cost-effectiveness of Phacoemulsification Versus Combined Phacotrabeculectomy for Treating Primary Angle Closure Glaucoma. J Glaucoma. 2017;26(10):911-22. https://doi.org/10.1097/IJG.0000000000000772
51. Sangtam T. Phacoemulsification versus trabeculectomy in medically uncontrolled chronic angle-closure glaucoma without cataract. Ophthalmology. 2013;120(7):e45. https://doi.org/10.1016/j.ophtha.2013.03.007
52. Mitchell WG, Azuara-Blanco A, Foster PJ, et al. Predictors of long-term intraocular pressure control after lens extraction in primary angle closure glaucoma: results from the EAGLE trial. Br J Ophthalmol. 2023;107(8):1072-8. https://doi.org/10.1136/bjophthalmol-2021-319765
53. Day AC, Cooper D, Burr J, et al. Clear lens extraction for the management of primary angle closure glaucoma: surgical technique and refractive outcomes in the EAGLE cohort. Br J Ophthalmol. 2018;102(12):1658-62. https://doi.org/10.1136/bjophthalmol-2017-311447
54. Javanbakht M, Azuara-Blanco A, Burr JM, et al. Early lens extraction with intraocular lens implantation for the treatment of primary angle closure glaucoma: an economic evaluation based on data from the EAGLE trial. BMJ Open. 2017;7(1):e013254. https://doi.org/10.1136/bmjopen-2016-013254
55. Levkovitch-Verbin H, Habot-Wilner Z, Burla N, et al. Intraocular pressure elevation within the first 24 hours after cataract surgery in patients with glaucoma or exfoliation syndrome. Ophthalmology. 2008;115(1):104-8. https://doi.org/10.1016/j.ophtha.2007.03.058
56. Husain R, Gazzard G, Aung T, et al. Initial management of acute primary angle closure: a randomized trial comparing phacoemulsification with laser peripheral iridotomy. Ophthalmology. 2012;119(11):2274-81. https://doi.org/10.1016/j.ophtha.2012.06.015
57. Zhang ZM, Niu Q, Nie Y, Zhang J. Reduction of intraocular pressure and improvement of vision after cataract surgeries in angle closure glaucoma with concomitant cataract patients. Int J Clin Exp Med. 2015;8(9):16557-63.

58. Holm JL, Bach-Holm D, Holm LM, Vestergaard AH. Prophylactic treatment of intraocular pressure elevation after uncomplicated cataract surgery in nonglaucomatous eyes - a systematic review. Acta Ophthalmol. 2019;97(6):545-57. https://doi.org/10.1111/aos.14092

59. Hayashi K, Yoshida M, Manabe SI, Yoshimura K. Prophylactic Effect of Oral Acetazolamide against Intraocular Pressure Elevation after Cataract Surgery in Eyes with Glaucoma. Ophthalmology. 2017;124(5):701-8. https://doi.org/10.1016/j.ophtha.2016.12.027

60. Bourne WM, Nelson LR, Hodge DO. Continued endothelial cell loss ten years after lens implantation. Ophthalmology .1994;101(6):1014-22; discussion 22-3. https://doi.org/10.1016/S0161-6420(94)31224-3

61. Liesegang TJ, Bourne WM, Ilstrup DM. Short- and long-term endothelial cell loss associated with cataract extraction and intraocular lens implantation. Am J Ophthalmol. 1984;97(1):32-9. https://doi.org/10.1016/0002-9394(84)90442-2

62. Traverso CE. Clear-lens extraction as a treatment for primary angle closure. Lancet. 2016;388(10052):1352-4. https://doi.org/10.1016/S0140-6736(16)31746-9

63. Kubota T, Toguri I, Onizuka N, Matsuura T. Phacoemulsification and intraocular lens implantation for angle closure glaucoma after the relief of pupillary block. Ophthalmologica. 2003;217(5):325-8. https://doi.org/10.1159/000071346

64. Lai JS, Tham CC, Chan JC. The clinical outcomes of cataract extraction by phacoemulsification in eyes with primary angle-closure glaucoma (PACG) and co-existing cataract: a prospective case series. J Glaucoma. 2006;15(1):47-52. https://doi.org/10.1097/01.ijg.0000196619.34368.0a

65. Tham CC, Kwong YY, Lai JS, Lam DS. Effect of a previous acute angle closure attack on the corneal endothelial cell density in chronic angle closure glaucoma patients. J Glaucoma. 2006;15(6):482-5. https://doi.org/10.1097/01.ijg.0000212273.73100.31

66. Khoramnia R, Auffarth G, Łabuz G, et al. Refractive Outcomes after Cataract Surgery. Diagnostics (Basel). 2022;12(2). https://doi.org/10.3390/diagnostics12020243

67. Koucheki B, Nouri-Mahdavi K, Patel G, et al. Visual field changes after cataract extraction: the AGIS experience. Am J Ophthalmol. 2004;138(6):1022-8. https://doi.org/10.1016/j.ajo.2004.08.006

68. Ang GS, Shunmugam M, Azuara-Blanco A. Effect of cataract extraction on the glaucoma progression index (GPI) in glaucoma patients. J Glaucoma. 2010;19(4):275-8. https://doi.org/10.1097/IJG.0b013e3181b21fb9

69. Mwanza JC, Bhorade AM, Sekhon N, et al. Effect of cataract and its removal on signal strength and peripapillary retinal nerve fiber layer optical coherence tomography measurements. J Glaucoma. 2011;20(1):37-43. https://doi.org/10.1097/IJG.0b013e3181ccb93b

70. Kim NR, Lee H, Lee ES, et al. Influence of cataract on time domain and spectral domain optical coherence tomography retinal nerve fiber layer measurements. J Glaucoma. 2012;21(2):116-22. https://doi.org/10.1097/IJG.0b013e31820277da

71. Dada T, Behera G, Agarwal A, et al. Effect of cataract surgery on retinal nerve fiber layer

thickness parameters using scanning laser polarimetry (GDxVCC). Indian J Ophthalmol. 2010;58(5):389-94. https://doi.org/10.4103/0301-4738.67048

72. Nakatani Y, Higashide T, Ohkubo S, et al. Effect of cataract and its removal on ganglion cell complex thickness and peripapillary retinal nerve fiber layer thickness measurements by fourier-domain optical coherence tomography. J Glaucoma. 2013;22(6):447-55. https://doi.org/10.1097/IJG.0b013e3182894a16

Goniosynechiolysis/phacoemulsification + goniosynechiolysis in the surgical management of primary angle-closure glaucoma

Dewang Angmo, Tanuj Dada

GSL

In cases of PACG with PAS, it is conceivable that IOP can be controlled by re-establishing the drainage angle and lysing of PAS with GSL.[1,2] In the absence of a visually significant cataract, GSL alone may be considered to preserve the accommodative function of the crystalline lens.

Indications

GSL is indicated in patients with PACD, including PAC, PACG, and post-acute angle-closure attack. The optimal timing for the operation is after the eye becomes quiet, typically 6 weeks after the acute attack.[3]

Contraindications

GSL is contraindicated in patients with secondary angle closure following uveitis, neovascular glaucoma, iridocorneal-endothelial syndrome, or posterior polymorphous dystrophy.

Mechanism

GSL is a surgical procedure designed to strip the PAS from the angle wall, thus restoring outflow through the TM. This procedure was first described by Shaffer in 1957,[3] and modified by Campbell and Vela in 1984 using OVD to maintain the AC.[4]

Technique

GSL is usually performed after Phaco and implantation of the IOL but prior to OVD removal. GSL should be performed under gonioscopic or endoscopic visualization. Thereafter, aspiration of the OVD is performed.

Gonioscopy-assisted GSL

GSL should be performed under the operating microscope with a surgical gonioscope. There are 2 major types of surgical gonioscopes that do not invert the image (an inverted image would make surgery next to impossible): the direct type and the double-mirrored, indirect type. The surgical settings are different between the 2 types of gonioscopes. To allow visualization during the operation under the direct-type gonioscope, the patient's head and eye should be rotated by 30°–45° away from the surgeon. Furthermore, the microscope should be tilted 30°–45° towards the surgeon, leading the angle between the ocular axis and the viewing direction to be close to 90° in total. Although the entire angular range cannot be observed, it is possible to focus on 4 clock hours (approximately 120°) of the angle. On the other hand, the double-mirrored indirect goniolens, which was reported in 2007,[5] is designed to directly observe the whole angle structure without tilting the patient's head or microscope.

Endoscopy-assisted GSL

GSL can also be performed under direct visualisation using an endoscopic probe.[6,7]

Instruments for performing GSL

GSL can be performed by injecting OVD to perform visco-dissection to release the PAS. For firm (long-standing) synechiae, separation with OVD alone is insufficient, and auxiliary separation with a blunt separator is required. Any blunt instrument or cannula can also be used for this, including Phaco choppers, microforceps, spatula, and some instruments specifically designed for GSL, such as the LAN Synechialyzer or the GSL spatula.

Results: IOP-lowering efficacy

In one of the first RCTs performed to evaluate the benefit of GSL, both Phaco and Phaco + GSL significantly lowered IOP by 26.5% and 27.8 % at 1 year, respectively, in patients with synechial PACD and cataract, and there was no significant difference in IOP outcomes or success rates.[8] In another RCT in PACG patients, adjunctive GSL did not show additional IOP-lowering effects to Phaco alone at 6 months of follow-up.[9]

Pearls and best practice

A clear, magnified and en face view of the angle structure is one of the most essential points in performing angle surgeries such as GSL or MIGS. A blind procedure can induce iatrogenic injury not only to the TM but also the nearby ocular structures, causing uncontrollable intraoperative hemorrhage or zonular/capsular damage of the lens. Pressure on the cornea can cause Descemet's folds and distortion. Ocular-surface conditions may also highly affect the visibility. When combining GSL with Phaco, GSL may be performed prior to or after cataract surgery, as per the choice of the surgeon. Performing GSL in an eye with a shallow AC requires surgical skill, but the visibility of the angle is much better before Phaco as there is no corneal edema. The use of cohesive viscoelastic and careful wound construction would avoid leakage and ease surgical manuverability.

Complications and management

Postoperative complications include a fibrinous AC reaction, an IOP spike, a limited hyphema, as well as the infrequent macular edema. A precise surgical technique, complete removal of viscoelastic, and frequent use of post-operative steroids can minimize these mild complications.

Comments

There is minimal evidence for the use of GSL alone to lower IOP in PACG. It should be performed along with Phaco lens extraction.

References

1. Tanihara H, Negi A, Akimoto M, Nagata M. Long-term results of non-filtering surgery for the treatment of primary angle-closure glaucoma. Graefes Arch Clin Exp Ophthalmol.1995;233(9):563-567. https://doi.org/10.1007/BF00404707
2. Lai JS, Tham CC, Chua JK, Lam DS. Efficacy and safety of inferior 180 degrees goniosynechialysis followed by diode laser peripheral iridoplasty in the treatment of chronic angle-closure glaucoma. J Glaucoma. 2000;9(5):388-391. https://doi.org/10.1097/00061198-200010000-00007
3. Shaffer RN. Operating room gonioscopy in angle closure glaucoma surgery. Trans Am Ophthalmol Soc. 1957;55:59-66.
4. Campbell DG, Vela A. Modern goniosynechialysis for the treatment of synechial angle-closure glaucoma. Ophthalmology. 1984;91:1052-1060. https://doi.org/10.1016/S0161-6420(84)34195-1
5. Mori K, Ikushima T, Ikeda Y, et al. Double-mirror goniolens with dual viewing system for

goniosurgery. Am J Ophthalmol. 2007;143:154-155. https://doi.org/10.1016/j.ajo.2006.07.034

6. Tang W, Zhang Z, Zhang Y, Yin X, Zhang Y, Li Q. Outcomes of effective goniosynechialysis under an endoscopic view combined with phacoemulsification in residual angle-closure glaucoma with lens opacity: 6-month results. Int Ophthalmol. 2020 Dec;40(12):3529-3538. https://doi.org/10.1007/s10792-020-01541-y
7. Qian Z, Huang J, Song B, et al. Cataract Surgery (Phacoemulsification with Intraocular Lens Implantation) Combined with Endoscopic Goniosynechialysis for Advanced Primary Angle-Closure Glaucoma. Ophthalmol Glaucoma. 2021 Jul-Aug;4(4):365-372. https://doi.org/10.1016/j.ogla.2020.11.003
8. Husain R, Do T, Lai J, et al. Efficacy of Phacoemulsification Alone vs Phacoemulsification With Goniosynechialysis in Patients With Primary Angle-Closure Disease: A Randomized Clinical Trial. JAMA Ophthalmol. 2019 Oct 1;137(10):1107-1113. https://doi.org/10.1001/jamaophthalmol.2019.2493
9. Angmo D, Shakarwal J, Gupta B, et al. Comparative Evaluation of Phacoemulsification Alone versus Phacoemulsification with Goniosynechialysis in Primary Angle-Closure Glaucoma. Ophthalmol Glaucoma. 2019 Sep-Oct;2(5):346-356. https://doi.org/10.1016/j.ogla.2019.05.004

Phaco + GSL

In the presence of a visually significant cataract, GSL can be combined with cataract extraction surgery.[1-3] Combined Phaco and GSL reduces circumferential ITC area more than Phaco alone.[4] While Phaco alone may reduce IOP, it is thought that in some cases Phaco + GSL may help further reduce IOP to a level needed for glaucoma control. However, the IOP-lowering effects of Phaco + GSL surgery may not differ significantly from those of Phaco alone in medically controlled PACG patients with visually significant cataract.[5]

Retrospective studies on Phaco + GSL

In a retrospective study on efficacy and safety of Phaco + GSL in advanced PACG with severe visual field loss, Qian *et al.* concluded that Phaco + GSL appeared safe and effective in treating advanced PACG cases with central or temporal field islands. However, caution is warranted when considering patients at high wipe-out risk or those with high expectations for visual outcomes.[6]

In a retrospective case series, Wu *et al.* concluded that Phaco + GSL is a safe and effective surgical management strategy for patients with refractory APAC and high IOP.[7] In their retrospective study about the efficacy of combined Phaco + GSL in PACG with different degrees of PAS (PAS < 180° and PAS > 180°), Wei *et al.* concluded that Phaco + GSL for the treatment of PACD showed equally effective IOP control regardless of the extent of preoperative PAS.[8]

A retrospective study of survival rate in surgical management of PACG showed that Phaco alone had a low survival rate of 13% at the 60-month follow-up whereas Phaco + GSL achieved the highest rate of 55%. Therefore, Phaco + GSL should be initially considered for management of PACG, since it can restore and sustain the physiologic aqueous pathway and preserve the conjunctiva for future filtering surgery if needed.[9]

RCTs on Phaco versus Phaco + GSL

In 2 RCTs of patients with synechial PACD and cataract, both Phaco and Phaco + GSL resulted in a significant decrease in IOP and number of medications at 1 year. However, Phaco + GSL did not result in additional IOP lowering compared to Phaco alone.[10,11]

In an RCT on AC angle evaluation by AS-OCT, the AC angle in eyes with PACG opened and widened significantly after Phaco + GSL as compared to the Phaco alone group.[12] However, in a RCT by Angmo *et al.*, a significant reduction in the ITC contact area using swept-source OCT was found in both the Phaco + GSL and Phaco alone groups.[11] Tun *et al.* noted that Phaco + GSL surgery resulted in a greater reduction in circumferential ITC area than Phaco alone.[4]

An RCT on aqueous outflow facility after Phaco with or without GSL in PAC by Rodrigues *et al.* noted that both groups had similar and good outcomes at 12 months. However, only eyes undergoing Phaco + GSL showed increased tonographic aqueous outflow, reduced glaucoma medication dependence, and reduced PAS postoperatively. GSL should therefore be considered in such patients.[13]

Studies on endoscopic Phaco + GSL

Two retrospective case series on Phaco with endoscopic GSL for PACG and advanced PACG concluded it to be an effective and safe surgical method.[2,3] However, both studies had limited follow-up.[14,15]

Studies on Phaco + GSL versus phacotrabeculectomy

In a multicenter RCT comparing the safety and efficacy of Phaco + GSL and phacotrabeculectomy, both were found to be effective in treating medically unresponsive cases of acute PACG with cataracts. However, Phaco + GSL showed better visual outcomes, wider drainage angles post-surgery, and fewer complications than phacotrabeculectomy.[16] Similar results were noted in 2 retrospective studies documenting the comparison of long-term effects following Phaco + GSL and trabeculectomy in PACG.[17,18]

Meta-analyses

A global meta-analysis based on RCTs on Phaco with or without GSL for PACG concluded there was low to moderate quality evidence that Phaco + GSL leads to an equivalent IOP-lowering effect.[19] The Phaco + GSL surgery may not help reduce long-term dependence on antiglaucoma eyedrops. A recent network meta-analysis of RCTs on the efficacy and safety of different types of IOP-lowering surgeries in PACG noted that Phaco + GSL (−1.73 [95% CI: −3.53 to −0.13]) provided better IOP-lowering effect than Phaco alone (−0.46 [95% CI: −0.79 to −0.13]).[20] In another meta-analysis, Liu *et al.* concluded that Phaco + GSL might be an optimal procedure to treat ACG with concomitant cataract due to its bleb-less nature, and its capacity for lowering IOP seemed superior to Phaco alone and comparable to phacotrabeculectomy.[21] In a meta-analysis of RCTs, Yu *et al.* showed that Phaco + GSL provides advantages over standalone Phaco treatment in PAS reduction. In terms of IOP and medication reduction, both groups were comparable. Thus, Phaco + GSL can be considered for the treatment of patients with ACG and cataract due to its ease, safety, and potential benefit for the AC angle.[22] A meta-analysis by Yao *et al.* showed that Phaco + GSL could result in significant reduction in IOP (mean difference, 1.81; $p = 0.002$) compared to Phaco alone.[23] In the subgroup where GSL was performed with an instrument, better reduction of IOP was shown in the Phaco + GSL group (mean difference, 2.11; $p = 0.02$). In the viscogonioplasty subgroup, there was no statistical difference between either (mean difference, 1.53; $p = 0.11$).[23]

Extent of GSL

Phaco combined with 120° of GSL has been shown to be effective in lowering IOP in PACG patients irrespective of the degree of PAS.[24] Although there are no studies comparing differences in efficacy with varying degrees of GSL, the above study suggested that 120° GSL may be the preferred extent as it was effective in lowering IOP in eyes even with 360° PAS while not requiring additional incisions or changes in surgeon positioning.[24]

Comments

Combined Phaco and GSL surgery can be considered when there are clinical indications to lower IOP in eyes with PAC, PACG, or post-acute angle-closure attack. The success of the procedure depends on the duration and recurrence of the synechia, and Phaco + GSL has been shown to be safe and effective procedure for lowering IOP, decreasing the need for medications and reducing the risk of synechial reformation. It is also an essential part of surgery to remove iridotrabecular adhesions when additional angle-based MIGS must be performed in PACG, which will be illustrated in other sections.

References

1. Teekhasaenee C, Ritch R. Combined phacoemulsification and goniosynechialysis for uncontrolled chronic angle-closure glaucoma after acute angle-closure glaucoma. Ophthalmology.1999;106(4):669-674. https://doi.org/10.1016/S0161-6420(99)90149-5
2. Lai JS, Tham CC, Lam DS. The efficacy and safety of combined phacoemulsification, intraocular lens implantation, and limited goniosynechialysis, followed by diode laser peripheral iridoplasty, in the treatment of cataract and chronic angle-closure glaucoma. J Glaucoma.2001;10(4):309-315. https://doi.org/10.1097/00061198-200108000-00011
3. Zhao XJ, Yang XX, Fan YP, Li BH, Li Q. Comparison of combined phacoemulsification, intraocular lens implantation, and goniosynechialysis with phacotrabeculectomy in the treatment of primary angle-closure glaucoma and cataract. Asia Pac J Ophthalmol (Phila). 2013;2(5):286-290. https://doi.org/10.1097/APO.0b013e318299df62
4. Tun TA, Baskaran M, Perera SA, Htoon HM, Aung T, Husain R. Swept-source optical coherence tomography assessment of iris-trabecular contact after phacoemulsification with or without goniosynechialysis in eyes with primary angle closure glaucoma. Br J Ophthalmol. 2015;99(7):927-931. https://doi.org/10.1136/bjophthalmol-2014-306223
5. Lee CK, Rho SS, Sung GJ, et al. Effect of goniosynechialysis during phacoemulsification on IOP in patients with medically well-controlled chronic angle-closure glaucoma. J Glaucoma.2015;24(6):405-409. https://doi.org/10.1097/IJG.0000000000000043
6. Qian Z, Pan W, Nie L, Lin L, Wei L. Efficacy and Safety of Phaco-Goniosynechialysis in Advanced Primary Angle-Closure Glaucoma with Severe Visual Field Loss. J Glaucoma. 2024 Aug 5. https://doi.org/10.1097/IJG.0000000000002474
7. Wu X, Liu X, Xiao S, et al. Efficacy and safety of primary customized phacoemulsification combined with goniosynechialysis for refractory acute primary angle closure. Int Ophthalmol. 2023 Dec;43(12):4515-4525. https://doi.org/10.1007/s10792-023-02852-6
8. Wei L, Fu L, Nie L, et al. Efficacy of combined phacoemulsification and goniosynechialysis in primary angle closure disease with different degrees of peripheral anterior synechiae. J Glaucoma. 2022 Jul 1;31(7):540-546. https://doi.org/10.1097/IJG.0000000000002050
9. Wanichwecharungruang B, Phumratprapin C, Kongsomboon K, Seresirikachorn K. Real-world Surgical Outcomes of Primary Angle-closure Glaucoma. Clin Ophthalmol. 2021 Jun 29;15:2823-2833. https://doi.org/10.2147/OPTH.S315747
10. Husain R, Do T, Lai J, et al. Efficacy of Phacoemulsification Alone vs Phacoemulsification With Goniosynechialysis in Patients With Primary Angle-Closure Disease: A Randomized Clinical Trial. JAMA Ophthalmol. 2019 Oct 1;137(10):1107-1113. https://doi.org/10.1001/jamaophthalmol.2019.2493

11. Angmo D, Shakarwal J, Gupta B, et al. Comparative Evaluation of Phacoemulsification Alone versus Phacoemulsification with Goniosynechialysis in Primary Angle-Closure Glaucoma. Ophthalmol Glaucoma. 2019 Sep-Oct;2(5):346-356. https://doi.org/10.1016/j.ogla.2019.05.004
12. Shao T, Hong J, Xu J, Le Q, Wang J, Qian S. Anterior Chamber Angle Assessment by Anterior-segment Optical Coherence Tomography After Phacoemulsification With or Without Goniosynechialysis in Patients With Primary Angle Closure Glaucoma. J Glaucoma. 2015 Dec;24(9):647-55. https://doi.org/10.1097/IJG.0000000000000061
13. Rodrigues IA, Alaghband P, Beltran Agullo L, et al. Aqueous outflow facility after phacoemulsification with or without goniosynechialysis in primary angle closure: a randomised controlled study. Br J Ophthalmol. 2017 Jul;101(7):879-885. https://doi.org/10.1136/bjophthalmol-2016-309556
14. Tang W, Zhang Z, Zhang Y, Yin X, Zhang Y, Li Q. Outcomes of effective goniosynechialysis under an endoscopic view combined with phacoemulsification in residual angle-closure glaucoma with lens opacity: 6-month results. Int Ophthalmol. 2020 Dec;40(12):3529-3538. https://doi.org/10.1007/s10792-020-01541-y
15. Qian Z, Huang J, Song B, et al. Cataract Surgery (Phacoemulsification with Intraocular Lens Implantation) Combined with Endoscopic Goniosynechialysis for Advanced Primary Angle-Closure Glaucoma. Ophthalmol Glaucoma. 2021 Jul-Aug;4(4):365-372. https://doi.org/10.1016/j.ogla.2020.11.003
16. Xuan HN, Dinh NN, Thu HN, et al. Comparing the Safety and Efficacy of Phacogoniosynechialysis with Phacotrabeculectomy in the Management of Refractory Acute Primary Closure Angle Glaucoma with Cataract: A Multicenter Randomized Trial. J Glaucoma 2021;30:552-558. https://doi.org/10.1097/IJG.0000000000001868
17. Zhang Y, Cheng G, Chen Y, et al. Comparison of long-term effects following phacoemulsification combined with goniosynechialysis and trabeculectomy in patients with primary angle-closure glaucoma and cataract. Ophthalmol Ther. 2024 Jan;13(1):423-434. https://doi.org/10.1007/s40123-023-00823-9
18. Zhao J, Zhang C, Pazo EE, et al. Phaco-goniosynechialysis versus phaco-trabeculectomy in patients with refractory primary angle-closure glaucoma: a comparative study. BMC Ophthalmol. 2023 Apr 6;23(1):144. https://doi.org/10.1186/s12886-023-02885-6
19. Wang N, Jia SB. Phacoemulsification with or without goniosynechialysis for angle-closure glaucoma: a global Meta-analysis based on randomized controlled trials. Int J Ophthalmol. 2019 May 18;12(5):826-833. https://doi.org/10.18240/ijo.2019.05.20
20. Sener H, Gulmez Sevim D, Evereklioglu C, et al. Efficacy and safety of different types of intraocular pressure-lowering surgeries in patients with Primary Angle Closure (PAC) or PAC Glaucoma: Systematic Review and Network Meta-Analysis of Randomized Clinical Trials. Semin Ophthalmol. 2024 Jan;39(1):17-26. https://doi.org/10.1080/08820538.2023.2223292
21. Liu Y, Li W, Jiu X, et al. Systematic Review and Meta-Analysis of Comparing Phacoemulsifi-

cation Combined with goniosynechialysis to other mainstream procedures in treating patients with angle-closure glaucoma. Medicine (Baltimore). 2019 Oct;98(42):e17654 https://doi.org/10.1097/MD.0000000000017654

22. Yu JG, Zhao F, Xiang Y. Phacoemulsification with Goniosynechialysis versus Phacoemulsification Alone in Angle-Closure Glaucoma: A Meta-Analysis of Randomized Controlled Trials. J Ophthalmol. 2021 Feb 15;2021:8831479. https://doi.org/10.1155/2021/8831479
23. Yao L, Wang H, Wang Y, Zhao P, Bai H. Phacoemulsification combined with goniosynechialysis versus phacoemulsification alone for patients with primary angle-closure disease: A meta-analysis. PLoS One. 2024 Feb 2;19(2):e0296849. https://doi.org/10.1371/journal.pone.0296849
24. Lin F, Zhang Y, Zhu X, et al. Impact of Peripheral Anterior Synechiae on the Outcome of Combined Phacoemulsification, Goniosynechialysis, and Goniotomy for Primary Angle Closure Glaucoma and Cataract: A Multicenter Observational Study. J Glaucoma. 2024 Aug1;33(8):587-593. https://doi.org/10.1097/IJG.0000000000002435

Phacoemulsification + goniosynechiolysis + minimally invasive glaucoma surgery in the surgical management of primary angle-closure glaucoma

Phaco ± GSL+ iStent

Bryan Ang, Benjamin Xu

The surgical management of PACG has traditionally focused on widening the angle and relieving PAS to restore aqueous outflow through the TM. Lens extraction, with and without GSL, achieves the above objectives, demonstrating good IOP-lowering effect.[1] However, long-term iridocorneal appositional disease may cause chronic damage to the TM, resulting in persistently impaired aqueous outflow and insufficient IOP lowering despite angle widening following cataract surgery.[2,3] While filtering surgeries such as trabeculectomy and glaucoma drainage device implantation have been shown to be efficacious in controlling IOP in angle-closure disease, they have risk of significant intra- and postoperative complications.

MIGS has gained widespread adoption for the treatment of OAG in recent years, demonstrating at least modest IOP-lowering efficacy and an excellent safety profile. Among MIGS devices are the iStent series (Glaukos Corporation, Laguna Hills, CA, USA), encompassing various iterations of trabecular microbypass devices placed through the TM, the major site of outflow resistance in OAG, into SC. The first-generation iStent (G1) comprises a single snorkel-shaped titanium stent. The second-generation iStent inject (G2) consists of 2 preloaded stents. Each stent has a flange that faces the AC, a head that resides in the SC, and a thorax that traverses the TM. The iStent inject W, the next iteration of the iStent series, comprises stents with wider flanges, intended to provide better visualization during surgery and improved predictability of implantation.[4] Finally, the iStent infinite was introduced in 2022 and consists of 3 stents placed over at least 4 clock hours of the angle for greater access to collector channels and increased aqueous outflow.[5]

The above iterations of the iStent have been given US Food and Drug Administration approval for use in the treatment of OAG across a range of severities.[6-10] However, the iStent series is considered off-label in the treatment of ACD.[11] PAS, if present, obscures visibility of the posterior pigmented TM and precludes the implantation of iStent devices. Furthermore, the efficacy of trabecular bypass devices may be limited due to damage to the TM and SC from chronic ITC and progressive PAS, resulting in both a reduced diameter of the SC and mechanical obstruction of the SC by pigmentary granules and TM endothelial cells.[12]

Nonetheless, since its introduction into clinical practice, the iStent series, particularly the G1 and G2 iStent inject, has been used off-label in the real-world treatment of ACD, with studies reporting favorable IOP and glaucoma medication-lowering outcomes following Phaco + iStent, performed with or without GSL.[13,14]

Mechanism

The iStent series are placed through the TM to gain access to the SC. The TM is considered the major site of outflow resistance in OAG and the iStent series enhance aqueous humor outflow from the AC directly into the SC and then out to the distal outflow collector channels of the episcleral venous system. When implanted in combination with cataract surgery, particularly in ACD, the resulting IOP reduction is likely due to both the implantation of the iStent series and cataract extraction. The overall extent of IOP reduction, however, is limited by resistance in the distal outflow capacity and the episcleral venous pressure. This constraint gives rise to a floor effect in IOP reduction.

Technique

All iterations of the iStent are implanted ab-interno under intraoperative gonioscopic guidance, usually through a clear temporal corneal incision (the Phaco wound if implanted in conjunction with cataract surgery). After intracameral miotic, OVD is used to deepen the angle, the injector is advanced toward the nasal angle, and the iStent devices are placed at least 2 clock hours apart in the TM, into the SC. Proper stent placement and seating are confirmed after implantation. OVD is removed, the wound is hydrated, and the corneal incision is sealed.

While implantation of iStent devices may be performed either before or after cataract extraction, implantation in angle-closure disease may be technically easier after lens removal, which allows deepening of the shallow AC and relief of angle crowding. In eyes with PAS, GSL would need to be performed at least in the quadrant of targeted implantation, to expose the posterior pigmented TM and enable the safe implantation of the iStent devices.

Results: IOP-lowering efficacy

In a prospective interventional case series of 37 eyes that underwent Phaco+iStent with the G1 iStent for PAC and PACG, at postoperative month (POM) 12 Hernstadt *et al.* reported a mean IOP reduction of 15.4% ($p = 0.008$) from baseline medicated IOP (17.50 ± 3.82 mmHg vs 14.80 ± 3.94 mmHg), and a mean IOP reduction of 39.8% ($p < 0.001$) from baseline unmedicated post-washout IOP (24.60 ± 3.40 mmHg vs 14.80 ± 3.94 mmHg). The mean number of glaucoma medications also decreased by 90.6%, from 1.49 ± 0.77 preoperatively to 0.14 ± 0.48 postoperatively ($p < 0.001$), with 89.2% of eyes remaining medication-free at 1 year. However, the authors did not describe the presence or extent of PAS at baseline, nor reported whether GSL was performed intraoperatively.[13]

In a 2-year retrospective multicenter study comparing the efficacy of Phaco + iStent with the G2 iStent inject across different glaucoma subtypes—including 35 eyes with appositional angle-closure glaucoma or angle-closure glaucoma suspects—Clement *et al.* successfully demonstrated a mean IOP reduction of 19% ($P < 0.001$) at POM24. Comparatively, mean IOP reduction following Phaco + iStent surgery was found to be 14% in eyes with POAG, 22% in eyes with ocular hypertension, and 13% in eyes with normal-tension glaucoma. The study also demonstrated a significant decrease in the mean number of glaucoma medications in angle-closure eyes (from 1.89 medications preoperatively to 0.49 medications postoperatively, $p < 0.001$). Comparatively, in normal-tension glaucoma eyes, there was a mean reduction from 1.05 medications preoperatively to 0.40 postoperatively; in ocular hypertension eyes, from 0.74 preoperatively to none postoperatively; and in POAG eyes, from 1.58 preoperatively to 0.55 postoperatively. Eyes with synechial angle closure were excluded in this study.[15]

Although it is established that standalone Phaco results in greater IOP lowering in eyes with ACD,[16,17] comparative studies have suggested that greater IOP-lowering may be achieved when Phaco is combined with iStent implantation.

In a 1-year retrospective, matched, cohort study of 158 eyes (79 eyes per group) comparing Phaco + iStent (with two G1 iStents or the G2 iStent inject) versus standalone Phaco in eyes with PACG, Salimi *et al.* found a 27% IOP reduction following Phaco + iStent (from 17.6 ± 3.2 mmHg preoperatively to 12.9 ± 2.3 mmHg postoperatively), compared to a 13% IOP reduction following standalone Phaco (from 16.8 ± 3.1 mmHg preoperatively to 14.6 ± 2.5 mmHg postoperatively) at POM12.[14] Ninety-seven percent (vs 89% in the Phaco group) of eyes that underwent Phaco + iStent achieved an IOP of ≤ 18 mmHg, 76% (vs 43%) achieved an IOP of ≤ 15 mmHg, and 24% (vs 16%) achieved an IOP of ≤ 12 mmHg. There was also a greater reduction in IOP medications following Phaco + iStent (2.2 ± 1.2 preoperatively to 1.2 ± 1.0 postoperatively, a 46% decrease) versus standalone Phaco (1.8 ± 1.3 preoperatively to 1.6 ± 1.4 postoperatively, an 11% decrease). Glaucoma medications were maintained or reduced in 96% of eyes which underwent Phaco+iStent compared to 81% in the Phaco group. Furthermore, eyes following Phaco+iStent surgery had fewer IOP spikes postoperatively (18% in the Phaco group vs 4% in Phaco + iStent group, $p = 0.005$). In this study, GSL was performed in both the Phaco and Phaco + iStent groups if PAS was present.

A single-masked, 1-year randomized controlled trial comparing Phaco and Phaco+iStent (G1) of 32 patients with PAC or PACG was performed by Chen *et al.*[18] While no significant difference in the postoperative IOP was found between groups, there was a higher rate of complete success in the Phaco+iStent group (14 eyes, 87.5%, 95% CI: 58.6 to 96.7) compared to the standalone Phaco group (7 eyes, 43.8%, 95% CI: 19.8 to 65.6). Eyes with PAS in the nasal quadrant were excluded from the study.

Complications and management

The excellent safety profile of the iStent series has been well established in the context of OAG.[19,20] Similarly, in ACD, sight-threatening complications are rare, and the overall rates of hyphema and stent malpositioning appear to be comparable to that in OAG. Postoperative stent occlusion by the iris may be of concern, particularly in ACD, given the associated increased incidence of PAS, high iris root insertion, and decreased axial length in these eyes.[21,22] Chen *et al.* reported stent occlusion in 5 eyes (31.3%), 2 of which required further glaucoma medications at POM12.[18] Risk factors for occlusion included a thick peripheral iris root, plateau iris configuration, and postoperative PAS secondary to angle trauma during iStent insertion. Hernstadt *et al.* reported stent occlusion in 10 eyes (27%) and found an increase in the risk of iStent occlusion by 1.33 times for every 1 mmHg rise in IOP ($p = 0.009$) and by 6.21 times for every 1 mm increase in AC depth ($p = 0.013$).[13] The risk of iStent occlusion appears to be greater in eyes with angle closure compared to eyes with OAG: iStent occlusion was reported to occur in only 5 out of 116 (4%) OAG subjects in a study by Craven *et al.*[23] and in 4 out of 111 (4%) OAG subjects in another study by Samuelson *et al.*[24]

Comments

Although considered off-label for the treatment of ACD, the literature shows good surgical outcomes of Phaco + iStent with both the G1 and G2 iStent inject, with studies demonstrating reduction in both mean IOP and number of glaucoma medications that persist up to 12 to 24 months postoperatively. Comparative studies have further shown that greater IOP lowering is achieved with Phaco + iStent, compared to standalone Phaco. However, the risk of stent occlusion by the iris may be greater than in eyes with OAG. The majority of studies have reported outcomes in eyes with mild to moderate ACG, with little evidence for iStent implantation in severe disease. More consistent reporting across studies—of the extent of PAS in eyes at baseline, whether or not GSL was performed, as well as the appropriate stage of PACG for its use (whether early or advanced) —would better contextualize outcomes of the iStent series in eyes with ACD.

References

1. Chen PP, Lin SC, Junk AK, et al. The Effect of Phacoemulsification on Intraocular Pressure in Glaucoma Patients: A Report by the American Academy of Ophthalmology. Ophthalmology. 2015;122(7):1294-307. https://doi.org/10.1016/j.ophtha.2015.03.021
2. Liton PB, Gonzalez P. Stress response of the trabecular meshwork. J Glaucoma. 2008;17(5):378-85. https://doi.org/10.1097/IJG.0b013e31815f52a8
3. Tham CC, Kwong YY, Leung DY, et al. Phacoemulsification versus combined phacotrabeculectomy in medically uncontrolled chronic angle closure glaucoma with cataracts. Ophthalmology. 2009;116(4):725-31, 31.e1-3. https://doi.org/10.1016/j.ophtha.2008.12.054
4. Glaukos istent inject W. OptoHellas. (2020, June 20). Available from: https://optohellas.com/product/ophthalmology/trabecular-micro-by-pass/glaukos-istent-inject-w/
5. Glaukos istent infinite. Available from: https://www.glaukos.com/glaucoma/products/istent-infinite/
6. Premarket approval (PMA). accessdata.fda.gov. (n.d.). Available from: https://www.accessdata.fda.gov/scripts/cdrh/cfdocs/cfPMA/pma.cfm?id=P080030
7. Premarket approval (PMA). accessdata.fda.gov. (n.d.-a). Available from: https://www.accessdata.fda.gov/scripts/cdrh/cfdocs/cfpma/pma.cfm?id=P170043
8. Voskanyan L, García-Feijoó J, Belda JI, et al. Prospective, unmasked evaluation of the iStent®

inject system for open-angle glaucoma: synergy trial. Adv Ther. 2014;31(2):189-201. https://doi.org/10.1007/s12325-014-0095-y

9. Buchacra O, Duch S, Milla E, Stirbu O. One-year analysis of the iStent trabecular microbypass in secondary glaucoma. Clin Ophthalmol. 2011;5:321-6. https://doi.org/10.2147/OPTH.S15025
10. Le K, Saheb H. iStent trabecular micro-bypass stent for open-angle glaucoma. Clin Ophthalmol. 2014;8:1937-45. https://doi.org/10.2147/OPTH.S45920
11. Summary of safety and Effectiveness Data (SSED). (n.d.). Available from: https://www.accessdata.fda.gov/cdrh_docs/pdf17/P170043B.pdf
12. Hamanaka T, Kasahara K, Takemura T. Histopathology of the trabecular meshwork and Schlemm's canal in primary angle-closure glaucoma. Invest Ophthalmol Vis Sci. 2011;52(12):8849-61. https://doi.org/10.1167/iovs.11-7591
13. Hernstadt DJ, Cheng J, Htoon HM, et al. Case Series of Combined iStent Implantation and Phacoemulsification in Eyes with Primary Angle Closure Disease: One-Year Outcomes. Adv Ther. 2019;36(4):976-86. https://doi.org/10.1007/s12325-019-00899-5
14. Salimi A, Abu-Nada M, Harasymowycz P. Matched Cohort Study of Cataract Surgery With and Without Trabecular Microbypass Stent Implantation in Primary Angle-Closure Glaucoma. Am J Ophthalmol. 2021;224:310-20. https://doi.org/10.1016/j.ajo.2020.12.032
15. Clement C, Howes F, Ioannidis AS, et al. Two-Year Multicenter Outcomes of iStent inject Trabecular Micro-Bypass Stents Combined with Phacoemulsification in Various Types of Glaucoma and Ocular Hypertension. Clin Ophthalmol. 2020;14:3507-17. https://doi.org/10.2147/OPTH.S271646
16. Masis M, Mineault PJ, Phan E, Lin SC. The role of phacoemulsification in glaucoma therapy: A systematic review and meta-analysis. Surv Ophthalmol. 2018;63(5):700-10. https://doi.org/10.1016/j.survophthal.2017.08.006
17. Poley BJ, Lindstrom RL, Samuelson TW, Schulze R, Jr. Intraocular pressure reduction after phacoemulsification with intraocular lens implantation in glaucomatous and nonglaucomatous eyes: evaluation of a causal relationship between the natural lens and open-angle glaucoma. J Cataract Refract Surg. 2009;35(11):1946-55. https://doi.org/10.1016/j.jcrs.2009.05.061
18. Chen DZ, Sng CCA, Sangtam T, et al. Phacoemulsification vs phacoemulsification with micro-bypass stent implantation in primary angle closure and primary angle closure glaucoma: A randomized single-masked clinical study. Clin Exp Ophthalmol. 2020;48(4):450-61. https://doi.org/10.1111/ceo.13721
19. Popovic M, Campos-Moller X, Saheb H, Ahmed IIK. Efficacy and Adverse Event Profile of the iStent and iStent Inject Trabecular Micro-bypass for Open-angle Glaucoma: A Meta-analysis. J Curr Glaucoma Pract. 2018;12(2):67-84. https://doi.org/10.5005/jp-journals-10028-1248
20. Agrawal P, Bradshaw SE. Systematic Literature Review of Clinical and Economic Outcomes of Micro-Invasive Glaucoma Surgery (MIGS) in Primary Open-Angle Glaucoma. Ophthalmol

Ther. 2018;7(1):49-73. https://doi.org/10.1007/s40123-018-0131-0

21. Sun X, Dai Y, Chen Y, et al. Primary angle closure glaucoma: What we know and what we don't know. Prog Retin Eye Res 2017;57:26-45. https://doi.org/10.1016/j.preteyeres.2016.12.003
22. George R, Paul PG, Baskaran M, et al. Ocular biometry in occludable angles and angle closure glaucoma: a population based survey. Br J Ophthalmol. 2003;87(4):399-402. https://doi.org/10.1136/bjo.87.4.399
23. Craven ER, Katz LJ, Wells JM, Giamporcaro JE. Cataract surgery with trabecular micro-bypass stent implantation in patients with mild-to-moderate open-angle glaucoma and cataract: two-year follow-up. J Cataract Refract Surg. 2012;38(8):1339-45. https://doi.org/10.1016/j.jcrs.2012.03.025
24. Samuelson TW, Katz LJ, Wells JM, et al. Randomized evaluation of the trabecular micro-bypass stent with phacoemulsification in patients with glaucoma and cataract. Ophthalmology. 2011;118(3):459-67. https://doi.org/10.1016/j.ophtha.2010.07.007

Phacogoniotomy (Phaco ± GSL+ GT)

Fei Li, Yunhe Song, Fengbin Lin, Syril Dorairaj, Ying Han, Masaki Tanito, Xiulan Zhang

Phaco alone or in conjunction with GSL has proven effective in reducing IOP in patients with mild or moderate PACG and cataract.[1-3] However, Phaco + GSL may not effectively reduce IOP to the requisite target level required for advanced PACG.[4,5] The pathological changes in the TM and SC in advanced PACG, with long-standing iridotrabecular adhesions preclude any significant lowering of IOP.[6] By incising/removing the damaged or dysfunctional TM and facilitating aqueous outflow, GT—or ab-interno trabeculotomy—provides additional IOP reduction required in advanced PACG.[7-9] Phacogoniotomy, a combination of Phaco, GSL, and GT has been demonstrated, to be a safe and effective procedure for the treatment of these patients across several studies.[10-22]

The incisional extent of GT procedures is variable and can range from 30° to 360° of circumferential incisions.[10-32] Zhang and Song *et al.* demonstrated that a 120° GT, whether used alone or combined with Phaco, is effective in treating POAG when compared to 240° and 360° GT approaches.[23-25] Regarding the extent of GSL, Lin *et al.* also showed that patients with various preoperative PAS ranges achieved comparable postoperative IOP levels and surgical success rates following Phaco combined with GSL (120°) and GT (120°) treatment.[16] Thus, the combination of Phaco, 120° GSL and 120° GT has proven to be safe and effective in managing advanced PACG with cataract.

Indications

Indications of phacogoniotomy are patients with advanced PACG and a visually significant cataract,[10-15] as well as patients with advanced PACG where early/CLE is indicated, including extremely shallow AC, a thick lens with a high vault, and any other high risk of malignant glaucoma following trabeculectomy.[33] Furthermore, phacogoniotomy may be considered for cases where previous treatments, such as laser or surgical peripheral iridectomy (LPI/SPI), or trabeculectomy, have failed, particularly when PACG is the underlying primary pathology.[34,35] Treatment can also be done in a graded manner, starting with Phaco + GSL and if IOP remains uncontrolled, proceeding to GT.

Contraindications

Phacogoniotomy is not recommended for patients with PACS, PAC, or early PACG. It is contraindicated in eyes with secondary angle closure resulting from uveitis, neovascular glaucoma, or iridocorneal-endothelial syndrome with extensive firm PAS formation.

Mechanism

The integrated approach of phacogoniotomy effectively addresses the pathogenesis of PACG. Phaco deepens the AC, thereby reducing angle crowding and alleviating pupillary block. Subsequently, GSL releases the PAS, while GT is utilized to remove or incise the dysfunctional TM,[6] thereby enhancing aqueous outflow and effectively reducing IOP.[10-15]

Technique

The surgical procedure is initiated with the Phaco, with the main incision positioned in the superior or temporal quadrant. With the surgeon sitting temporally, GSL and GT procedures are conducted in the nasal quadrant from the temporal clear corneal main incision. For maximal and optimal visualization of the nasal angle, the patient's head is rotated 35°–45° away from the surgeon, and the surgical microscope is tilted 35°–45° toward the surgeon. A surgical goniolens is subsequently placed on the cornea to visualize the angle and TM. GSL is performed by gently depressing the synechiae with a blunt chopper or a synechialyzer at the angle wall to enable the scleral spur and TM to be clearly visualized, covering a range of 120°. GT is performed using the tip of a microhook or a microblade inserted into SC and moved to incise the inner wall of SC and TM 120°.[10-15] The nasal and inferior quadrants are recommended as the preferred sites for GSL and GT. This is because these regions contain nearly 80% of the collector channels, which are responsible for the majority of aqueous humor outflow.[36]

Multiple tools are available for performing 120° GT: the Kahook Dual Blade (New World Medical & Co., Ltd., FL, USA), non-device reuseable instruments including the Tanito Microhook (TMH; Inami & Co., Ltd., Tokyo, Japan), the LAN microhook (Belle Healthcare Technology Co., Ltd., Suzhou, China), microvitreoretinal blades, and even 25-G/26-G bent needles. The TMH or LAN microhook, featuring a curved-blade design, enable an extra 120° incision in the supranasal sector. This design significantly eases the process of 2-site GT, ultimately achieving a total incision of 240°. Additionally, the bent needle ab-interno goniotomy (BANG) technique is unique in its affordability, convenience, and wide availability and can be used in combination with viscodilation of the canal.[30-32]

Results: IOP-lowering efficacy

A growing body of evidence has consistently demonstrated that phacogoniotomy achieves statistically and clinically significant reductions of IOP in eyes with advanced PACG and cataract.[10-22] In a series of prospective multicenter studies, Song *et al.* reported that this combination strategy controlled IOP to below 18 mmHg with or without medications in 94%, 95.2%, 90.5%, and 88.6% of eyes at 6-, 12-, 24-, and 36-month follow-ups, respectively.[10-13] The corresponding average percentage reductions in IOP were 51.1%, 44.8%, 54.9%, and 53.9%, respectively.[10-13] Similarly, Gupta *et al.* reported in a prospective study a cumulative qualified success rate (IOP < 18 mmHg, with or without medications) of 87.8% at 22 months, with a median IOP reduction of 36.4%.[20] Additionally, in their retrospective case series, Dorairaj *et al.* demonstrated that this approach effectively maintained IOP below 18 mmHg, with or without medication, in 92.9%, 92.9%, and 95.2% of eyes at the 6, 12, and 24-month follow-up points, respectively.[17-19] The average IOP reductions were 48.8%, 47.2%, and 47.1%, respectively, at the same time points.[17-19] A recent meta-analysis summarized that Phaco with IOL implantation ± GSL + angle-based MIGS decreased both IOP and the number of antiglaucoma medications while providing a favorable safety profile in treating patients with PACG. The subgroup analysis revealed no significant difference between gonioscopy-assisted transluminal trabeculotomy (GATT) and GT in terms of IOP-lowering effect. Additionally, both GATT and GT were found to be more effective in reducing IOP compared to the iStent.[9]

Complications and management

The reported postoperative complications consist of a fibrinous aqueous reaction, IOP spikes, and mild hyphema.[10-22] Elevated IOP is chiefly attributed to the postoperative application of steroid eye drops. Song *et al.* and Lin *et al.* reported that the incidence of IOP spikes associated with this approach ranges from 6.2% to 16%,[10-16] closely mirroring the rates observed in their studies on GT with or without Phaco for POAG, which ranged from 6.3% to 15.3%.[23-25] However, this figure is significantly lower than those documented in studies on other ab-interno trabeculotomy procedures, where rates exceeded 30%.[37,38] This discrepancy may be attributed to the timely discontinuation of steroid eye drops within the first 7 days by Song *et al.* and Lin *et al.*[10-16] Hyphema, linked to the incised TM and occurring at rates between 6.2% and 18%, tends to resolve within the initial postoperative week for the vast majority of patients.[10-16] Reports indicate that the incidence of hyphema in 120° GT is significantly lower compared to 360° GT (60% to 84.9%).[23-25] Most cases of fibrinous aqueous reactions also typically resolve within this initial postoperative period. There is a risk of recurrence of PAS and closure of the goniotomy cleft over time with a rebound increase in IOP. The use of pilocarpine in the initial postoperative period may help prevent PAS recurrence, although evidence to support this is lacking.

Can phacogoniotomy replace traditional phacotrabeculectomy?

A multicenter, randomized, non-inferiority trial has demonstrated that phacogoniotomy is non-inferior to phacotrabeculectomy in reducing IOP for advanced PACG and cataracts.[14,15] This was consistent at both the 12-month postoperative interval, where mean IOP reductions were 26.1 mmHg for phacogoniotomy compared to 25.7 mmHg for phacotrabeculectomy ($P = 0.383$),[15] and over a 24-month follow-up period, with reductions of 25.6 mmHg versus 24.7 mmHg, respectively ($P = 0.417$).[14] Moreover, no differences in complete (78.0% vs 84.6%, respectively; $P = 0.47$) or qualified (89.8% vs 88.5%, respectively; $P = 0.30$) surgical success at the 2-year mark were noted between the groups, nor were differences in postoperative complications or safety outcomes noted.[14] Additionally, phacogoniotomy provided a shorter surgical time, lower postoperative complication rate, fewer postoperative interventions, and better postoperative quality of life.[15]

Any other options for clear lens or mild cataract in advanced PACG?

The concept of CLE to treat patients with PACG has been well established in the EAGLE study. For patients without visually significant cataract, phacogoniotomy can serve as a viable alternative for advanced PACG patients, particularly those with an extremely shallow AC or a thick lens with a high vault, which heightens the risk of malignant glaucoma following trabeculectomy. For patients who are reluctant to undergo CLE, Lin *et al.* and Gao *et al.* demonstrated that a combination of SPI, GSL (120° degree), and GT (120 degree) effectively reduces IOP and eliminates the challenges associated with trabeculectomy in patients with advanced PACG without cataracts.[39-43] Furthermore, a RCT study has shown that this approach is not inferior to trabeculectomy in maintaining IOP levels with fewer postoperative complications and a reduced need for postoperative interventions (including bleb massage, suture lysis, or releasable suture removal) over a 12-month follow-up period.[39,43] Further research with longer follow-up is essential to determine whether this procedure can effectively serve as a substitute for trabeculectomy for patients with advanced PACG who do not have visually significant cataract and decline phacogoniotomy.

Comments

Phacogoniotomy, the combination of Phaco, GSL, and GT, offers a high safety profile and effective IOP management for advanced PACG with cataract. This approach could emerge as the preferred first-line treatment option, potentially as an alternative to phacotrabeculectomy for patients with advanced PACG and cataract.

References

1. Thomas R, Walland M, Thomas A, Mengersen K. Lowering of Intraocular Pressure After Phacoemulsification in Primary Open-Angle and Angle-Closure Glaucoma: A Bayesian Analysis. Asia Pac J Ophthalmol (Phila). 2016;5(1):79-84. https://doi.org/10.1097/APO.0000000000000174
2. Husain R, Do T, Lai J, et al. Efficacy of Phacoemulsification Alone vs Phacoemulsification With Goniosynechialysis in Patients With Primary Angle-Closure Disease: A Randomized Clinical Trial. JAMA Ophthalmol. 2019;137(10):1107-13. https://doi.org/10.1001/jamaophthalmol.2019.2493
3. Angmo D, Shakrawal J, Gupta B, et al. Comparative Evaluation of Phacoemulsification Alone versus Phacoemulsification with Goniosynechialysis in Primary Angle-Closure Glaucoma: A Randomized Controlled Trial. Ophthalmol Glaucoma. 2019;2(5):346-56. https://doi.org/10.1016/j.ogla.2019.05.004
4. Senthil S, Rao HL, Choudhari N, Garudadri C. Phacoemulsification versus Phacotrabeculectomy in Medically Controlled Primary Angle Closure Glaucoma with Cataract in an Indian Cohort: A randomized controlled trial. Int Ophthalmol. 2022;42(1):35-45. https://doi.org/10.1007/s10792-021-01997-6
5. Tian T, Li M, Pan Y, et al. The effect of phacoemulsification plus goniosynechialysis in acute and chronic angle closure patients with extensive goniosynechiae. BMC Ophthalmol. 2019;19(1):65. https://doi.org/10.1186/s12886-019-1070-9

6. Hamanaka T, Kasahara K, Takemura T. Histopathology of the trabecular meshwork and Schlemm's canal in primary angle-closure glaucoma. Invest Ophthalmol Vis Sci. 2011;52(12):8849-61. https://doi.org/10.1167/iovs.11-7591
7. Chan PPM, Larson MD, Dickerson JE, Jr., et al. Minimally Invasive Glaucoma Surgery: Latest Developments and Future Challenges. Asia Pac J Ophthalmol (Phila). 2023;12(6):537-64. https://doi.org/10.1097/APO.0000000000000646
8. Song Y, Zhang H, Zhang Y, et al. Minimally Invasive Glaucoma Surgery in Primary Angle-Closure Glaucoma. Asia Pac J Ophthalmol (Phila). 2022;11(5):460-9. https://doi.org/10.1097/APO.0000000000000561
9. Fang Z, Song Y, Jin L, Han Y, Zhang X. Phacoemulsification combined with trabecular meshwork-Schlemm canal-based minimally invasive glaucoma surgery in primary angle-closure glaucoma: a systematic review and meta-analysis. BMC Ophthalmol. 2025;25(1):168. https://doi.org/10.1186/s12886-025-04005-y
10. Song Y, Tang Li, Fan F, Zhu X, et al. Three-year Outcome of Phacogoniotomy for Advanced Primary Angle-closure Glaucoma with Cataracts: a Multicenter Study. J Glaucoma. 2025. https://doi.org/10.1136/bjo-2024-325375
11. Song Y, Xie L, Zhu X, et al. Two-year Outcome of Phacogoniotomy for Advanced Primary Angle-closure Glaucoma with Cataracts: a Multicenter Study. Br J Ophthalmol. 2025 Jun 23;109(7):770-774. https://doi.org/10.1136/bjo-2024-325375
12. Song Y, Zhang Y, Li F, et al. One-Year Results of a Multicenter Study: Intraocular Pressure-Lowering Effect of Combined Phacoemulsification, Goniosynechialysis, and Goniotomy for Cases of Advanced Primary Angle-Closure Glaucoma With Cataract. Asia Pac J Ophthalmol (Phila). 2022;11(6):529-35. https://doi.org/10.1097/APO.0000000000000579
13. Song Y, Zhang Y, Lin F, et al. Outcomes and safety of phacoemulsification combined with intraocular lens implantation plus goniosynechialysis and goniotomy for advanced primary angle-closure glaucoma. Chin J Exp Ophthalmol. 2022;40(4):334-9.
14. Song Y, Fan S, Tang L, et al. Two-Year Outcomes of Phacogoniotomy vs Phacotrabeculectomy for Advanced Primary Angle-Closure Glaucoma With Cataract: A Noninferiority Randomized Clinical Trial. JAMA Ophthalmol. 2025 Jun 1;143(6):462-469. https://doi.org/10.1001/jamaophthalmol.2025.0685
15. Song Y, Lin F, Lv A, et al. Phacogoniotomy versus phacotrabeculectomy for advanced primary angle-closure glaucoma with cataract: A randomized non-inferiority trial. Asia Pac J Ophthalmol (Phila). 2024;13(1):100033. https://doi.org/10.1016/j.apjo.2023.100033
16. Lin F, Zhang Y, Zhu X, et al. Impact of Peripheral Anterior Synechiae on the Outcome of Combined Phacoemulsification, Goniosynechialysis, and Goniotomy for Primary Angle Closure Glaucoma and Cataract: A Multicenter Observational Study. J Glaucoma. 2024;33(8):587-93. https://doi.org/10.1097/IJG.0000000000002435
17. Dorairaj S, Tam MD, Balasubramani GK. Two-Year Clinical Outcomes of Combined Phacoemul-

sification, Goniosynechialysis, and Excisional Goniotomy For Angle-Closure Glaucoma. Asia Pac J Ophthalmol (Phila) 2020;10(2):183-7. https://doi.org/10.1097/APO.0000000000000321

18. Dorairaj S, Tam MD, Balasubramani GK. Twelve-month outcomes of excisional goniotomy using the Kahook Dual Blade(®) in eyes with angle-closure glaucoma. Clin Ophthalmol. 2019;13:1779-85. https://doi.org/10.2147/OPTH.S221299
19. Dorairaj S, Tam MD. Kahook Dual Blade Excisional Goniotomy and Goniosynechialysis Combined With Phacoemulsification for Angle-closure Glaucoma: 6-Month Results. J Glaucoma. 2019;28(7):643-6. https://doi.org/10.1097/IJG.0000000000001256
20. Gupta S, Sethi A, Yadav S, et al. Safety and efficacy of incisional goniotomy as an adjunct with phacoemulsification in primary angle-closure glaucoma. J Cataract Refract Surg. 2021;47(4):504-11. https://doi.org/10.1097/j.jcrs.0000000000000481
21. Tanito M, Sugihara K, Tsutsui A, et al. Midterm Results of Microhook ab Interno Trabeculotomy in Initial 560 Eyes with Glaucoma. J Clin Med. 2021;10(4). https://doi.org/10.3390/jcm10040814
22. Shokoohi-Rad S, Karimi F, Zarei-Ghanavati S, Tireh H. Phacoemulsification, visco-goniosynechialysis, and goniotomy in patients with primary angle-closure glaucoma: A comparative study. Eur J Ophthalmol. 2021;31(1):88-95. https://doi.org/10.1177/1120672119879331
23. Zhang Y, Yu P, Zhang Y, et al. Influence of Goniotomy Size on Treatment Safety and Efficacy for Primary Open-Angle Glaucoma: A Multicenter Study. Am J Ophthalmol. 2023;256:118-25. https://doi.org/10.1016/j.ajo.2023.08.002
24. Song Y, Zhu X, Zhang Y, et al. Outcomes of Partial Versus Complete Goniotomy With or Without Phacoemulsification for Primary Open Angle Glaucoma: A Multicenter Study. J Glaucoma. 2023;32(7):563-8. https://doi.org/10.1097/IJG.0000000000002210
25. Song Y, Ye X, Yang M, et al. Outcomes of Phacogoniotomy for Medically Controlled and Uncontrolled Primary Open Angle Glaucoma With Cataract: A Multicenter Study. J Glaucoma. 2025;34(8):591-7. https://doi.org/10.1097/IJG.0000000000002598
26. El Sayed YM, Mettias NM, Elghonemy HME, Mostafa YSE. Phacoemulsification with gonioscopy-assisted transluminal trabeculotomy versus phacoemulsification alone in primary angle closure glaucoma: A randomized controlled study. Acta Ophthalmol. 2024;102(2):e195-e203. https://doi.org/10.1111/aos.15733
27. Sharkawi E, Artes PH, Lindegger DJ, et al. Gonioscopy-assisted transluminal trabeculotomy in primary angle-closure glaucoma. Graefes Arch Clin Exp Ophthalmol. 2021;259(10):3019-26. https://doi.org/10.1007/s00417-021-05244-7
28. Fontana L, De Maria M, Iannetta D, Moramarco A. Gonioscopy-assisted transluminal trabeculotomy for chronic angle-closure glaucoma: preliminary results. Graefes Arch Clin Exp Ophthalmol. 2022;260(2):545-51. https://doi.org/10.1007/s00417-021-05400-z
29. Chira-Adisai T, Mori K, Kobayashi A, et al. Outcomes of combined gonioscopy-assisted transluminal trabeculotomy and goniosynechialysis in primary angle closure: a retrospective

case series. Int Ophthalmol. 2021;41(4):1223-31. https://doi.org/10.1007/s10792-020-01676-y

30. Dada T, Bukke AN, Huang AS, et al. Recruitment of Temporal Aqueous Outflow Channels After Bent Needle Ab-Interno Goniectomy Demonstrated by Aqueous Angiography. J Glaucoma. 2023;32(2):e15-e8. https://doi.org/10.1097/IJG.0000000000002131
31. Dada T, Beri N, Sethi A, Sharma N. Viscodilation of Schlemm's Canal Combined with Goniectomy Using a 30 G Needle (Visco-Bent Ab Interno Needle Goniectomy). J Curr Glaucoma Pract. 2023;17(4):210-3. https://doi.org/10.5005/jp-journals-10078-1424
32. Shute T, Green W, Liu J, Sheybani A. An Alternate Technique for Goniotomy: Description of Procedure and Preliminary Results. J Ophthalmic Vis Res. 2022;17(2):170-5. https://doi.org/10.18502/jovr.v17i2.10787
33. Azuara-Blanco A, Burr J, Ramsay C, et al. Effectiveness of early lens extraction for the treatment of primary angle-closure glaucoma (EAGLE): a randomised controlled trial. Lancet. 2016;388(10052):1389-97. https://doi.org/10.1016/S0140-6736(16)30956-4
34. Lin F, Nie X, Shi J, et al. Safety and Efficacy of Goniotomy following Failed Surgery for Glaucoma. J Glaucoma. 2023;32(11):942-7. https://doi.org/10.1097/IJG.0000000000002301
35. Lin F, Li L, Fan F, Xiaokaiti D, et al. Two-year outcomes of goniotomy following failed surgery for glaucoma: A multicenter study. Ophthalmol Sci. 2025 Aug 20;6(1):100922. https://doi.org/10.1016/j.xops.2025.100922
36. Huang AS, Penteado RC, Saha SK, et al. Fluorescein Aqueous Angiography in Live Normal Human Eyes. J Glaucoma. 2018;27(11):957-964. https://doi.org/10.1097/IJG.0000000000001042
37. Lai J, Qiao Y, Tan C, Chen J. Outcomes of gonioscopy-assisted transluminal trabeculotomy in primary congenital glaucoma treatment: a retrospective study. BMC Ophthalmol. 2024;24(1):88. https://doi.org/10.1186/s12886-024-03351-7
38. Sato T, Kawaji T, Hirata A, Mizoguchi T. 360-degree suture trabeculotomy ab interno to treat open-angle glaucoma: 2-year outcomes. Clin Ophthalmol. 2018;12:915-23. https://doi.org/10.2147/OPTH.S161238
39. Gao X, Lv A, Lin F, et al. Efficacy and safety of trabeculectomy versus peripheral iridectomy plus goniotomy in advanced primary angle-closure glaucoma: study protocol for a multicentre, non-inferiority, randomised controlled trial (the TVG study). BMJ Open. 2022;12(7):e062441. https://doi.org/10.1136/bmjopen-2022-062441
40. Lin F, Li L, Lu P, et al. Two-Year Outcomes of Combined Surgical Peripheral Iridectomy, Goniosynechialysis, and Goniotomy for Advanced Primary Angle-Closure Glaucoma Without Cataract: A Multicenter Study. Asia Pac J Ophthalmol (Phila). 2025 Feb 26:100166. https://doi.org/10.1016/j.apjo.2025.100166
41. Gao X, Lin F, Lu P, et al. Efficacy and Safety of Surgical Peripheral Iridectomy, Goniosynechialysis, and Goniotomy for Advanced Primary Angle-closure Glaucoma without Cataract: One-year Results of a Multicenter Study. J Glaucoma. 2024 Sep 1;33(9):632-639. https://doi.

org/10.1097/IJG.0000000000002443

42. Lin F, Lu P, Song Y, et al. Surgical outcome and safety of peripheral iridectomy plus goniosynechialysis and goniotomy in the treatment of advanced primary angle-closure glaucoma. Chin J Exp Ophthalmol. 2023;41(2):134-9.
43. Lin F, Lv A, Li F, et al. Peripheral Iridectomy with Goniosynechialysis and Goniotomy vs. Trabeculectomy for Advanced PACG: A Randomized Controlled Trial. JAMA Ophthalmol. 2025 Jun 1;143(6):472-479. https://doi.org/10.1001/jamaophthalmol.2025.0757

Phaco ± GSL+ XEN

Bryan Ang, Benjamin Xu

Surgical management of eyes with moderate to advanced PACG has traditionally relied upon filtering surgeries such as trabeculectomy and glaucoma drainage devices.[1,2] Despite their long history,[3,4] and continued improvements in surgical technique and postoperative management,[5,6] these incisional surgeries are still associated with considerable risk of complications such as aqueous misdirection and higher re-operation rates in eyes with ACD.[7] In recent years, traditional filtering surgeries have been challenged by promising surgical alternatives with potentially lower surgical risk. Minimally invasive bleb surgery (MIBS) has emerged as a viable surgical option in the treatment of OAG. Among the emerging MIBS devices is the XEN45 Gel Stent (XEN; Allergan Inc., Irvine, CA, USA). The XEN is a 6-mm biocompatible, hydrophilic, non-inflammatory stent, composed of porcine gelatin cross-linked with glutaraldehyde. It is highly flexible and expands when hydrated by aqueous fluid, to adapt to the shape of surrounding tissues, thereby reducing the risk of device migration and erosion. The XEN has demonstrated an overall superior safety profile compared to conventional filtering surgeries.[8-10]

The pivotal trial leading to US FDA approval of the XEN excluded eyes with ACG.[11,12] Implantation of this stent requires a sufficiently open angle in the specific quadrant of implantation. A shallow AC may also further increase the risk of stent occlusion.[13] Nonetheless, since its introduction, the XEN has been used in the real-world treatment of ACD, both as a standalone procedure and in combination with Phaco surgery (Phaco + XEN).[14-22]

Mechanism

XEN implantation is a bleb-forming procedure that lowers IOP by establishing a permanent filtration channel from the AC to the subconjunctival space, bypassing any diseased TM, SC, and distal collector channels. The stent's internal diameter, external diameter, and length are approximately 45 μm, 150 μm, and 6mm, respectively, facilitating its passage into the subconjunctival space and providing a steady flow resistance of approximately 6 mmHg to 8 mmHg to reduce the risk of postoperative hypotony.[12,23,24]

Technique

The following describes the ab-interno, open-conjunctival XEN implantation technique described in the FDA pivotal trial by Grover *et al.*[12] Viscoelastic is first used to maintain the AC depth. The target area is pre-treated with subconjunctival MMC, following which the needle tip of the preloaded XEN delivery device is advanced through a peripheral incision 1–2 mm anterior to the limbus, through the AC towards the target quadrant. The needle tip is then advanced through the TM and sclera under gonioscopic guidance. As the needle tip exits the sclera, the entire bevelled tip is visualized within the subconjunctival space. The XEN is then implanted into the subconjunctival space, and if properly positioned, should have approximately 2 mm and 1 mm of its length visible in the subconjunctival space and AC, respectively. The conjunctiva is sutured closed, and the viscoelastic is irrigated and aspirated. In Phaco + XEN surgery, Phaco is performed before implantation of the XEN.

Following FDA approval, the device manufacturer's usage directions described an ab-interno, closed-conjunctival procedure with pretreatment of the surgical site with MMC.[11] Further variations in surgical technique have since been described with the aim of improving outcomes and lowering postoperative needling rates. These include the ab-externo closed-conjunctival and ab-externo open-conjunctival approaches,[5,25,26] as well as primary intraoperative needling and adoption of the XEN Air implantation technique, among others.[27]

In angle-closure disease, if PAS is present in the target quadrant, GSL would need to be performed before XEN implantation to facilitate the entry of the needle tip of the XEN delivery device through the TM and out into the subconjunctival space.

Results: IOP-lowering efficacy

In a prospective, single-arm study of 19 Chinese eyes with PACG undergoing Phaco + XEN, Sng *et al.* found a mean IOP reduction from 15.2 ± 3.0 mmHg (preoperative, medicated) and 21.7 ± 3.7 mmHg (preoperative, unmedicated), to 11.7 ± 3.0 mmHg at 12 months postoperative (combined medicated and unmedicated) ($p < 0.001$). This study also found a decrease in the mean number of glaucoma medications from 1.4 ± 0.7 medications at baseline to 0.2 ± 0.5 medications at 12 months postoperative ($p < 0.001$). There was no significant difference in the IOP reduction and reduction in number of glaucoma medications at 12 months postoperative between eyes with PACG and POAG.[14]

Wanichwecharungruang *et al.* conducted a retrospective cohort study comparing 15 PACG eyes which underwent Phaco + XEN or XEN with 15 PACG eyes which underwent trabeculectomy surgery. The study found a significant mean IOP reduction from 20.3 ± 4.8 mmHg preoperatively to 14.4 ± 5.3 mmHg at 12 months postoperative and 13.3 ± 3.5 mmHg at 24 months postoperative in eyes following Phaco + XEN/XEN surgery. IOP reduction was significant at all timepoints (all $p < 0.001$). In comparison, in eyes which underwent trabeculectomy surgery, there was a significant mean IOP reduction from 21.2 ± 4.9 mmHg preoperatively to 13.0 ± 3.9 mmHg at POM12 and 12.4 ± 3.3 mmHg at POM24. This reduction in mean IOP was significant at all timepoints as well ($p < 0.001$). Mean IOP was lower in the Phaco + XEN/XEN group at POD1 ($p = 0.041$), while it was lower in the trabeculectomy group at POM9 ($p = 0.047$); differences between both groups at other timepoints failed to reach statistical significance (all $p > 0.05$).[15]

In terms of reduction in the mean number of glaucoma medications, there was a decrease from 2.1 ± 1.2 medications preoperatively in the Phaco + XEN/XEN group to 0.7 ± 1.1 medications at POM12, and 0.5 ± 0.9 medications at POM24 ($p < 0.001$). This was compared to a decrease from 2.2 ± 1.0 medications preoperatively in the trabeculectomy group to 0.5 ± 0.7 medications at both POM12 and POM24 ($p < 0.001$). There was no statistically significant difference in the extent of medication reduction between the 2 groups at all timepoints (all $p > 0.05$). Both Phaco + XEN/XEN and trabeculectomy groups had complete success (defined as achieving at least 20% IOP reduction from baseline without glaucoma medication) rates of 66.7% at POM12 and 60.0% at POM24, with no statistically significant difference identified between the 2 groups at all timepoints (all $p > 0.05$).[15]

This study also included analysis of 42 eyes with POAG which underwent Phaco + XEN or XEN, and found the efficacy of pooled Phaco + XEN and XEN surgery, in terms of reduction in mean IOP, mean number of glaucoma medications and complete success rates, to be comparable between PACG and POAG eyes, with no statistically significant differences between these 2 groups at all timepoints (all $p > 0.05$), up to POM24.[15]

Complications and management

XEN implantation has demonstrated an overall excellent intraoperative and postoperative safety profile across the various glaucoma subtypes, with sight-threatening complications rare, and complications such as hypotony and hyphema mostly self-limiting.[12-16,28] Safety outcomes in angle-closure subgroups have seldom been reported specifically in studies. However, there remains theoretical concern of higher rates of certain complications in the context of angle-closure disease, such as internal stent occlusion, hyphema from angle trauma during stent insertion, and aqueous misdirection. Asanad *et al.* published a case report of an 86-year-old man with PACG who underwent Phaco + XEN and developed a raised IOP of 24 mmHg at approximately POM2, which was found to be a result of stent occlusion by iris pigmentary deposits that had traversed to the distal conjunctival end of the stent within the bleb.[29] The occluded stent was successfully extracted from the AC via an ab-interno approach, with the IOP decreasing to 10 mmHg and remaining adequately controlled without medications up to 1 month later.

In terms of postoperative bleb needling, Sng *et al.* found that bleb needling was required in a total of 11 eyes (32.3% across both PACG and POAG groups) that underwent Phaco + XEN.[14] Wanichwecharungruang *et al.* reported bleb needling in a total of 10 patients (17.5% across both PACG and POAG groups) in the Phaco + XEN/XEN group compared to a total of 11 patients (19.3% across both PACG and POAG groups) in the trabeculectomy group, over 24 months postoperatively.[15] Eyes in the trabeculectomy group, however, appeared to require needling earlier in their postoperative course compared to eyes which underwent Phaco + XEN/XEN (mean = 98 ± 93 days, median = 68 days vs mean = 132 ± 130 days, median = 89 days). No subgroup analysis for bleb needling rates nor the timing of needling was performed specifically for PACG eyes in either study.

Comments

Overall, current literature suggests good surgical outcomes of Phaco+XEN and standalone XEN in terms of safety and surgical success rates in eyes with angle-closure disease of at least moderate severity. Both Phaco + XEN and XEN have demonstrated reduction in both the mean IOP and number of glaucoma medications up to 24 months postoperatively. However, there remains a paucity of literature and an absence of high-quality RCTs in this area. Outside those referenced above, other studies on the XEN also included eyes with angle-closure disease: Nicolaou *et al.* (32 eyes, 17%);[16] Hengerer *et al.* (21 eyes, 8.7%);[18] Hu *et al.* (11 eyes, 16.5%);[17] Smith *et al.*[19] (3 patients, 4.4%); and Heidinger *et al.*[20] (2 patients, 1.0%). However, these studies did not report outcomes or perform subgroup analysis, likely owing to the small numbers of angle-closure eyes in these studies. The extent of PAS in eyes at baseline and whether GSL was performed, as well as the appropriate stage of PACG for its use (whether early or advanced), have not been consistently reported across studies. Finally, although standalone Phaco is known to result in significant IOP reduction in eyes with angle-closure disease, there is little comparative data on outcomes following Phaco + XEN and standalone Phaco. There is also a lack of comparative trials examining the outcomes of XEN versus other surgical alternatives in PACG. All the above may limit the conclusiveness of current evidence regarding the role of Phaco + XEN and XEN in the treatment of angle-closure disease.

References

1. Caprioli J, de Leon JM, Azarbod P, et al. Trabeculectomy Can Improve Long-Term Visual Function in Glaucoma. Ophthalmology. 2016;123(1):117-28. https://doi.org/10.1016/j.ophtha.2015.09.027
2. Sihota R, Sood A, Gupta V, et al. A prospective longterm study of primary chronic angle closure glaucoma. Acta Ophthalmol. 2004;82(2):209-13. https://doi.org/10.1046/j.1600-0420.2004.00218.x
3. Cairns JE. Trabeculectomy. Preliminary report of a new method. Am J Ophthalmol. 1968;66(4):673-9. https://doi.org/10.1016/0002-9394(68)91288-9
4. Ashburn FS, Netland PA. The Evolution of Glaucoma Drainage Implants. J Ophthalmic Vis Res. 2018;13(4):498-500. https://doi.org/10.4103/jovr.jovr_26_18
5. Ang BCH, Lim SY, Betzler BK, et al. Recent Advancements in Glaucoma Surgery-A Review. Bioengineering (Basel) 2023;10(9). https://doi.org/10.3390/bioengineering10091096
6. Khodeiry M, Sayed MS. New glaucoma drainage implants available to glaucoma surgeons. Curr Opin Ophthalmol. 2023;34(2):176-80. https://doi.org/10.1097/ICU.0000000000000936
7. Hall NE, Chang EK, Samuel S, et al. Risk Factors for Glaucoma Drainage Device Revision or Removal Using the IRIS Registry. Am J Ophthalmol. 2022;240:302-20. https://doi.org/10.1016/j.ajo.2022.03.029
8. Saheb H, Ahmed, II. Micro-invasive glaucoma surgery: current perspectives and future directions. Curr Opin Ophthalmol. 2012;23(2):96-104. https://doi.org/10.1097/ICU.0b013e32834ff1e7
9. Gedde SJ, Schiffman JC, Feuer WJ, et al. Three-year follow-up of the tube versus trabeculectomy study. Am J Ophthalmol. 2009;148(5):670-84. https://doi.org/10.1016/j.ajo.2009.06.018
10. Chaudhary A, Salinas L, Guidotti J, et al. XEN Gel Implant: a new surgical approach in glaucoma. Expert Rev Med Devices. 2018;15(1):47-59. https://doi.org/10.1080/17434440.2018.1419060
11. Xen Gel Stent. Available from: https://www.rxabbvie.com/pdf/xen_dfu.pdf
12. Grover DS, Flynn WJ, Bashford KP, et al. Performance and Safety of a New Ab Interno Gelatin Stent in Refractory Glaucoma at 12 Months. Am J Ophthalmol. 2017;183:25-36. https://doi.

org/10.1016/j.ajo.2017.07.023

13. Gan L, Wang L, Chen J, Tang L. Complications of XEN gel stent implantation for the treatment of glaucoma: a systematic review. Front Med (Lausanne). 2024;11:1360051. https://doi.org/10.3389/fmed.2024.1360051
14. Sng CCA, Chew PTK, Htoon HM, et al. Case Series of Combined XEN Implantation and Phacoemulsification in Chinese Eyes: One-Year Outcomes. Adv Ther. 2019;36(12):3519-29. https://doi.org/10.1007/s12325-019-01127-w
15. Wanichwecharungruang B, Ratprasatporn N. 24-month outcomes of XEN45 gel implant versus trabeculectomy in primary glaucoma. PLoS One. 2021;16(8):e0256362. https://doi.org/10.1371/journal.pone.0256362
16. Nicolaou S, Khatib TZ, Lin Z, et al. A retrospective review of XEN implant surgery: efficacy, safety and the effect of combined cataract surgery. Int Ophthalmol. 2022;42(3):881-9. https://doi.org/10.1007/s10792-021-02069-5
17. Hu JY, Ang BCH, Yip LW. Efficacy of the XEN gel stent on intraocular pressure lowering in East Asian eyes. Int Ophthalmol. 2020;40(5):1191-9. https://doi.org/10.1007/s10792-020-01284-w
18. Hengerer FH, Kohnen T, Mueller M, Conrad-Hengerer I. Ab Interno Gel Implant for the Treatment of Glaucoma Patients With or Without Prior Glaucoma Surgery: 1-Year Results. J Glaucoma. 2017;26(12):1130-6. https://doi.org/10.1097/IJG.0000000000000803
19. Smith M, Charles R, Abdel-Hay A, et al. 1-year outcomes of the Xen45 glaucoma implant. Eye (Lond). 2019;33(5):761-6. https://doi.org/10.1038/s41433-018-0310-1
20. Heidinger A, Schwab C, Lindner E, et al. A Retrospective Study of 199 Xen45 Stent Implantations From 2014 to 2016. J Glaucoma 2019;28(1):75-9. https://doi.org/10.1097/IJG.0000000000001122
21. Gillmann K, Bravetti GE, Rao HL, et al. Combined and stand-alone XEN 45 gel stent implantation: 3-year outcomes and success predictors. Acta Ophthalmol. 2021;99(4):e531-e9. https://doi.org/10.1111/aos.14605
22. José P, Teixeira FJ, Barão RC, et al. Needling after XEN gel implant: What's the efficacy? A 1-year analysis. Eur J Ophthalmol. 2021;31(6):3087-92. https://doi.org/10.1177/1120672120963447
23. De Gregorio A, Pedrotti E, Stevan G, et al. XEN glaucoma treatment system in the management of refractory glaucomas: a short review on trial data and potential role in clinical practice. Clin Ophthalmol. 2018;12:773-82. https://doi.org/10.2147/OPTH.S146919
24. Lewis RA. Ab interno approach to the subconjunctival space using a collagen glaucoma stent. J Cataract Refract Surg. 2014;40(8):1301-6. https://doi.org/10.1016/j.jcrs.2014.01.032
25. El Helwe H, Ingram Z, Neeson CE, et al. Comparing Outcomes of 45 Xen Implantation Ab Interno With Closed Conjunctiva to Ab Externo With Open Conjunctiva Approaches. J Glaucoma. 2024;33(2):116-25. https://doi.org/10.1097/IJG.0000000000002320
26. Birnbaum FA, Neeson C, Solá-Del Valle D. Microinvasive Glaucoma Surgery: An Evi-

dence-Based Review. Semin Ophthalmol. 2021;36(8):772-86. https://doi.org/10.1080/08820538.2021.1903513
27. Vera V, Gagne S, Myers JS, Ahmed IIK. Surgical Approaches for Implanting Xen Gel Stent without Conjunctival Dissection. Clin Ophthalmol. 2020;14:2361-71. https://doi.org/10.2147/OPTH.S265695
28. Betzler BK, Lim SY, Lim BA, et al. Complications and post-operative interventions in XEN45 gel stent implantation in the treatment of open angle glaucoma-a systematic review and meta-analysis. Eye (Lond). 2023;37(6):1047-60. https://doi.org/10.1038/s41433-022-02022-5
29. Asanad S, Kalarn S, Kaleem MA. Postoperative complications of Ab-Interno XEN implantation in primary angle closure glaucoma. Am J Clin Exp Immunol. 2021;10(1):44-7.

Phaco ± GSL+ other MIGS

Fengbin Lin, Xiulan Zhang

When combined with Phaco, the Trabectome (MicroSurgical Technology, Redmond, WA, USA) offers a viable alternative for patients with PACG. Wu *et al.* reported that the combined approach of Phaco, GSL, and Trabectome effectively controlled IOP to below 21 mmHg with or without medication in 88.9% and 90.0% of eyes at the 12-month and 36-month follow-ups, respectively.[1,2] Similarly, Bussel *et al.* documented a 24% reduction in mean IOP and a 0.8% decrease in medication use following Phaco combined with Trabectome in patients with narrow angles.[3] The procedure was associated with only mild complications, such as hyphema (up to 100%), PAS (6.4% to 9.1%), and IOP spikes (4.3% to 8%).[1-3]

The Hydrus microstent (Alcon, Geneva, Switzerland) has been utilized for angle closure. A case report highlighted a patient with mixed-mechanism glaucoma and a clear lens who benefited significantly from cataract extraction, GSL, and Hydrus stent placement. The IOP was reduced from 18 mmHg on 1 medication to 12 mmHg without any medication.[4] However, no additional clinical studies have examined the implantation of the Hydrus microstent in PACG.

The PRESERFLO MicroShunt (Santen Pharmaceutical, Osaka, Japan) has also been employed for ACG cases. In 1 case, a patient with secondary ACG related to iridocorneal endothelial syndrome who consented to surgical intervention underwent combined cataract surgery and PRESERFLO MicroShunt implantation. The IOP dropped from 22 mmHg while on 3 classes of glaucoma medications to 12 mmHg while on 2 medications after 5 months follow-up.[5] In another instance, a case reported the occurrence of aqueous misdirection immediately following the implantation of a PRESERFLO MicroShunt device for the treatment of advanced ACG, which was further complicated by the subsequent development of persistent uveal effusion.[6] Nevertheless, no additional clinical studies have been conducted to assess the implantation of the PRESERFLO MicroShunt in PACG.

References

1. Yang F, Ma Y, Liang Z, et al. Combined Phacoemulsification, Goniosynechialysis and Ab Interno Trabeculectomy in Primary Angle-closure Glaucoma: Long-term Results. Int J Med Sci. 2025;22: 451-459. https://doi.org/10.7150/ijms.103795
2. Wang Y, Liang ZQ, Zhang Y, et al. Efficacy and safety of phacoemulsification plus goniosynechialysis and Trabectome in patients with primary angle-closure glaucoma. Sci Rep. 2021;11:13921. https://doi.org/10.1038/s41598-021-92972-9
3. Bussel, II, Kaplowitz K, Schuman JS, et al. Outcomes of ab interno trabeculectomy with the trabectome by degree of angle opening. Br J Ophthalmol. 2015;99: 914-919. https://doi.org/10.1136/bjophthalmol-2014-305577
4. Laroche D, Brown A, Ng C. Clear Lensectomy, Goniosynechiolysis and Hydrus Microstent in a Patient with Mixed Mechanism Glaucoma. J Natl Med Assoc. 2020;112: 339-343. https://doi.org/10.1016/j.jnma.2020.04.003
5. Ruparelia S, Darwich R, Eadie BD. PreserFlo Microshunt for the management of intraocular pressure elevation in iridocorneal endothelial syndrome. Am J Ophthalmol Case Rep. 2023;32:101932. https://doi.org/10.1016/j.ajoc.2023.101932
6. Malick H, Wilde C, Stead RE. Combined aqueous misdirection and persistent choroidal effusions following implantation of a Preserflo MicroShunt. Int J Ophthalmol. 2023;16(4):652-655. https://doi.org/10.18240/ijo.2023.04.21

Filtering surgery in the surgical treatment for primary angle-closure glaucoma

Do Tan, Rahat Husain, Claire Peterson, Dang Phuong Anh, Shamira Perera, Joseph Anthony Tumbocon, Benjamin Xu

Trabeculectomy

Do Tan, Dang Phuong Anh, Shamira Perera

Trabeculectomy has been the gold standard for the surgical management of severe glaucoma for more than 50 years. The indications for trabeculectomy in PACG are like to those in POAG, including inadequate control of IOP and/or continuing optic disc/visual field damage (despite medical therapy and LPI), as well as intolerance or poor compliance to medical therapy. A successful trabeculectomy benefits patients as it eliminates adverse side effects from long-term topical and systemic glaucoma medications, reduces the overall number of visits needed to control IOP, and is more cost-effective in the longer term. Recent studies showed that trabeculectomy slows the rate of visual field loss and provides sustained, long-term improvement of visual function in glaucoma.[1]

Although trabeculectomy might offer better control of IOP and hence prevent or slow down progression of glaucoma, it might be challenging to perform in PACG eyes, especially as experienced trabeculectomy surgeons are gradually retiring and exposure to trabeculectomy in residency and fellowship has decreased.[2] In addition to the common complications of intraocular surgery, trabeculectomy is associated with a considerable risk of postoperative flat AC, malignant glaucoma,[3] early as well as delayed leaks, hypotony, and cataract development and progression, which may require additional surgery. These potential complications, along with the growing use of primary tube shunts and MIGS as well as the advances in Phaco technology and techniques may explain why the number of trabeculectomies performed has continued to decline.[4] However, trabeculectomy remains crucial for its ability to achieve very low, sometimes single-digit target IOP. It is the most reasonable choice in managing certain types of glaucoma cases, such as advanced and refractory cases. A real-world retrospective study demonstrated that the survival rate of trabeculectomy in PACG eyes was 43% after 5 years of follow-up, which was comparable to phacotrabeculectomy (42%), but slightly worse than Phaco combined with GSL (53%), though much better than standalone Phaco (13%).[5]

PACG is traditionally classified as acute or chronic according to the presence of symptoms. The conventional management of APAC is to reduce the IOP medically, followed by LPI to relieve pupillary block. However, in medically unresponsive cases, many ophthalmologists consider surgery as the definitive treatment of APAC, such as Phaco or SPI. However, in some cases, trabeculectomy may be required in APAC, but results are modest. A study by Aung *et al.* showed a total success rate of 65.6% after 22 months of follow-up, while 10 patients (31.3%) encountered early postoperative complications, such as shallow AC.[6] Similarly, in a retrospective study from Taiwan, the results showed a relatively low rate of success of 60% with relatively high rate of postoperative complications (40%) such as shallow AC, hypotony, encapsulated blebs, increased cataract, among others, after 40 months of follow-up.[7] Another study of APAC eyes from Vietnam, an RCT comparing trabeculectomy with combined SPI plus argon LPI, found that the trabeculectomy group had a success rate of 92.7% with a mean IOP of 16.1

mmHg, showing that trabeculectomy in APAC eyes can obtain good results.[8]

In an RCT by Tham *et al.* comparing Phaco alone with trabeculectomy in medically uncontrolled chronic ACG without cataract, trabeculectomy with MMC reduced the mean IOP from a preoperative level of 24.8 ± 3.4 mmHg to 15.8 ± 4.3 mmHg (36% reduction) at 24 months after surgery ($p = 0.001$, paired t test). The trabeculectomy group required fewer IOP-lowering drugs (mean of 0.4 medications) compared to the Phaco group (mean of 1.5 medications), but resulted in more postoperative complications, such as cataract, wound leak, shallow AC, and choroidal detachment, than the Phaco group (46% vs 23% $p = 0.001$).[9]

Another question is whether combining lens extraction with trabeculectomy provides superior IOP lowering compared to trabeculectomy alone in PACG eyes. Few studies have compared the long-term outcomes of trabeculectomy with MMC with and without simultaneous lens extraction in the setting of PACG. Findings from these studies report similar success rates ranging from 54% to 78% for trabeculectomy in PACG and 56% to 88% for phacotrabeculectomy at follow-up intervals of 10 months to 3 years.[10,11] In another more recent retrospective study, Cox hazard regression analysis found no benefit of concurrent lens extraction on long-term IOP control after trabeculectomy in PACG patients. In this study, there were no significant differences in mean IOP ($p = 0.42$), number of glaucoma medications ($p = 0.85$), or logMAR visual acuity ($p = 0.42$) between the trabeculectomy and phacotrabeculectomy groups after 12 months.[12] In theory, lens extraction can open the drainage angle so that aqueous outflow pathways are more accessible. However, this anatomical benefit may be offset by the deleterious effects of combined surgery on bleb function.

It is important to note that if the PACG eye has significant (*e.g.*, > 270°) synechial angle closure and elevated IOP, LPI is unlikely to be effective and the patient will likely require filtering surgery. An RCT of established PACG eyes, defined as having PAS ≥ 6 clock hours and glaucomatous optic neuropathy and visual field defects, found that primary trabeculectomy was more effective than LPI for lowering IOP.[13] Trabeculectomy is also better for achieving long-term IOP control in PACG eyes.[14]

Studies have also shown that, even in chronic PACG, TM function can recover when the angle is opened by GSL.[15] However, PAS tends to recur after GSL in phakic eyes. Therefore, GSL should be performed with Phaco to open the angle, help the TM to recover, and reduce the IOP effectively in the long run. In one study of this combined surgery, the rate of complete surgical success was 90.4% after up to 6 years of follow-up.[16] Posterior chamber intraocular lens (PCIOL

When compared with trabeculectomy, in a retrospective study, Phaco combined with GSL showed similar mean postoperative IOP but with fewer number of topical IOP medications (0.36 ± 0.59 versus 1.05 ± 0.99, $p = 0.02$) after 10 months of follow-up.[17] On the other hand, this surgical modality seems to have some advantages over trabeculectomy, such as avoidance of bleb-related complications and the need for additional surgical procedures to maintain the artificial fistulae.

Tips when performing trabeculectomy in PACG eyes

Trabeculectomy augmentation with antimetabolites (5-fluorouracil and MMC)

The use of antimetabolites such as MMC and 5-fluorouracil to modulate wound healing and reduce bleb failure from scarring has become routine in trabeculectomy, although their use is still off-label.[12] In trabeculectomy surgery for PACG eyes, there are no specific recommendations for altering the dose or application method of MMC during routine trabeculectomy surgery in PACG eyes compared to POAG eyes. However, general precautions include more posterior scleral application of MMC-soaked sponges to reduce MMC-related complications.[18-20]

Sutures: fixed versus releasable/adjustable

Similar to trabeculectomy surgery in POAG eyes, at least two 10-0 nylon sutures are typically used to close the scleral flap in PACG eyes. While there are no specific recommendations for using fixed or releasable sutures when performing trabeculectomy in PACG eyes from literature review, some surgeons suggest that care must be taken when performing a trabeculectomy on patients with angle closure as they are at greater risk of having AC flattening in the absence of adequate resistance to outflow. However, a study by Tan *et al.* in Singapore found no difference.[21] On the other hand, extra consideration should be given when performing trabeculectomy in PACG eyes of high myopes, who have thinner sclera, and younger patients, who have highly elastic sclera, as they are at higher risk of early postoperative hypotony.[22-24] In such patients, tying tighter sutures may mitigate flap gape and prevent postoperative hypotony.

Comments

It should be highlighted that the lens plays a key role in the pathogenesis of PACG, and its removal should be considered in the overall management of PACG. When performing trabeculectomy alone in PACG eyes, it may be worthwhile considering cataract removal before trabeculectomy to reduce complications.

References

1. Caprioli J, de Leon JM, Azarbod P, et al. Trabeculectomy Can Improve Long-Term Visual Function in Glaucoma. Ophthalmology. 2016;123(1):117-128. https://doi.org/10.1016/j.ophtha.2015.09.027
2. Singh K, Sherwood MB, Pasquale LR. Trabeculectomy Must Survive! Ophthalmology Glaucoma. 2021;4(1):1-2. https://doi.org/10.1016/j.ogla.2020.08.009
3. Tang J, Du E, Li X. Combined Surgical Techniques for the Management of Malignant Glaucoma. J Ophthalmol. 2018;2018:9189585. https://doi.org/10.1155/2018/9189585
4. Jayaram RH, Maheshwari A, Sarrafpour S, Liu J, Teng C. Trends for Glaucoma Surgeries in the United States from 2011 and 2021 - A National Study. Invest Ophthalmol Vis Sci. 2024;65(7):4641.
5. Wanichwecharungruang B, Phumratprapin C, Kongsomboon K, Seresirikachorn K. Real-world Surgical Outcomes of Primary Angle-closure Glaucoma. Clin Ophthalmol. 2021;15:2823-2833. https://doi.org/10.2147/OPTH.S315747
6. Aung T, Tow SL, Yap EY, Chan SP, Seah SK. Trabeculectomy for acute primary angle closure. Ophthalmology. 2000;107(7):1298-1302. https://doi.org/10.1016/S0161-6420(00)00137-8
7. Chen YH, Lu DW, Cheng JH, Chen JT, Chen CL. Trabeculectomy in patients with primary angle-closure glaucoma. J Glaucoma. 2009;18(9):679-683. https://doi.org/10.1097/IJG.0b013e31819c4a07
8. Nguyen HX, Nguyen ND, Nguyen HT, et al. Comparing combined laser iridoplasty and surgical iridectomy with trabeculectomy in treatment of refractory acute primary angle closure without significant cataract: a randomized controlled trial. Eye (Lond). 2023;37(10):2139-2144. https://doi.org/10.1038/s41433-022-02311-z
9. Tham CCY, Kwong YYY, Baig N, Leung DYL, Li FCH, Lam DSC. Phacoemulsification versus trabeculectomy in medically uncontrolled chronic angle-closure glaucoma without cataract. Ophthalmology. 2013;120(1):62-67. https://doi.org/10.1016/j.ophtha.2012.07.021
10. Wang M, Fang M, Bai Y jing, et al. Comparison of combined phacotrabeculectomy with trabeculectomy only in the treatment of primary angle-closure glaucoma. Chin Med J (Engl). 2012;125(8):1429-1433.
11. Tsai HY, Liu CJ, Cheng CY. Combined trabeculectomy and cataract extraction versus trabeculectomy alone in primary angle-closure glaucoma. Br J Ophthalmol. 2009;93(7):943-948. https://doi.org/10.1136/bjo.2008.151803
12. Song BJ, Ramanathan M, Morales E, et al. Trabeculectomy and combined phacoemulsification-trabeculectomy: outcomes and risk factors for failure in primary angle closure glaucoma. J Glaucoma. 2016;25(9):763-769. https://doi.org/10.1097/IJG.0000000000000493
13. Chen YY, Fan SJ, Liang YB, et al. Laser Peripheral Iridotomy versus Trabeculectomy as an Initial Treatment for Primary Angle-Closure Glaucoma. J Ophthalmol. 2017;2017:2761301. https://doi.org/10.1155/2017/2761301

14. Romero P, Hirunpatravong P, Alizadeh R, et al. Trabeculectomy with mitomycin-C: outcomes and risk factors for failure in primary angle-closure glaucoma. Journal of glaucoma. 2018;27(2):101-107. https://doi.org/10.1097/IJG.0000000000000842

15. Rodrigues IA, Alaghband P, Beltran Agullo L, et al. Aqueous outflow facility after phacoemulsification with or without goniosynechialysis in primary angle closure: a randomised controlled study. Br J Ophthalmol. 2017;101(7):879-885. https://doi.org/10.1136/bjophthalmol-2016-309556

16. Teekhasaenee C, Ritch R. Combined phacoemulsification and goniosynechialysis for uncontrolled chronic angle-closure glaucoma after acute angle-closure glaucoma. Ophthalmology. 1999;106(4):669-674; discussion 674-675. https://doi.org/10.1016/S0161-6420(99)90149-5

17. Tang Y, Qian S, Wang J, et al. Effects of combined phacoemulsification and viscogoniosynechialysis versus trabeculectomy in patients with primary angle-closure glaucoma and coexisting cataract. Ophthalmologica. 2012;228(3):167-173. https://doi.org/10.1159/000338241

18. Zhang X, Song Y, Liebmann J, Weinreb RN. A Modified Technique in Applying Sponge Soaked with Mitomycin C in Trabeculectomy. Asia Pac J Ophthalmol (Phila). 2021;10(6):548. https://doi.org/10.1097/APO.0000000000000438

19. Hu K, Song YH, Lin FB, et al. Posterior scleral application of a mitomycin C-soaked sponge during trabeculectomy. International Journal of Ophthalmology. 2023;16(7):1071. https://doi.org/10.18240/ijo.2023.07.11

20. Hu K, Lin F, Song Y, et al. Two-year outcomes of anterior versus posterior scleral application of mitomycin C-soaked sponge in trabeculectomy. Jpn J Ophthalmol. 2024;68(2):126-133. https://doi.org/10.1007/s10384-023-01043-1

21. Tan YL, Tsou PF, Tan GS, et al. Postoperative Complications After Glaucoma Surgery for Primary Angle-Closure Glaucoma vs Primary Open-Angle Glaucoma. Archives of Ophthalmology. 2011;129(8):987-992. https://doi.org/10.1001/archophthalmol.2011.71

22. Seah SKL, Prata JAJ, Minckler DS, Baerveldt G, Lee PP, Heuer DK. Hypotony Following Trabeculectomy. J Glaucoma. 1995;4(2):73. https://doi.org/10.1097/00061198-199504000-00002

23. Fannin LA, Schiffman JC, Budenz DL. Risk factors for hypotony maculopathy. Ophthalmology. 2003;110(6):1185-1191. https://doi.org/10.1016/S0161-6420(03)00227-6

24. Saeedi OJ, Jefferys JL, Solus JF, Jampel HD, Quigley HA. Risk Factors for Adverse Consequences of Low Intraocular Pressure After Trabeculectomy. J Glaucoma. 2014;23(1):e60. https://doi.org/10.1097/IJG.0000000000000008

Phacotrabeculectomy

Rahat Husain, Claire Peterson, Shamira Perera

Is there a role for phacotrabeculectomy in PACG?

Cataract and glaucoma, both being aging-related conditions that tend to affect older people, are often seen in the same patient in glaucoma clinics. If a patient needs surgery to lower IOP, and if trabeculectomy is deemed to be the most appropriate technique to lower IOP to the desired level, it is practical to perform both surgeries together. This is even more reasonable in PACG, where a crowded AC contributes to the disease mechanism, and deepening the AC with lens extraction combined with trabeculectomy ought to improve vision, lower IOP, and deepen the AC all in a single procedure: phacotrabeculectomy.

The main concern with trabeculectomy is that scarring at the outflow site may lead to surgical failure. This is also the main concern with phacotrabeculectomy: does combining the surgeries reduce the longevity or effectiveness of the trabeculectomy? Some data that support this concern is that the prolonged inflammation in the AC that results from Phaco exacerbates the natural scarring that occurs after trabeculectomy, thereby adversely impacting long-term functionality. According to one study, compared to the inflammation after trabeculectomy, which lasts approximately 1 month, the inflammation after Phaco can last 6 months.[1]

A few clinical studies support this hypothesis. The Singapore 5-FU study by Wong *et al.* assessed the timing of cataract surgery on IOP control in eyes that previously had a trabeculectomy. They found that the time between surgeries was inversely proportional to the trabeculectomy failure rate, *i.e.*, the sooner cataract surgery was performed, the worse the IOP control. Extrapolating these results, if the time between surgeries was essentially nil (*i.e.*, the procedures were performed simultaneously) it ought to make the trabeculectomy fail earlier. It should be noted that only approximately half of the Singapore 5-FU study were PACG.[2–4]

One aspect of combined phacotrabeculectomy is that it precludes the need for cataract surgery later, which has been shown to have deleterious effects that precipitate bleb failure[5] due to cytokine upregulation in the AC following Phaco, which leads to bleb fibrosis.[6,7]

In a retrospective analysis of a prospective trial, Hansapinyo *et al.* reported 5-year data on phacotrabeculectomy and found a 29.5% reduction of IOP at 5-year compared to baseline compared to 20% in the standalone Phaco group, which was statistically significant.[8] However, the complication rate in the phacotrabeculectomy group was also significantly higher than the standalone Phaco group. A 2-year study comparing phacotrabeculectomy versus sequential surgery in PACG subjects found similar success rates and complications between the 2 groups; however, in this retrospective analysis, trabeculectomy was performed before Phaco in the sequential group.[9] A retrospective study of over 700 Singaporean eyes with primary glaucoma reported a success rate of 97% at 3 years, with success defined as IOP < 21 mmHg.[10]

The studied conducted by Tham and colleagues on phacotrabeculectomy versus Phaco alone in medically controlled and uncontrolled glaucoma found that although phacotrabeculectomy resulted in lower IOPs (marginal in the case of medically controlled), the complication rate in the former group was higher.[11] Additionally, a study by Ong *et al.* found that combined phacotrabeculectomy resulted in greater myopic refractive prediction error compared to Phaco performed at least 3 months after trabeculectomy and Phaco alone. This may be secondary to fluctuations in AC depth, axial length, and cornea curvature after combined phacotrabeculectomy, which affect the refractive outcome.[12]

Phaco, if combined with GSL, might be the preferred option in specific cases where there is more than 180° of PAS.[13] There is emerging evidence that Phaco plus angle-based MIGS may be effective in PACG.[14-19] Another recent RCT showed phacogoniotomy was non-inferior to phacotrabeculectomy in IOP lowering even in patients with advanced PACG and cataract while providing other advantages, such as improved quality of life.[20,21]

Standalone trabeculectomy has been performed in cases of acute angle closure with some success.[22] However, trabeculectomy alone carries the risk of cataract progression, and subsequent cataract surgery and its associated release of inflammatory mediators can precipitate bleb scarring.[23-25] Additionally, performing trabeculectomy alone can lead to further shallowing of the AC in PACG. A study comparing trabeculectomy alone versus combined phacotrabeculectomy in PACG eyes found that the long-term IOP-lowering effects and surgical complications were similar between both groups; however, the combined phacotrabeculectomy group required fewer subsequent surgical interventions.[26] Another study comparing Phaco and phacotrabeculectomy with MMC in chronic PACG eyes with cataracts found that combined phacotrabeculectomy with MMC is slightly more effective than Phaco alone in controlling IOP and reducing drop dependence at 24 months.[11]

The most pertinent question facing most glaucoma specialists in dealing with patients with cataract and PACG who require surgery is whether to perform a phacotrabeculectomy or Phaco first followed by trabeculectomy, if need be. To our knowledge, there have been no large long-term studies comparing MMC-augmented phacotrabeculectomy to trabeculectomy in pseudophakic PACG eyes—the biological plausibility argument outlined above suggests that the latter strategy ought to perform better. Hence, if longstanding IOP lowering is the objective, then it would be preferable to perform trabeculectomy after cataract surgery (and preferably as long as possible after the surgery, certainly after 6 months), rather than phacotrabeculectomy. However, there are situations where phacotrabeculectomy may still have a role:

- Cost: Depending on the health care system, separating cataract surgery from trabeculectomy is often more expensive than combining them.
- Convenience: If patients live far away from the surgical center, it may be more convenient for them to have the surgery simultaneously, particularly if follow up can be performed by clinicians closer to their home.
- Advanced glaucoma: Wipe-out, although thankfully rare, does occur. Pressure spikes can occur after Phaco, and this can result in wipe-out in cases with very advanced glaucoma.[27,28] Similarly, some patients may not be able to tolerate the somewhat modest IOP-lowering effect of Phaco alone for 6 months before the trabeculectomy is performed.

Tips when performing phacotrabeculectomy in PACG eyes

MMC

Combined surgery with adjunctive use of MMC in PACG eyes has also been associated with a higher risk of hypotony.[29,30] Chen *et al.* examined outcomes of primary phacotrabeculectomy with MMC in a multi-ethnic Asian population.[31] They found that the most common postoperative complications were hypotony (defined as IOP < 6 mmHg), hyphema, and shallow AC. In addition, there was a trend toward PACG eyes having higher complication rates than POAG eyes, although the difference was not statistically significant.[31] However, another study from Singapore found no difference in complications between POAG and PACG eyes undergoing phacotrabeculectomy and trabeculectomy.[32]

When applying MMC during phacotrabeculectomy for PACG, a few considerations should be made:

- Copiously irrigate the area after MMC treatment to remove residual MMC
- The location of improved MMC applications is worth considering.Posterior scleral application of MMC-soaked sponges can greatly reduce MMC-related complications.[33-35]
- If Phaco is performed first:

- Consider suturing the main wound: a firm eye helps with flap creation and prevents the possibility of MMC entering the eye, which causes endothelial damage and increased AC inflammation.[36]
- Be aware that MMC is toxic to the ciliary body, which can lead to cases of late hypotony from aqueous hyposecretion.[37]

One site versus two sites

Phacotrabeculectomy can be done using a 1-site or 2-site approach. In the 1-site technique, the surgeon operates superiorly and Phaco is performed under the scleral flap. Alternatively, a scleral tunnel can be created first, followed by Phaco through it, with the tunnel sides incised to form a flap afterwards. The first method risks wound leakage due to the shorter entry, while the second may hinder probe maneuverability and pose a risk of wound burn from the tight tunnel.

In the 2-site technique, Phaco is performed through a temporal clear corneal incision, and the trabeculectomy is created superiorly. To prevent antimetabolite from entering the AC, the scleral flap and antimetabolite application can be performed prior to Phaco. However, some surgeons prefer performing Phaco first in case of complications during cataract surgery, such as posterior capsule rupture or dropped nucleus, which may necessitate abandoning the trabeculectomy. If Phaco is performed first, the corneal wound should be sutured and the pupil constricted to avoid a broad iridectomy.

Overall, both techniques seem to yield similar results and outcomes and are effective in treating PACG patients with cataract.[38,39] Tow *et al.* compared the IOP outcomes at a mean follow-up duration of 22.0 +/- 5.6 months of 1-site versus separate-site phacotrabeculectomy in chronic PACG eyes and found no significant difference between both groups.[40] Another study by Koh *et al.* studied the 3-year data for 2-site phacotrabeculectomy with MMC in Asian eyes and found it to be a good surgical approach for PACG and POAG eyes with cataracts, with PACG eyes having a more significant IOP reduction than POAG eyes at 3 years.[41] However, 2-site surgery has also been shown to have more corneal endothelial cell loss, likely due to the introduction of a second surgical wound and longer surgery duration.[42,43] Tehran, Iran Therefore, care must be taken during Phaco to stay near the pupil plane or within the bag, especially in eyes with a shallow AC, to reduce damage to corneal endothelial cells. Regardless, for both techniques, use of intensive topical steroids is recommended as there will be increased intraocular inflammation from the concurrent cataract surgery.

Comments

In PACG patients who require filtering surgery, one may consider performing concurrent cataract surgery and mitigate the scarring risk via intraoperative and postoperative measures to yield good long-term results. An alternative is performing Phaco alone, or combined with GSL, and trabeculectomy later if need be.

In many Western countries, phacotrabeculectomy is not commonly performed, as it is presumed that inflammation from concurrent cataract surgery may adversely affect the success of the trabeculectomy. However, in Asian eyes with PACG, there is good evidence that phacotrabeculectomy has good long-term success, particularly for end-stage disease.

In countries with limited access to specialist ophthalmic care and high incidences of ACD with high IOP, a single procedure such as Phaco combined with GSL, with or without goniotomy, with less intensive follow-up may be favored over phacotrabeculectomy.

References

1. Siriwardena D, Kotecha A, Minassian D, et al. Anterior chamber flare after trabeculectomy and after phacoemulsification. Br J Ophthalmol. 2000;84(9):1056-7. https://doi.org/10.1136/bjo.84.9.1056
2. Wong MH, Husain R, Ang BC, et al. The Singapore 5-fluorouracil trial: intraocular pressure outcomes at 8 years. Ophthalmology. 2013;120(6):1127-34. https://doi.org/10.1016/j.ophtha.2012.12.004
3. Wong TT, Khaw PT, Aung T, et al. The singapore 5-Fluorouracil trabeculectomy study: effects on intraocular pressure control and disease progression at 3 years. Ophthalmology. 2009;116(2):175-84. https://doi.org/10.1016/j.ophtha.2008.09.049
4. Husain R, Liang S, Foster PJ, et al. Cataract surgery after trabeculectomy: the effect on trabeculectomy function. Arch Ophthalmol. 2012;130(2):165-70. https://doi.org/10.1001/archophthalmol.2011.329
5. Arimura S, Iwasaki K, Gozawa M, et al. Trabeculectomy followed by phacoemulsification versus trabeculectomy alone: The Collaborative Bleb-Related Infection Incidence and Treatment Study. PLoS One. 2019;14(10):e0223439. https://doi.org/10.1371/journal.pone.0223439
6. Kawai M, Inoue T, Inatani M, et al. Elevated levels of monocyte chemoattractant protein-1 in the aqueous humor after phacoemulsification. Invest Ophthalmol Vis Sci. 2012;53(13):7951-60. https://doi.org/10.1167/iovs.12-10231
7. Inoue T, Kawaji T, Inatani M, et al. Simultaneous increases in multiple proinflammatory cytokines in the aqueous humor in pseudophakic glaucomatous eyes. J Cataract Refract Surg. 2012;38(8):1389-97. https://doi.org/10.1016/j.jcrs.2012.04.028

8. Hansapinyo L, Choy BNK, Lai JSM, Tham CC. Phacoemulsification Versus Phacotrabeculectomy in Primary Angle-closure Glaucoma With Cataract: Long-Term Clinical Outcomes. J Glaucoma. 2020;29(1):15-23. https://doi.org/10.1097/IJG.0000000000001397
9. Li HJ, Xuan J, Zhu XM, Xie L. Comparison of phacotrabeculectomy and sequential surgery in the treatment of chronic angle-closure glaucoma coexisted with cataract. Int J Ophthalmol. 2016;9(5):687-92.
10. Chew AC, Htoon HM, Perera SA, et al. Long-term Outcomes of Combined Phacotrabeculectomy Surgery in a Singapore Tertiary Hospital. Asia Pac J Ophthalmol (Phila). 2024;13(5):100102. https://doi.org/10.1016/j.apjo.2024.100102
11. Tham CC, Kwong YY, Leung DY, et al. Phacoemulsification versus combined phacotrabeculectomy in medically controlled chronic angle closure glaucoma with cataract. Ophthalmology. 2008;115(12):2167-73.e2. https://doi.org/10.1016/j.ophtha.2008.06.016
12. Ong C, Nongpiur M, Peter L, Perera SA. Combined Approach to Phacoemulsification and Trabeculectomy Results in Less Ideal Refractive Outcomes Compared With the Sequential Approach. J Glaucoma. 2016;25(10):e873-e8. https://doi.org/10.1097/IJG.0000000000000489
13. Nguyen Xuan H, Nguyen Dinh N, Nguyen Thu H, et al. Comparing the Safety and Efficacy of Phacogoniosynechialysis With Phacotrabeculectomy in the Management of Refractory Acute Primary Closure Angle Glaucoma With Cataract: A Multicenter Randomized Trial. J Glaucoma. 2021;30(7):552-8. https://doi.org/10.1097/IJG.0000000000001868
14. Salimi A, Abu-Nada M, Harasymowycz P. Matched Cohort Study of Cataract Surgery With and Without Trabecular Microbypass Stent Implantation in Primary Angle-Closure Glaucoma. Am J Ophthalmol. 2021;224:310-20. https://doi.org/10.1016/j.ajo.2020.12.032
15. Song Y, Xie L, Zhu X, et al. Two-year outcome of phacogoniotomy for advanced primary angle-closure glaucoma with cataracts: a multicentre study. Br J Ophthalmol. 2025;109(7):770-4. https://doi.org/10.1136/bjo-2024-325375
16. Song Y, Zhang Y, Li F, et al. One-Year Results of a Multicenter Study: Intraocular Pressure-Lowering Effect of Combined Phacoemulsification, Goniosynechialysis, and Goniotomy for Cases of Advanced Primary Angle-Closure Glaucoma With Cataract. Asia Pac J Ophthalmol (Phila). 2022;11(6):529-35. https://doi.org/10.1097/APO.0000000000000579
17. Dorairaj S, Tam MD, Balasubramani GK. Two-Year Clinical Outcomes of Combined Phacoemulsification, Goniosynechialysis, and Excisional Goniotomy For Angle-Closure Glaucoma. Asia Pac J Ophthalmol (Phila). 2020;10(2):183-7. https://doi.org/10.1097/APO.0000000000000321
18. Wang Y, Liang ZQ, Zhang Y, et al. Efficacy and safety of phacoemulsification plus goniosynechialysis and Trabectome in patients with primary angle-closure glaucoma. Sci Rep. 2021;11(1):13921. https://doi.org/10.1038/s41598-021-92972-9
19. Laroche D, Brown A, Ng C. Clear Lensectomy, Goniosynechiolysis and Hydrus Microstent in a Patient with Mixed Mechanism Glaucoma. J Natl Med Assoc. 2020;112(4):339-43. https://doi.org/10.1016/j.jnma.2020.04.003

20. Song Y, Fan S, Tang L, et al. Two-Year Outcomes of Phacogoniotomy vs Phacotrabeculectomy for Advanced Primary Angle-Closure Glaucoma With Cataract: A Noninferiority Randomized Clinical Trial. JAMA Ophthalmol. 2025;143(6):462-9. https://doi.org/10.1001/jamaophthalmol.2025.0685
21. Song Y, Lin F, Lv A, et al. Phacogoniotomy versus phacotrabeculectomy for advanced primary angle-closure glaucoma with cataract: A randomized non-inferiority trial. Asia Pac J Ophthalmol (Phila). 2024;13(1):100033. https://doi.org/10.1016/j.apjo.2023.100033
22. Nguyen HX, Nguyen ND, Nguyen HT, et al. Comparing combined laser iridoplasty and surgical iridectomy with trabeculectomy in treatment of refractory acute primary angle closure without significant cataract: a randomized controlled trial. Eye (Lond). 2023;37(10):2139-44. https://doi.org/10.1038/s41433-022-02311-z
23. Costa VP, Smith M, Spaeth GL, et al. Loss of visual acuity after trabeculectomy. Ophthalmology. 1993;100(5):599-612. https://doi.org/10.1016/S0161-6420(93)31597-6
24. Sharma TK, Arora S, Corridan PG. Phacoemulsification in patients with previous trabeculectomy: role of 5-fluorouracil. Eye (Lond). 2007;21(6):780-3. https://doi.org/10.1038/sj.eye.6702327
25. Nishi O, Nishi K, Ohmoto Y. Synthesis of interleukin-1, interleukin-6, and basic fibroblast growth factor by human cataract lens epithelial cells. J Cataract Refract Surg. 1996;22 Suppl 1:852-8. https://doi.org/10.1016/S0886-3350(96)80174-X
26. Tsai HY, Liu CJ, Cheng CY. Combined trabeculectomy and cataract extraction versus trabeculectomy alone in primary angle-closure glaucoma. Br J Ophthalmol. 2009;93(7):943-8. https://doi.org/10.1136/bjo.2008.151803
27. Fu L, Chan YK, Li J, et al. Long term outcomes of cataract surgery in severe and end stage primary angle closure glaucoma with controlled IOP: a retrospective study. BMC Ophthalmol. 2020;20(1):160. https://doi.org/10.1186/s12886-020-01434-9
28. Ramsden C, Shweikh Y, Kam R, et al. Estimating the rate of severe visual loss (wipe-out) following cataract surgery, a British Ophthalmological Surveillance Unit (BOSU) study. Eye (Lond). 2023;37(18):3787-92. https://doi.org/10.1038/s41433-023-02606-9
29. El Sayed YM, Elhusseiny AM, Albalkini AS, et al. Mitomycin C-augmented Phacotrabeculectomy Versus Phacoemulsification in Primary Angle-closure Glaucoma: A Randomized Controlled Study. J Glaucoma. 2019;28(10):911-5. https://doi.org/10.1097/IJG.0000000000001345
30. Kupin TH, Juzych MS, Shin DH, et al. Adjunctive mitomycin C in primary trabeculectomy in phakic eyes. Am J Ophthalmol. 1995;119(1):30-9. https://doi.org/10.1016/S0002-9394(14)73810-3
31. Chen DZ, Koh V, Sng C, et al. Complications and outcomes of primary phacotrabeculectomy with mitomycin C in a multi-ethnic Asian population. PLoS One. 2015;10(3):e0118852. https://doi.org/10.1371/journal.pone.0118852
32. Tan YL, Tsou PF, Tan GS, et al. Postoperative complications after glaucoma surgery for primary

angle-closure glaucoma vs primary open-angle glaucoma. Arch Ophthalmol. 2011;129(8):987-92. https://doi.org/10.1001/archophthalmol.2011.71

33. Zhang X, Song Y, Liebmann J, Weinreb RN. A Modified Technique in Applying Sponge Soaked with Mitomycin C in Trabeculectomy. Asia Pac J Ophthalmol (Phila) 2021;10(6):548-52. https://doi.org/10.1097/APO.0000000000000438
34. Hu K, Song YH, Lin FB, et al. Posterior scleral application of a mitomycin C-soaked sponge during trabeculectomy. Int J Ophthalmol. 2023;16(7):1071-7. https://doi.org/10.18240/ijo.2023.07.11
35. Hu K, Lin F, Song Y, et al. Two-year outcomes of anterior versus posterior scleral application of mitomycin C-soaked sponge in trabeculectomy. Jpn J Ophthalmol. 2024;68(2):126-33. https://doi.org/10.1007/s10384-023-01043-1
36. Swogger J, Conner IP, Rosano M, et al. Injected Versus Sponge-Applied Mitomycin C (MMC) During Modified Trabeculectomy in New Zealand White Rabbit Model. Transl Vis Sci Technol. 2020;9(11):23. https://doi.org/10.1167/tvst.9.11.23
37. Nuyts RM, Felten PC, Pels E, et al. Histopathologic effects of mitomycin C after trabeculectomy in human glaucomatous eyes with persistent hypotony. Am J Ophthalmol 1994;118(2):225-37. https://doi.org/10.1016/S0002-9394(14)72903-4
38. Wyse T, Meyer M, Ruderman JM, et al. Combined trabeculectomy and phacoemulsification: a one-site vs a two-site approach. Am J Ophthalmol. 1998;125(3):334-9. https://doi.org/10.1016/S0002-9394(99)80143-3
39. Borggrefe J, Lieb W, Grehn F. A prospective randomized comparison of two techniques of combined cataract-glaucoma surgery. Graefes Arch Clin Exp Ophthalmol. 1999;237(11):887-92. https://doi.org/10.1007/s004170050381
40. Tow SL, Aung T, Oen FT, Seah SK. Combined phacoemulsification, intraocular lens implantation and trabeculectomy for chronic angle closure glaucoma. Int Ophthalmol. 2001;24(5):283-9. https://doi.org/10.1023/A:1025478923950
41. Koh V, Chen D, Aquino CM, et al. Success rates of 2-site phacoemulsification combined with fornix-based trabeculectomy using mitomycin C for primary angle-closure glaucoma and primary open-angle glaucoma in an Asian population. Jpn J Ophthalmol. 2017;61(3):245-52. https://doi.org/10.1007/s10384-017-0502-4
42. Nassiri N, Nassiri N, Rahnavardi M, Rahmani L. A comparison of corneal endothelial cell changes after 1-site and 2-site phacotrabeculectomy. Cornea. 2008;27(8):889-94. https://doi.org/10.1097/ICO.0b013e31817618b0
43. Buys YM, Chipman ML, Zack B, et al. Prospective randomized comparison of one- versus two-site Phacotrabeculectomy two-year results. Ophthalmology. 2008;115(7):1130-3.e1. https://doi.org/10.1016/j.ophtha.2007.09.007

GDD/Phaco + GDD in the surgical treatment of primary angle-closure glaucoma

Joseph Anthony Tumbocon, Benjamin Xu

An aqueous tube shunt to an extraocular equatorial plate, also referred to as GDD or tube, is usually indicated in eyes with high risk for failure or complications with other types of glaucoma surgeries or procedures.[1-4] In PACG, the pupillary block component should be corrected by LPI, SPI, or lens extraction to allow aqueous to flow from the posterior chamber to the AC. If IOP remains medically uncontrolled or if there is presence of extensive PAS, then other interventions should be considered.

Potential indications for GDD implantation in PACG

GDD implantation is indicated in more refractory and/or complicated forms of PACG unresponsive to other types of treatment, or those with comorbidities/ conditions that increase the risk of failure with other management options[1,2,4], such as presence of:

- Extensive conjunctival scarring.
- Previous failed trabeculectomy with MMC.
- Anterior segment neovascularization.
- Active, recurrent or chronic AC inflammation.
- Aphakia.
- Epithelial ingrowth.
- Vitreoretinal pathology that required pars plana vitrectomy or scleral buckling.
- Intravitreal silicone oil.
- Thin superior sclera.
- Severe periocular disease.

Types of devices

This group of devices have a common design: a tube that shunts aqueous from the eye to an extraocular equatorial plate located in sub-Tenon's space. Commonly used glaucoma drainage devices are the Ahmed Glaucoma Valve (New World Medical, Rancho Cucamonga, CA, USA), Baerveldt (Johnson & Johnson Surgical Vision, Irvine, CA, USA), PAUL Glaucoma Implant (Advanced Ophthalmic Innovations, Singapore), Molteno 3 (Molteno Ophthalmic Limited, Dunedine, New Zealand), Aurolab Aqueous Drainage Implant (AADI; Aravind Eye Care System, Madurai, India), and Ahmed ClearPath (New World Medical) implants.[1,5-7]

The Ahmed Glaucoma Valve has a flow restricting mechanism that allows for immediate and controlled IOP reduction with lower incidence of hypotony, but tends to have higher postoperative IOPs compared to the Baerveldt 350 mm^2 implant.[1-3] The PAUL Glaucoma Implant has a small internal tube diameter that may help prevent excessive aqueous outflow.[5] The non-valved implants such as the Baerveldt, Molteno 3, Ahmed ClearPath, and AADI implants require external tube ligation with an absorbable suture ± intraluminal stent to prevent early postoperative hypotony.

Considerations in the choice of GDD

- In eyes that require low target IOPs, a non-valved GDD with larger surface area is preferred since it will have a better chance of achieving lower postoperative IOPs compared to devices with smaller plates, but this is true only up to a certain extent.[1-3,8-10]
- In eyes with very high IOPs despite maximum medical therapy or those at higher risk for hypotony-related complications, a valved GDD can achieve immediate and controlled IOP reduction with less risk of hypotony.[1-3] Another possible option is to use a device with a small internal tube diameter together with an intraluminal stent. Fenestrations or venting slits may be used in ligated non-valved implants for early postoperative IOP control, but the results may sometimes be unpredictable.
- The amount of conjunctival scarring or presence of impediments to GDD implantation may influence the location and size of the implant.
- Availability.
- Experience with the device(s).
- Cost, especially in healthcare systems where GDDs are an out-of-pocket expense for the patient.

Review of evidence of GDDs in PACG

There are case series, retrospective and non-randomized comparative studies describing short and intermediate-term outcomes of GDDs specifically in PACG eyes.[11-13] However, the literature is sparse and lacks higher-level studies. It has been suggested that the success rate of GDD implantation in primary glaucoma is higher than in secondary glaucoma.[11] This is probably due to less risk factors for failure in primary versus secondary glaucoma.

A retrospective comparative study by Helwe *et al.* showed that GDD surgery in ACG eyes produced similar IOP reduction,[12] complication rates, and qualified success rates compared to trabeculectomy with MMC. However, more eyes in the GDD group had prior Phaco and/or trabeculectomy (67%) compared to the trabeculectomy with MMC group (17%). The difference in the baseline characteristics may influence the accuracy in the comparison of outcomes between the 2 interventions.

PACG eyes were included in the Ahmed Baerveldt Comparison (ABC) and Ahmed Versus Baerveldt (AVB) RCTs.[1,2] However, they comprised a small proportion of the study population at 6% to 7%, and subgroup analysis was not conducted. In retrospective studies on GDD implantation in ACG patients, the probability of success was estimated to range from 67% to 75% at 2 years.[12,13] The results seem to parallel the results of the pooled analysis of the ABC, AVB, and Tube Versus Trabeculectomy (TVT) studies, which showed a 38.3% cumulative probability of failure at 5 years after GDD surgery,[14] although the pooled analysis had a more heterogenous study population and longer observation period.

The chance of re-operation after GDD implantation in PACG may be higher due to potential technical difficulties in this group of eyes. In an analysis of cases that underwent repeat GDD surgery, revision, or removal of implant in the Intelligent Research in Sight (IRIS) registry, it was observed that the diagnosis of chronic angle closure increased the risk by a factor of 1.32 compared to other diagnostic entities. It is hypothesized that shallower AC depth, tendency to insert the tube more anteriorly, more obtuse angle of entry, and corneal compromise by the tube may be some reasons for this finding.[15]

Preoperative evaluation

PACG eyes that require GDD surgery are usually those that have a higher risk for failure or complications with other types of intervention. Careful preoperative examination and planning is essential to increase the chance of successful outcomes. The conjunctiva, AC depth, iridocorneal angle, lens status, presence of comorbidities, and impediments to plate and/or tube insertion should be meticulously evaluated. This will help determine the ideal location for plate implantation and tube insertion as well as type of GDD to use. Combined Phaco with IOL and GDD implantation can be considered in eyes with significant cataract or very shallow AC due to a thick crystalline lens.

Surgical considerations

A challenge for conventional AC tube placement in PACG is the presence of PAS and/or a shallow AC. In eyes with PAS, but with resolved pupillary block and relatively deep AC, an OVD can be injected in the AC to push the peripheral iris posteriorly and the tube inserted into the AC through the PAS (Fig. 1) or GSL performed prior to tube insertion. Other options include placing the tip of the tube

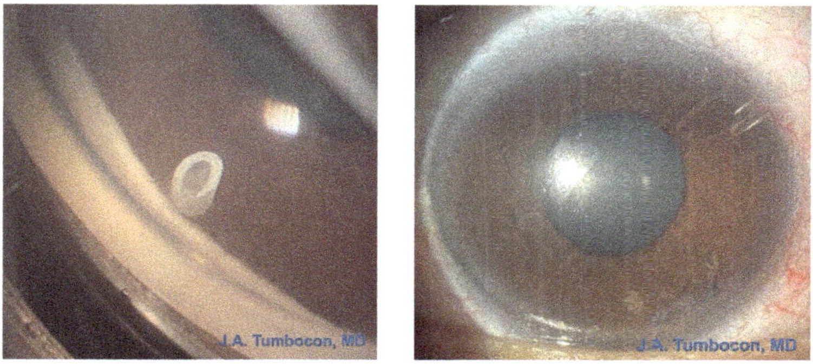

Fig. 1. Tube insertion into the anterior chamber and through the peripheral anterior synechiae in an eye with primary angle-closure glaucoma with failed trabeculectomy. Intraoperative deepening of the peripheral anterior chamber was performed using ophthalmic viscosurgical device to push the peripheral iris posteriorly prior to tube insertion in the anterior chamber.

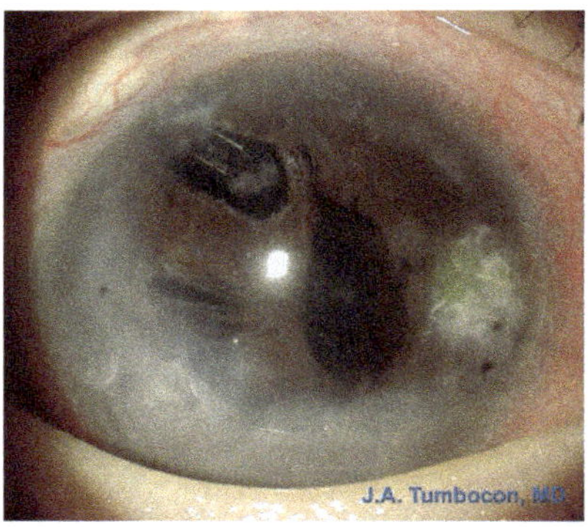

Fig. 2. A surgical peripheral iridectomy was created to make more space for anterior chamber tube insertion in an eye that previously underwent multiple complicated ocular surgeries, had shallow anterior chamber, and high peripheral anterior synechiae/peripheral iridocorneal adhesions.

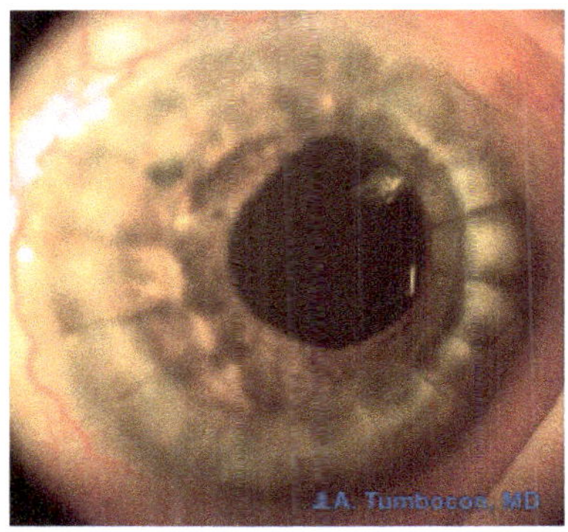

Fig. 3. Tube insertion through the ciliary sulcus in an eye with primary angle-closure glaucoma with failed trabeculectomy and post-penetrating keratoplasty for pseudophakic bullous keratopathy. The tip of the tube is visible through a pharmacologically dilated pupil.

at the area of a SPI whether pre-existing or created intraoperatively prior to tube insertion (Fig. 2); ciliary sulcus tube insertion in pseudophakic eyes (Fig. 3); or pars plana insertion in vitrectomized eyes (Fig. 4). In eyes with shallow AC due to a thick lens and presence of extensive PAS, a combined Phaco/tube with sulcus tube insertion is a viable alternative to avoid corneal damage. It is important to keep the tube as far away from the corneal endothelium as possible to decrease the chance of significant corneal endothelial cell loss. The aforementioned techniques can help achieve this in PACG eyes with shallow AC and/or PAS.[16,17]

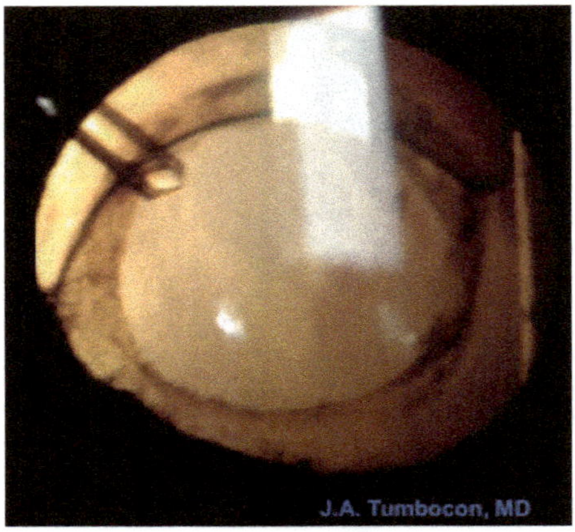

Fig. 4. Pars plana tube insertion in a vitrectomized pseudophakic eye with the tube visible through a pharmacologically dilated pupil.

Areas for future investigation

There are gaps in knowledge regarding GDD implantation in PACG eyes. Future research studies that can be considered are:

- RCTs and non-randomized cohort studies comparing AC versus ciliary sulcus insertion of GDD tubes in pseudophakic PACG eyes that include corneal endothelial cell count as well as complete and qualified success rates as outcome measures.
- RCTs, non-randomized cohort, and cross-sectional studies comparing success rates of GDD implantation in phakic and pseudophakic PACG eyes.
- RCTs and non-randomized cohort studies comparing non-valved versus valved GDDs in PACG.
- Network meta-analyses to investigate safety and efficacy of various GDDs in PACG and other types of glaucoma.

Comments

GDD implantation is a useful tool for managing refractory and complicated forms of PACG that have a high risk of failure with other types of interventions. Meticulous preoperative evaluation, familiarity with the available devices, careful attention to details, modification of surgical technique when needed, and proper postoperative care will help achieve favorable outcomes.

References

1. Budenz DL, Barton K, Gedde SJ, et al. Five-year treatment outcome in the Ahmed Baerveldt comparison study. Ophthalmology. 2015:122:308-316 https://doi.org/10.1016/j.

ophtha.2014.08.043

2. Christakis PG, Kalenak JW, Tsai JC, et al. The Ahmed versus Baerveldt study: Five-year treatment outcomes. Ophthalmology. 2016:123:2093-2102. https://doi.org/10.1016/j.ophtha.2016.06.035
3. Christakis PG, Zhang D, Budenz DL, et al. Five-year pooled data analysis of the Ahmed Baerveldt comparison study and Ahmed versus Baerveldt study. Am J Ophthalmol. 2017;176:118-126. https://doi.org/10.1016/j.ajo.2017.01.003
4. Gedde SJ, Schiffman JC, Feuer WJ, et al Treatment outcomes in tube versus trabeculectomy (TVT) study after five years of follow up. Am J Ophthalmol. 2012;153:789-803. https://doi.org/10.1016/j.ajo.2011.10.026
5. Tan MCJ, Ong CW, Aquino MC, et al. Three-year outcome of Paul Glaucoma Implant for treatment of glaucoma. J Glaucoma. 2024; 33: 478-405. https://doi.org/10.1097/IJG.0000000000002369
6. Grover DS, Kahook MY, Seibod LK, et al. Clinical outcomes of Ahmed ClearPath implantation in glaucomatous eyes: A novel valveless glaucoma drainage Device. J Glaucoma. 2022;31:335-339. https://doi.org/10.1097/IJG.0000000000002013
7. Hong M, Peng Y, Lai Yuan, et al. Comparison of Aurolab aqueous drainage implant with Ahmed glaucoma valve for refractory glaucoma: A meta-analysis. Ophthalmic Res. 2023;66:457-464. https://doi.org/10.1159/000529039
8. Meyer AM, Rodgers CD, Zou B, et al. Retrospective comparison of Intermediate-term efficacy 350 mm2 and glaucoma drainage device implant and medium-sized 230-250mm2 implants, J Curr Glaucoma Pract. 2017;11:8-15. https://doi.org/10.5005/jp-journals-10008-1214
9. Heuer DK, Lloyd MA, Abrams DA, et al. Whis is better? One or two? A randomized clinical trial of single-plate versus double plate Molteno implantation for glaucoma in aphakia and pseudophakia. Ophthalmogy .1992; 99: 1512-1519. https://doi.org/10.1016/S0161-6420(92)31772-5
10. Britt MT, LaBree LD, Llloyd MA, et al. Randomized clinical trial of 350mm2 versus the 500 mm2 Baerveldt implant longer term results. Is bigger better? Ophthalmology. 1999;106:2312-2318. https://doi.org/10.1016/S0161-6420(99)90532-8
11. Rojananuangnit K, Jiaranaisilawong P, Rattanaphaithun O, et al. Surgical outcomes of glaucoma drainage device implantation in refractory glaucoma patients in Thailand. Clin Ophthalmol. 2022:16:4163-4178. https://doi.org/10.2147/OPTH.S393730
12. Helwe HE, Samuel S, Falah H, et al. Comparing outcomes of tube vs trabeculectomy among patients with angle closure glaucoma. Ophthalmol Glaucoma. 2024;7(5):476-484. https://doi.org/10.1016/j.ogla.2024.04.005
13. Huang KH, Chen CL, Lu DW, et al. Outcomes of small size Ahmed glaucoma valve implantation in Asian chronic angle-closure glaucoma. J Clin Med. 2021;10:813. https://doi.org/10.3390/jcm10040813

14. Bowden EC, Choudhury A, Gedde SJ, et al. Risk factors for failure of tube shunt surgery: A pooled data analysis. Am J Ophthalmol. 2022;204:217-224. https://doi.org/10.1016/j.ajo.2022.02.027
15. Hall NE, Chang Ek, Samuel S, et al. Risk factors for glaucoma drainage device revision or removal using the IRIS registry. Am J Ophthalmol. 2022:240:302-320. https://doi.org/10.1016/j.ajo.2022.03.029
16. Tan AN, Webers CAB, Berendschot TTJM, et al. Corneal endothelial cell loss after Baervedlt glaucoma drainage implantation in the anterior chamber. Acta Ophthalmol. 2017:95:91-96. https://doi.org/10.1111/aos.13161
17. Hau S, Bunce C and Barton K. Corneal endothelial cell loss after Baerveldt glaucoma implant surgery. Ophthalmol Glaucoma. 2021;4(1):20-31. https://doi.org/10.1016/j.ogla.2020.06.012

Cycloablation procedures

Parul Ichhpujani, Tanuj Dada

Introduction

Cycloablation therapeutics for reducing IOP in glaucoma act by inducing the coagulative necrosis of secretory ciliary epithelium either using laser (trans-scleral/endoscopic), focused ultrasound, or cryotherapy, thus partially damaging the CB and reducing aqueous production. However, non-selectivity for the target tissue, an unpredictable dose-effect relationship, and sight threatening complications have been the major drawbacks of these techniques.

UCP

UCP is a non-invasive MIGS which uses high-intensity focused ultrasound and has proven to be a precise method of CB coagulation resulting in a significant IOP reduction. This technique involves 6 active transducers which treat 6 separate areas of the CB, covering approximately 40% of the total surface area, thereby reducing the risk of hypotony. The temperature with diode cyclophotocoagulation may vary from 60°C to over 100°C, whereas UCP causes smaller temperature variation between 70° and 80°C, which eliminates the risks of tissue explosion. UCP induces a remodeling of the CB by removal of epithelial cell layers.[1] Since there is no tissue explosion, re-treatment is feasible after UCP in cases where the desired IOP reduction is not reached. UCP results in reduction of aqueous humor production as well as increase in the uveoscleral outflow. A recent meta-analysis has shown that UCP is a safe and effective procedure that may help in reduction of antiglaucoma medications.[2]

Standalone UCP

Several studies have demonstrated positive outcomes of UCP for IOP reduction in patients with different types of glaucoma. However, the literature is sparse regarding UCP for PACG. Luo *et al.* reported results of UCP in 23 eyes of Chinese glaucoma patients, of which only 9 had PACG. Mean IOP reduced from 43.3 ± 13 mmHg at baseline to 22.8 ± 10.7 mmHg. The PACG eyes had 41% IOP reduction and 78% success rate at 6 months.[3] Hu *et al.* also evaluated UCP in Chinese glaucoma patients and found that PACG responded better than other types of glaucoma, achieving an IOP reduction of 36.1% ($N = 18$).[4]

A retrospective cohort study by Almobarak *et al.* evaluated the 2-year outcomes of UCP in uncontrolled glaucoma.[5] They evaluated 66 eyes with PACG of a total of 182 eyes. At 1 year and 2 years, the overall success rates were 78% (143/182 eyes) and 85.6% (95/111 eyes), respectively, and the failure rates were 21.4% (39/182 eyes) and 14.4% (16/111 eyes), respectively. The most common complications were cataract development/progression and AC reaction. However, the reduction in IOP and the complication profiles were not reported for different types of glaucoma. In a subsequent retrospective cohort study, Almobarak *et al.* studied the efficacy of UCP in 62 eyes with angle closure.[6] There was a significant IOP reduction from a baseline value of 23.0 ± 6.4 mmHg to a mean value of 15.6 ± 8.0 mmHg at 1 year and 14.2 ± 5.0 mmHg at 2 years. The authors found that a high baseline IOP was associated with a higher risk of failure.

Complications such as AC reaction, cataract development or progression, IOP spikes, and macular edema have been reported post-UCP. These can be attributed to the possible disruption of the blood-aqueous barrier following coagulative necrosis of the ciliary epithelium. Inflammatory mediators released due to the compromised blood-aqueous barrier result in inflammation, fibrinous reaction, aggravation of cataractogenesis, and in cases with transvitreal spread of these mediators, macular edema. Other mild and temporary adverse effects include transient mild mydriasis, conjunctival hyperemia, and superficial punctate keratitis.[7]

Phaco + UCP

Combined Phaco with UCP (Phaco+UCP) has also been found to be effective for the management of coexisting cataract and OAG.[8] However, no study has reported outcomes of Phaco + UCP exclusively for PACG.

Comments

- UCP is an effective technique to lower IOP in eyes with PACG. However, there is paucity of studies on its utility in PACG patients.
- No study has reported on the efficacy of combined Phaco + UCP for PACG.

MP-TLT

MP-TLT is a variation of continuous trans-scleral cyclophotocoagulation that delivers energy in a pulsatile manner. The Cyclo G6 Laser with the MicroPulse P3 Delivery Device (Iridex, Mountain View, CA, USA) uses an infrared diode laser with a wavelength of 810 nm in which the continuous energy wave is divided into a series of pulses, minimizing tissue temperature elevation and coagulative damage. MP-TLT does not generate any macroscopic or microscopic alterations to TM cells, resulting in reduced inflammation and adverse effects.[9] Johnstone *et al.* have suggested that MP-TLT acts on the longitudinal fibers of the ciliary muscle, causing a displacement of the scleral spur in an inward and posterior direction, which modifies the configuration of the TM and improves the aqueous outflow akin to pilocarpine.[10]

Standalone MP-TLT

The treatment protocols in the literature have been very heterogeneous, especially after introduction of the revised MP3 probe. A dosimetry study for OAG patients comparing 100-seconds (total energy: 78.25 J, fluence: 109.2 J/cm^2) versus 120-seconds (total energy: 93.9 J, fluence: 131.0 J/cm^2) total treatment duration, delivering 2.5 W energy, 31.3% duty cycle, applied in 3 sweeps per hemisphere using the revised MP3 probe, showed that significantly greater IOP reduction was noted in the 120-seconds group.[11]

Grippo *et al.* have highlighted sweep velocity as an important parameter to be considered.[12] Consensus recommendations for standard MP-TLT settings using the revised MicroPulse P3 Probe are 2,500 mW, 4 sweeps at a sweep velocity of 20 seconds each per hemisphere, and 31.3% duty cycle.[13]

In an Indian study, 33 phakic PACG eyes with a patent laser iridotomy and uncontrolled IOP despite maximum ocular hypotensive medications underwent MP-TLT using power of 2,000 mW for a duration of 180 seconds.[14] Twenty eyes (62.5%) achieved qualified success, while only 1 eye (3.12%) attained absolute success at 1 year with IOP $\leq$ 18 mmHg. There was a significant reduction of IOP from baseline, from 25.7 $\pm$ 5.3 mmHg to 17.9 $\pm$ 4.6 mmHg at the end of 1 year ($p < 0.0001$). The number of antiglaucoma medications also decreased significantly from 4.4 $\pm$ 0.8 at baseline to 2.9 $\pm$ 1.1 at 1 year ($p < 0.0001$). Five eyes (15.6%)

received additional treatment. No major post-laser complications were noted.

Waldo *et al.* described a modified technique, Cyclo Mix, where MP-TLT was performed with continuous energy in the inferior hemifield (Thermo Cyclo mode; 1,000 mW with exposure of 2 seconds per spot) and micropulse energy in the superior hemifield (Subcyclo; 2,000 mW at a duty cycle of 35% for 80–150 seconds). Of 23 eyes that were evaluated, only 4 eyes had advanced PACG with visual potential. The authors did not stratify their results based on types of glaucoma included. However, they found that the Cyclo Mix effectively reduced IOP and glaucoma medications for a period of up to 6 months.[15]

A histological study has shown that MP-TLT causes conjunctival inflammation and scarring, both of which are risk factors for fibrosis of the conjunctival bleb in case of a subsequent filtration surgery.[16] Neurotrophic keratitis, although rare, has been reported after MP-TLT in patients with underlying corneal pathologies for decreased corneal sensation.[17] Conjunctival laceration has been reported in a case with significant subconjunctival hemorrhage.[18]

Phaco + MP-TLT

Daas *et al.* were the first to evaluate the effect of Phaco combined with MP-TLT (Phaco + MP-TLT) in glaucoma patients.[19] However, only 4 out of 42 eyes had PACG. Glaucoma filtration surgery was in 5 patients, 2 of which had PACG.

Habash *et al.* conducted a retrospective review of 22 eyes of 19 patients that underwent combined Phaco + MP-TLT, of which 9 eyes had chronic PACG.[20] They reported no significant difference in IOP reduction between POAG (34.0% ± 10.1%), PACG (48.8% ± 10.4%), and pseudoexfoliation glaucoma (45.7% ± 0.2%) ($p = 0.077$). There was no significant difference in antiglaucoma medication or best-corrected visual acuity, implying that the combined approach was suitable for different glaucoma subtypes.

No RCT has been conducted comparing MP-TLT with any other glaucoma surgery in individuals with PACG and good visual acuity.[21] Evidence supporting a wider use of standalone MP-TLT or combined with Phaco in the earlier stages of PACG is lacking.

Comments

- MP-TLT can be used as an interim treatment to lower IOP in eyes with PACG before definitive treatments, such as lens extraction with or without glaucoma surgery, is performed.
- Limited literature exists regarding MP-TLT as a standalone or combined procedure with Phaco in PACG patients.

- Prospective trials with standardized parameters are needed for evaluating the safety and efficacy of MP-TLT in PACG

ECP

ECP) uses laser photocoagulation to ablate the ciliary processes under direct visualization, thus reducing aqueous production. An 810 nm diode laser is commonly used as a light source; however, recently, a 532 nm green laser with lower penetration depth has also been utilized.[22] ECP can be used as a standalone procedure only in eyes that have previously undergone lens extraction in PACG as there is risk of lenticular injury if performed in phakic PACG eyes. It is usually combined with lens extraction/cataract surgery and performed after IOL insertion through the same clear corneal incision used for Phaco.[23] A slow, continuous wave application of the laser treatment to individual ciliary processes for 180°–270° provides optimal IOP reduction.

Standalone ECP

While ECP can be effective in managing PACG, it is not used as a standalone procedure in PAC/PACG as it is not possible to perform this procedure in phakic eyes with a shallow AC.

Phaco + ECP

Combined Phaco and ECP (Phaco + ECP) has primarily been used in patients with plateau iris to shrink the ciliary processes and open the angle.[24] ECP has also been tried in non-plateau iris cases of chronic PACG considering that shrinkage of the ciliary processes creates a space that will accommodate the thickened peripheral iris without blocking the TM during pupillary dilation.

Lin *et al.* have shown that Phaco + ECP reduced IOP to a greater degree in ACG as compared to OAG.[25] Twenty-two eyes with chronic PACG had greater IOP reduction (6.4 mmHg versus 2.1 mmHg, $p = 0.01$) and reduction of antiglaucoma medications (0.9 versus 0.2, $p = 0.04$) than the 41 eyes with POAG at 1 year. They reported that ECP caused significant reduction in aqueous production in eyes with any amount of damage, unlike most MIGS procedures that target the TM, which are effective mostly in mild to moderate glaucomatous damage.

In a study by Pathak-Ray, 32 eyes underwent Phaco +ECP, with ECP performed for 180° to 210°. The median IOP pre-Phaco + ECP was 20.5 mmHg, which decreased significantly post-procedure at last follow-up to 16 mmHg ($p < 0.001$).[26] There was a significant decrease in the number of antiglaucoma medications from a median of 3 to a median of none at the last follow-up ($p <$

0.001). There were no serious sight-threatening complications. In a subsequent study, the author also compared the efficacy and safety of Phaco + ECP (25 eyes) versus phacotrabeculectomy (20 eyes) in medically controlled or uncontrolled PAC or PACG after laser iridotomy.[27] Mean preoperative and postoperative IOP, antiglaucoma medications, and best-corrected visual acuity did not differ between the groups. However, the rate of complications ($p = 0.011$) and interventions ($p = 0.047$) was greater in the phacotrabeculectomy group.

No significant differences were noted in reduction of IOP and antiglaucoma medications when combined Phaco and visco-GSL with and without ECP were compared in PACG patients.[28] In a RCT by Lai *et al.*, 27 PACG eyes received Phaco + ECP while 21 PACG eyes underwent Phaco alone. Combined Phaco + ECP resulted in lower mean IOP and antiglaucoma medications than Phaco alone at all follow-up visits, but the differences did not reach statistical significance.[29]

A systematic meta-analysis of 9 studies with data from 5,389 eyes compared Phaco +ECP with Phaco alone in different types of glaucoma patients. Phaco + ECP showed sustained IOP reduction and decreased antiglaucoma medication dependence when compared with Phaco alone in all forms of glaucoma. However, the combined group had higher complication rates. This meta-analysis did not analyze the response of Phaco + ECP in terms of POAG versus PACG.[30]

Comments

- ECP has been found to be effective in reducing IOP in both plateau and non-plateau iris cases of chronic PACG. Phaco + ECP has the potential to lower IOP and reduce the need for medications much more than Phaco alone.
- Prospective studies are needed to compare Phaco +ECP versus Phaco alone and its utility when combined with other MIGS procedures performed in conjunction with Phaco in patients with PACG.

References

1. Roquancourt T, Aptel F, Rouland JF. UBM evaluation of mechanisms that drive intraocular pressure (IOP) decrease after ultrasound ciliary plasty (UCP) with high intensity focused ultrasound (HIFU), towards a new explanation of the role of uveoscleral pathway outflow. Presented at the 20th European Association for Vision and Eye Research Conference. Acta Ophthalmol. 2017;95. https://doi.org/10.1111/j.1755-3768.2017.0S055
2. Wu TH, Yin X, Li JQ, Lu PR. Efficacy and safety of ultrasound cycloplasty for the treatment of glaucoma: a Meta-analysis. Int J Ophthalmol. 2023 Aug 18;16(8):1317-1325. https://doi.org/10.18240/ijo.2023.08.19

3. Luo Q, Xue W, Wang Y, et al. Ultrasound Cycloplasty in Chinese Glaucoma Patients: Results of a 6-Month Prospective Clinical Study. Ophthalmic Res. 2022;65(4):466-473. https://doi.org/10.1159/000515013
4. Hu D, Tu S, Zuo C, Ge J. Short-Term Observation of Ultrasonic Cyclocoagulation in Chinese Patients with End-Stage Refractory Glaucoma: A Retrospective Study. J Ophthalmol. 2018 Sep 6;2018:4950318. https://doi.org/10.1155/2018/4950318
5. Almobarak FA, Alrubean A, Alsarhani WK, Aljenaidel A, Osman EA. Ultrasound Cyclo Plasty in Glaucoma: 2-Year Outcomes. J Glaucoma. 2022 Oct 1;31(10):834-838. https://doi.org/10.1097/IJG.0000000000002078
6. Almobarak FA, Alrubean A, Alsarhani WK, Aljenaidel A, Osman EA. Outcomes of Ultrasound Cyclo Plasty in Primary Angle Closure Glaucoma. J Glaucoma. 2023 May 1;32(5):407-413. https://doi.org/10.1097/IJG.0000000000002182
7. Nardi M, Denis P, Stalman I, Pinto LA,Morselli S, Gregorio AD. What's New with Focused Ultrasound Glaucoma Therapy - Efficacy and Safety in Surgery-naive Patients and of Multiple Ultrasound Treatments. European Ophthalmic Review. 2018;12(Suppl 1):3-9.
8. Torky MA, Alzafiri YA, Abdelhameed AG, Awad EA. Phaco-UCP; combined phacoemulsification and ultrasound ciliary plasty versus phacoemulsification alone for management of coexisting cataract and open angle glaucoma: a randomized clinical trial. BMC Ophthalmol. 2021 Jan 21;21(1):53. https://doi.org/10.1186/s12886-021-01818-5
9. Ma A, Yu SWY, Wong JKW. Micropulse laser for the treatment of glaucoma: A literature review. Surv Ophthalmol. 2019 Jul-Aug;64(4):486-497. https://doi.org/10.1016/j.survophthal.2019.01.001
10. Johnstone M, MJ. Transcleral Laser Induces Aqueous Outflow Pathway Motion & Reorganization. 2017. Poster presentation at the American Glaucoma Society; Coronado, CA: 2017.
11. Balendiran V, Landreneau J, An J. MicroPulse Transscleral Laser Therapy Dosimetry Utilizing the Revised P3 Delivery Device: A Randomized Controlled Trial. Ophthalmol Glaucoma. 2023 May-Jun;6(3):283-290. https://doi.org/10.1016/j.ogla.2022.09.004
12. Grippo TM, Sanchez FG, Stauffer J, Marcellino G. MicroPulse transscleral laser therapy - fluence may explain variability in clinical outcomes; a literature review. Clin Ophthalmol. 2021;15:2411-2419. https://doi.org/10.2147/OPTH.S313875
13. Grippo TM, de Crom RMPC, Giovingo M, et al. Evidence-Based Consensus Guidelines Series for MicroPulse Transscleral Laser Therapy: Dosimetry and Patient Selection. Clin Ophthalmol. 2022 Jun 7;16:1837-1846. https://doi.org/10.2147/OPTH.S365647
14. Chauhan D, Midha N, Mahalingam K, et al. Efficacy of Micropulse Laser Cyclophotocoagulation Therapy in Primary Angle Closure Glaucoma. J Glaucoma. 2023 Dec 1;32(12):1011-1017. https://doi.org/10.1097/IJG.0000000000002322
15. Waldo LG, Julio HQ, Jennifer CV, et al. Combined Technique for the Application of Micropulse Cyclophotocoagulation in Patients with Uncontrolled Glaucoma: Cyclo Mix. J Curr

Glaucoma Pract. 2020 Sep-Dec;14(3):93-97. https://doi.org/10.5005/jp-journals-10078-1289

16. Tan NYQ, Ang M, Chan ASY, et al. Transscleral cyclophotocoagulation and its histological effects on the conjunctiva. Sci Rep. 2019 Dec 10;9(1):18703. https://doi.org/10.1038/s41598-019-55102-0
17. Perez CI, Han Y, Rose-Nussbaumer J, Ou Y, Hsia YC. Neurotrophic keratitis after micropulse transscleral diode laser cyclophotocoagulation. Am J Ophthalmol Case Rep. 2019 May 20;15:100469. https://doi.org/10.1016/j.ajoc.2019.100469
18. Kiyama Y, Nakashima KI, Inoue T. A Case of Primary Open-angle Glaucoma With Conjunctival Laceration After Micropulse Transscleral Cyclophotocoagulation. J Glaucoma. 2020 Dec;29(12):e135-e137. https://doi.org/10.1097/IJG.0000000000001658
19. Daas A, Sherman T, Danieliute L, et al. Phacoemulsification combined with micropulse cyclodiode laser in glaucoma patients: efficacy and safety. Eye (Lond). 2022 Nov;36(11):2188-2191. https://doi.org/10.1038/s41433-021-01826-1
20. Habash AA, Otaif W. Surgical Outcome of Combined MicroPulse Transscleral Laser Therapy with Phaco Emulsification in Patients with Cataract and Glaucoma. The Open Ophthalmology Journal 2022; 16:e187436412209260. https://doi.org/10.2174/18743641-v16-e2209260
21. Quigley HA. The Need for Rigor in Evaluating Micropulse and Other New Procedures. Ophthalmol Glaucoma. 2020 May-Jun;3(3):171-173. https://doi.org/10.1016/j.ogla.2020.04.004
22. Tanito M, Manabe SI, Hamanaka T, Sato H, Mori K. A case series of endoscopic cyclophotocoagulation with 532-nm laser in Japanese patients with refractory glaucoma. Eye (Lond). 2020 Mar;34(3):507-514. doi: 10.1038/s41433-019-0538-4. Epub 2019 Jul 22. https://doi.org/10.1038/s41433-019-0538-4
23. Uram M. Combined phacoemulsification, endoscopic ciliary process photocoagulation, and intraocular lens implantation in glaucoma management. Ophthalmic Surg. 1995;26:346-352. https://doi.org/10.3928/1542-8877-19950701-17
24. Francis BA, Pouw A, Jenkins D, et al. Endoscopic cycloplasty (ECPL) and lens extraction in the treatment of severe plateau iris syndrome. J Glaucoma. 2016;25:e128-e133. https://doi.org/10.1097/IJG.0000000000000156
25. Lin MM, Rageh A, Turalba AV, et al. Differential Efficacy of Combined Phacoemulsification and Endocyclophotocoagulation in Open-angle Glaucoma Versus Angle-closure Glaucoma. J Glaucoma. 2019 May;28(5):473-480. https://doi.org/10.1097/IJG.0000000000001225
26. Pathak-Ray V. Intermediate results of phaco-endocycloplasty in an exclusive cohort of angle closure glaucoma: potential for change. Int Ophthalmol. 2019 Oct;39(10):2257-2265. https://doi.org/10.1007/s10792-018-01062-9
27. Pathak-Ray V, Choudhari N. Phaco-endocycloplasty versus Phacotrabeculectomy in Primary Angle-Closure Glaucoma: A Prospective Randomized Study. Ophthalmol Glaucoma. 2020 Nov-Dec;3(6):434-442. https://doi.org/10.1016/j.ogla.2020.06.006
28. Mohammadi M, Daraby M, Eslami Y, et al. One-year outcomes of combined phacoemul-

sification and viscogoniosynechialysis with and without endoscopic cyclophotocoagulation in primary angle-closure glaucoma. Int Ophthalmol. 2023 Sep;43(9):3227-3236. https://doi.org/10.1007/s10792-023-02723-0

29. Lai ISW, Chan NCY, Ling A, et al. Combined Phacoemulsification-Endoscopic Cyclophotocoagulation versus Phacoemulsification Alone in Primary Angle-Closure Glaucoma: A Pilot Randomized Controlled Trial. Ophthalmol Glaucoma. 2021 Nov-Dec;4(6):589-596. https://doi.org/10.1016/j.ogla.2021.03.007
30. Amaral DC, Louzada RN, Moreira PHS, et al. Combined Endoscopic Cyclophotocoagulation and Phacoemulsification Versus Phacoemulsification Alone in the Glaucoma Treatment: A Systematic Review and Meta-Analysis. Cureus. 2024 Mar 9;16(3):e55853. https://doi.org/10.7759/cureus.55853

Future directions

Fei Li, Benjamin Xu, Xiulan Zhang

In the surgical management of PACG, “less is more” signifies a future trend toward simpler surgeries with fewer complications. Traditional surgical approaches for PACG, such as trabeculectomy and phacotrabeculectomy, have dominated the field for several decades. However, these procedures are often complex, carry a higher risk of complications, and require extensive surgical expertise.[1,2] This has raised interest in simpler and more effective surgical alternatives, particularly MIGS, which represent a promising shift in the surgical management of PACG. These procedures are less invasive, associated with fewer complications, and simpler to master, making them especially appealing to early-career ophthalmologists. The widespread adoption of techniques such as Phaco and GSL under surgical gonioscopy has further facilitated the integration of MIGS into the PACG treatment paradigm. Although there is increasing evidence that procedures combining Phaco, GSL, and various MIGS are promising,[3-25] several important issues still need to be addressed.

Comprehensive treatment guidelines

Despite the availability of various surgical options, there remains a lack of standardized guidelines for managing PACG. Current treatments, including lens extraction, LPI/SPI, and filtering surgeries, often yield variable outcomes depending on patient demographics, disease severity, and the presence of comorbidities. Developing a consensus on treatment algorithms that integrate these factors could significantly enhance patient outcomes and facilitate clinical decision-making.

The surgical management of PACG can be customized according to the specific stage of the disease. For PACS, PAC and early PACG, interventions such as LPI, SPI, and Phaco, with or without GSL, are effective. Conversely, advanced stages of PACG may require more sophisticated MIGS strategies, such as the combination of Phaco ± GSL with various kinds of MIGS and traditional filtering surgeries (Table 1 and Figure 1).

Table 1. Surgical options for PACG based on disease severity

Disease stage	**Other conditions**	**General surgical categories**	**Specific surgical procedures**
PACS, PAC and early PACG	With or without PAS	LPI, SPI	
	Shallow anterior chamber, thick lens with a high vault, high risk of malignant glaucoma	Phaco	Clear lens extraction
	With cataract	Phaco	
	With extensive PAS	Phaco + GSL	
Advanced PACG	With cataract	Phaco ± GSL + MIGS	iStent/GT/ Hydrus/ Trabectome/XEN
		Phaco + Filtering surgery	Trab/GDD
		Phaco + Ciliary body ablation	UCP/MP-TLT/ECP
	Without cataract	Phaco ± GSL + MIGS	Clear lens extraction SPI + GSL + GT
		Filtering surgery	Trab
		Ciliary body ablation	UCP/MP-TLT/ECP

PACS: primary angle-closure suspect; PAC: primary angle-closure; PACG: primary angle-closure glaucoma; PAS: peripheral anterior synechiae; LPI: laser peripheral iridectomy; SPI: surgical peripheral iridectomy; Phaco: phacoemulsification or phacoemulsification with intraocular lens implantation; GSL: goniosynechialysis; MIGS: minimally invasive glaucoma surgery; GT: goniotomy/ab interno trabeculotomy; UCP: ultrasound cycloplasty; MP-TLT: micropulse trans-scleral laser therapy; ECP: endoscopic cyclophotocoagulation; Trab: trabeculectomy; GDD: glaucoma drainage device

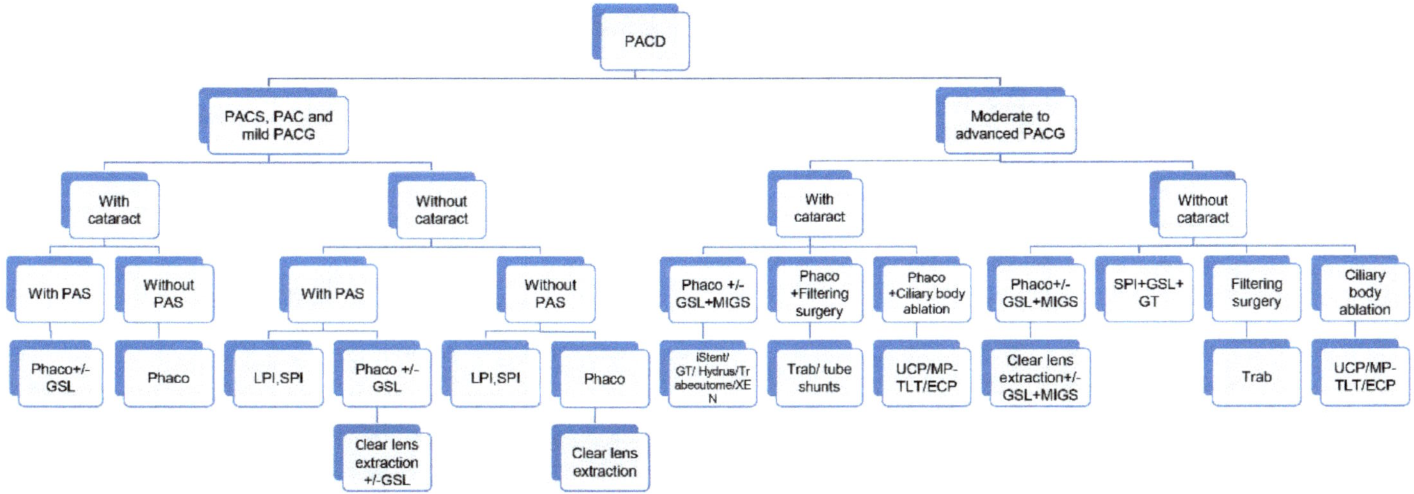

Fig. 1. Surgical options (strategies) for PACG based on disease severity. PACD: primary angle-closure diseases; PACS: primary angle-closure suspect; PAC: primary angle-closure; PACG: primary angle-closure glaucoma; PAS: peripheral anterior synechia; LPI: laser peripheral iridectomy; SPI: surgical peripheral iridectomy; Phaco: phacoemulsification or phacoemulsification with intraocular lens implantation; GSL: goniosynechialysis; MIGS: minimally invasive glaucoma surgery; GT: goniotomy/ab interno trabeculotomy; UCP: ultrasound cycloplasty; MP-TLT: micropulse transscleral laser therapy; ECP: endoscopic cyclophotocoagulation; Trab: trabeculectomy; Tube shunt: glaucoma drainage device

Long-term efficacy and safety

While many surgical interventions effectively lower IOP in the short term, there is a need for comprehensive studies evaluating long-term efficacy and safety. For example, phacogoniotomy combines Phaco, GSL, and GT to safely manage IOP in advanced PACG with cataracts,[3,6-16,20] potentially replacing phacotrabeculectomy.[14,15] These techniques have the potential to become the future standard. However, the follow-up period has not yet been long enough to confirm this. Therefore, it is recommended that future research focuses on extended follow-up periods to understand the durability of surgical outcomes and the incidence of late-onset complications.

Novel technologies

Advancements in surgical technology, including the development of new devices and techniques for angle widening and aqueous drainage, hold promise for improving surgical outcomes. Innovations such as robotic-assisted surgery and artificial intelligence-based surgical navigation systems are poised to increase the precision of surgical interventions.[26]

Personalized approaches

Current surgical management strategies often do not adequately address the individual needs of patients, particularly regarding postoperative quality of life and visual function. Future strategies should incorporate the development of patient-reported outcome measures, allowing for the evaluation of the impact of surgical interventions on patients' daily activities. This approach can help tailor treatments to individual preferences, ensuring that surgical management aligns with patients' expectations and lifestyle.

Enhanced postoperative care and monitoring

The integration of technology in postoperative care, including telemedicine and remote monitoring, can facilitate better management of PACG patients after surgery. This advanced monitoring is instrumental in early detection of complications, enabling timely interventions and ultimately improving patient outcomes.

References

1. Jampel HD, Solus JF, Tracey PA, et al. Outcomes and bleb-related complications of trabeculectomy. Ophthalmology. 2012; 119:712-722. https://doi.org/10.1016/j.ophtha.2011.09.049
2. MR, Havens SJ, Katz LJ. Trabeculectomy bleb-associated infections. Surv Ophthalmol. 2017;62:591-610. https://doi.org/10.1016/j.survophthal.2017.01.009

3. Song Y, Zhang H, Zhang Y, et al. Minimally Invasive Glaucoma Surgery in Primary Angle-Closure Glaucoma. Asia Pac J Ophthalmol (Phila). 2022; 11:460-469. https://doi.org/10.1097/APO.0000000000000561
4. Hernstadt DJ, Cheng J, Htoon HM, et al. Case Series of Combined iStent Implantation and Phacoemulsification in Eyes with Primary Angle Closure Disease: One-Year Outcomes. Adv Ther 2019;36(4):976-986. https://doi.org/10.1007/s12325-019-00899-5
5. Salimi A, Abu-Nada M, Harasymowycz P. Matched Cohort Study of Cataract Surgery With and Without Trabecular Microbypass Stent Implantation in Primary Angle-Closure Glaucoma. Am J Ophthalmol. 2021 Apr; 224:310-320. https://doi.org/10.1016/j.ajo.2020.12.032
6. Dorairaj S, Tam MD. Kahook Dual Blade Excisional Goniotomy and Goniosynechialysis Combined with Phacoemulsification for Angle-closure Glaucoma: 6-Month Results. J Glaucoma 2019;28(7):643-646. https://doi.org/10.1097/IJG.0000000000001256
7. Dorairaj S, Tam MD, Balasubramani GK. Twelve-month outcomes of excisional goniotomy using the Kahook Dual Blade(®) in eyes with angle-closure glaucoma. Clin Ophthalmol 2019; 13:1779-178. https://doi.org/10.2147/OPTH.S221299
8. Dorairaj S, Tam MD, Balasubramani GK. Two-Year Clinical Outcomes of Combined Phacoemulsification, Goniosynechialysis, and Excisional Goniotomy For Angle-Closure Glaucoma. Asia Pac J Ophthalmol (Phila) 2020;10(2):183-187. https://doi.org/10.1097/APO.0000000000000321
9. Gupta S, Sethi A, Yadav S, et al. Safety and efficacy of incisional goniotomy as an adjunct with phacoemulsification in primary angle-closure glaucoma. J Cataract Refract Surg 2021;47(4):504-511. https://doi.org/10.1097/j.jcrs.0000000000000481
10. Tanito M, Sugihara K, Tsutsui A, et al. Midterm Results of Microhook ab Interno Trabeculotomy in Initial 560 Eyes with Glaucoma. J Clin Med 2021; Feb 17;10(4):814. https://doi.org/10.3390/jcm10040814
11. Shokoohi-Rad S, Karimi F, Zarei-Ghanavati S, et al. Phacoemulsification, visco-goniosynechialysis, and goniotomy in patients with primary angle-closure glaucoma: A comparative study. Eur J Ophthalmol 2021;31(1):88-95. https://doi.org/10.1177/1120672119879331
12. Song Y, Zhang Y, Li F, et al. One-Year Results of a Multicenter Study: Intraocular Pressure-Lowering Effect of Combined Phacoemulsification, Goniosynechialysis, and Goniotomy for Cases of Advanced Primary Angle-Closure Glaucoma with Cataract. Asia Pac J Ophthalmol (Phila) 2022;11(6):529-535. https://doi.org/10.1097/APO.0000000000000579
13. Song Y, Xie L, Zhu X, et al. Two-year Outcome of Phacogoniotomy for Advanced Primary Angle-closure Glaucoma with Cataracts: A Multicenter Study. Br J Ophthalmol. 2025 Jun 23;109(7):770-774. https://doi.org/10.1136/bjo-2024-325375
14. Song Y, Lin F, Lv A, et al. Phacogoniotomy versus phacotrabeculectomy for advanced primary angle-closure glaucoma with cataract: A randomized non-inferiority trial. Asia Pac J Ophthalmol (Phila) 2023:100033. https://doi.org/10.1016/j.apjo.2024.100076

15. Song Y, Fan S, Tang L, et al. Two-Year Outcomes of Phacogoniotomy vs Phacotrabeculectomy for Advanced Primary Angle-Closure Glaucoma With Cataract: A Noninferiority Randomized Clinical Trial. JAMA Ophthalmol. 2025 Jun 1;143(6):462-469. https://doi.org/10.1001/jama-ophthalmol.2025.0685
16. Lin F, Zhang Y, Zhu X, et al. Impact of peripheral anterior synechiae on the outcome of combined phacoemulsification, goniosynechialysis and goniotomy for primary angle-closure glaucoma and cataract: a multicenter observational study. J Glaucoma 2024;33(8):587-593. https://doi.org/10.1097/IJG.0000000000002435
17. Gao X, Lin F, Lu P, et al. Efficacy and Safety of Surgical Peripheral Iridectomy, Goniosynechialysis, and Goniotomy for Advanced Primary Angle Closure Glaucoma Without Cataract: 1-Year Results of a Multicenter Study. J Glaucoma. 2024 Sep 1;33(9):632-639. https://doi.org/10.1097/IJG.0000000000002443
18. Lin F, Li L, Lu P, et al. Two-Year Outcomes of Combined Surgical Peripheral Iridectomy, Goniosynechialysis, and Goniotomy for Advanced Primary Angle-Closure Glaucoma Without Cataract: A Multicenter Study. Asia Pac J Ophthalmol (Phila), 2025 Feb 26:100166.doi: 10.1016/j.apjo.2025.100166. https://doi.org/10.1016/j.apjo.2025.100166
19. Lin F, Lv A, Li F, et al. Peripheral Iridectomy with Goniosynechialysis and Goniotomy vs. Trabeculectomy for Advanced PACG: A Randomized Controlled Trial. JAMA Ophthalmol. 2025 Jun 1;143(6):472-479. https://doi.org/10.1001/jamaophthalmol.2025.0757
20. El SY, Mettias NM, Elghonemy H, et al. Phacoemulsification with gonioscopy-assisted transluminal trabeculotomy versus phacoemulsification alone in primary angle closure glaucoma: A randomized controlled study. Acta Ophthalmol 2024;102(2):e195-e203. https://doi.org/10.1111/aos.15733
21. Fontana L, De Maria M, Iannetta D, et al. Gonioscopy-assisted transluminal trabeculotomy for chronic angle-closure glaucoma: preliminary results. Graefes Arch Clin Exp Ophthalmol 2022;260(2):545-551. https://doi.org/10.1007/s00417-021-05400-z
22. Sng C, Chew P, Htoon HM, et al. Case Series of Combined XEN Implantation and Phacoemulsification in Chinese Eyes: One-Year Outcomes. Adv Ther 2019;36(12):3519-3529. https://doi.org/10.1007/s12325-019-01127-w
23. Gabbay IE, Allen F, Morley C, et al. Efficacy and safety data for the XEN45 implant at 2 years: a retrospective analysis. Br J Ophthalmol 2020;104(8):1125-1130. https://doi.org/10.1136/bjophthalmol-2019-313870
24. Lai ISW, Chan NCY, Ling A, et al. Combined Phacoemulsification-Endoscopic Cyclophotocoagulation versus Phacoemulsification Alone in Primary Angle-Closure Glaucoma: A Pilot Randomized Controlled Trial. Ophthalmol Glaucoma. 2021; 4:589-596. https://doi.org/10.1016/j.ogla.2021.03.007
25. Daas A, Sherman T, Danieliute L, et al. Phacoemulsification combined with micropulse cyclodiode laser in glaucoma patients: efficacy and safety. Eye (Lond). 2022; 36:2188-2191. https://

doi.org/10.1038/s41433-021-01826-1

26. Zhang X. Development of a general visual foundation model for ophthalmic surgeries. Research Registry. Available from: https://www.researchregistry.com/browse-the-registry/#home/registrationdetails/684c27a1bf5fca02cc9d2243/

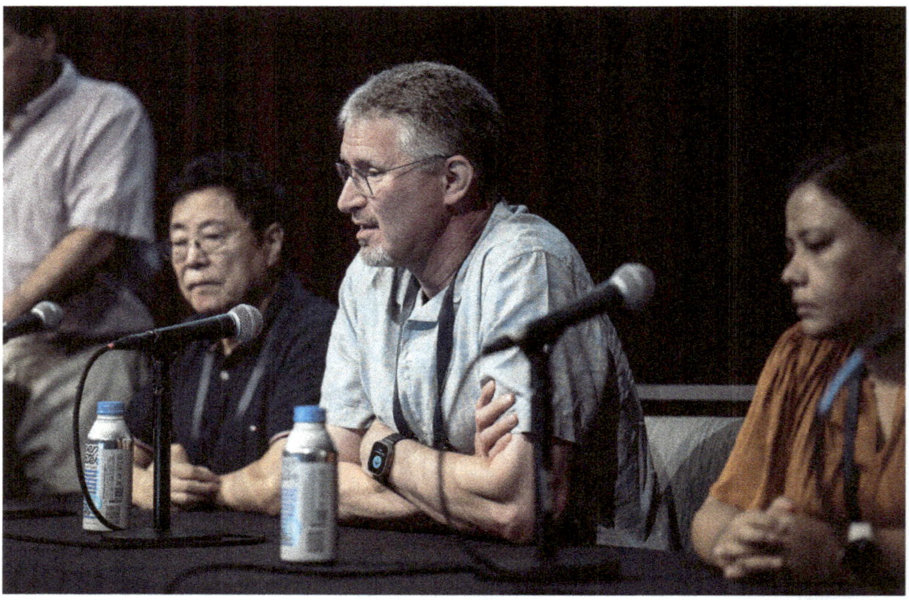

Ningli Wang, Paul Foster and Monisha Nongpiur

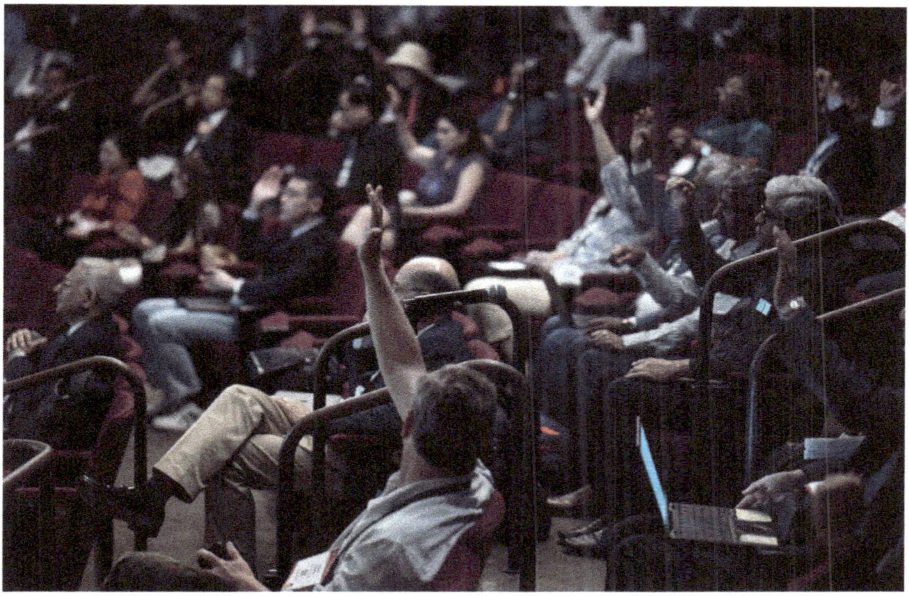

Consensus audience rasing hands

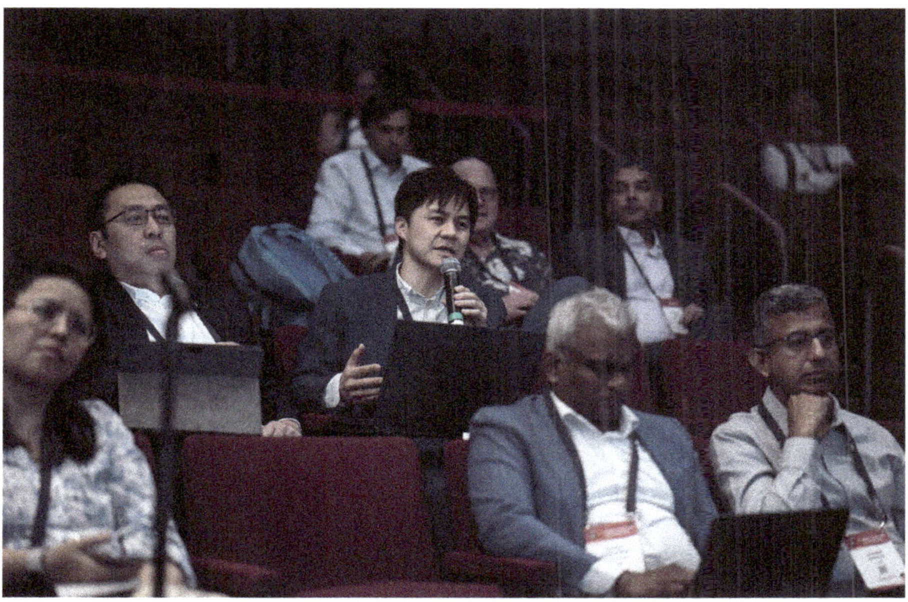

Poemen Chan

Section Leaders

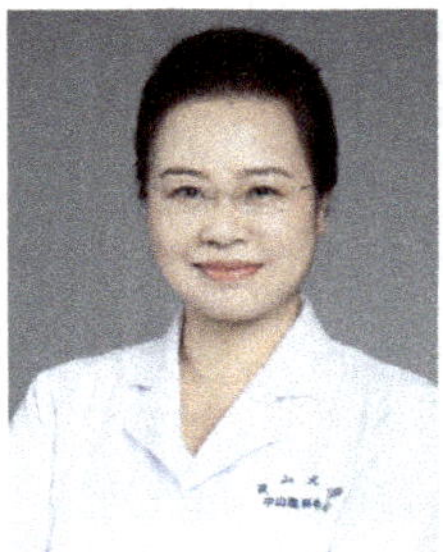

Xiulan Zhang

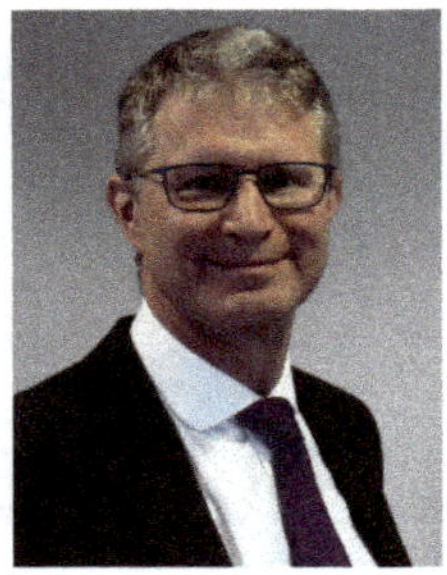

Paul Foster

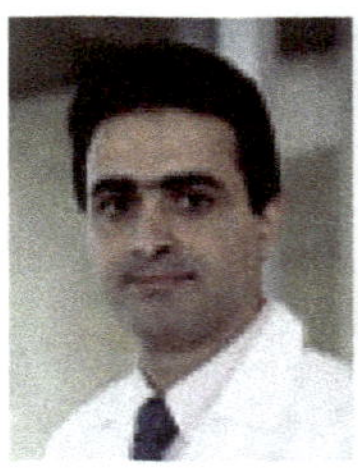

Sasan Moghimi

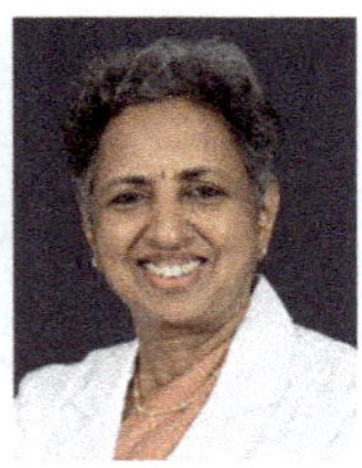

Vijaya Lingham

6. ACUTE PRIMARY ANGLE CLOSURE

Xiulan Zhang, Paul Foster, Sasan Moghimi, Vijaya Lingam

Abbreviations
ALPI: argon laser peripheral iridoplasty
APAC: acute primary angle closure
GSL: goniosynechialysis
IOP: intraocular pressure
LPI: laser peripheral iridotomy
LPIP laser peripheral iridoplasty
LPP: laser pupilloplasty
OCT: optical coherence tomography
PAC: primary angle closure
PACD: primary angle-closure disease
PACG: primary angle-closure glaucoma
PACS: primary angle-closure suspect
PAS: peripheral anterior synechiae
RCT: randomized controlled trial
SPI: surgical peripheral iridectomy
UBM: ultrasound biomicroscopy
ZAP: Zhongshan Angle-Closure Progression Trial

Consensus statements

1. APAC is an ophthalmic emergency that can cause sudden, pronounced, but typically transient reduction in vision.
    - APAC typically presents with severe ocular pain, headache, nausea, and a fixed mid-dilated pupil.
    - Secondary causes of angle closure should be excluded.

Angle Closure and Angle Closure Glaucoma, pp 1-19
Edited by Robert N. Weinreb, Benjamin Xu, David Friedman, Paul Foster, Tin Aung, Xiulan Zhang
2026 © Kugler Publications, Amsterdam, The Netherlands

- APAC more commonly affects older individuals, women, and those of Asian descent.
- A range of medications may precipitate APAC, including those with adrenergic or anticholinergic effects. Careful medication review should be performed in at-risk individuals.
- APAC usually occurs unilaterally. Systemic medications (such as anticonvulsants and antidepressants) and systemic disease (such as Vogt-Koyanagi-Harada syndrome) may cause bilateral APAC.

2. Initial treatment with topical and systemic medications can lower the IOP, relieve pain, improve corneal clarity, and reduce inflammation.
   - Miotics should be used in cases of APAC but may not be effective due to iris ischemia while the IOP is high.
   - Early administration of anti-inflammatory agents may facilitate a more rapid reduction in IOP.
3. LPI should be performed as soon as possible.
   - If LPI is not possible due to corneal edema, anterior chamber paracentesis, diode laser, or LPIP, with or without LPP, can be performed.
   - If the iris is thick and there are no convenient iris crypts, argon laser pretreatment should be considered, followed by YAG:Nd LPI.
4. Anterior chamber paracentesis is an option for immediate IOP reduction and symptom relief in APAC.
   - It is particularly useful when systemic IOP-lowering agents such as mannitol or acetazolamide are contraindicated or when LPI or LPIP cannot be performed. However, the procedure carries risks and should be performed with caution.
5. Lens extraction (once IOP and inflammation have been controlled) is the definitive treatment for APAC, as it alleviates pupillary block, deepens the anterior chamber angle, lowers IOP, and improves vision.
   - Surgical challenges include corneal edema, a shallow anterior chamber, intraocular inflammation, and zonular weakness or dehiscence.
6. SPI can be performed in eyes with medically uncontrolled APAC when an appropriate laser is unavailable, when LPI is not possible, or in cases with both severe corneal edema and a clear lens.
7. Trabeculectomy can be considered for uncontrolled IOP after APAC resolution if there are extensive PAS after iridectomy or if the iridectomy could not be performed.
   - Phacoemulsification and combined GSL with or without goniotomy is an alternative to trabeculectomy.

8. Patients with spectrum of primary angle closure should be educated about APAC symptoms and the need to see an eye care specialist urgently if they present.
9. There is no effective method to identify individuals at high risk for APAC.
   - The use of anterior segment imaging or polygenic risk score is unproven.
10. Additional research is needed to identify anatomical features predictive of APAC.

Definition

Paul Foster

APAC is a symptomatic variant of PACD. It results from sudden, total occlusion of the trabecular meshwork as a result of complete iridotrabecular contact. It is a relatively uncommon presentation of PACD accounting for between 15% and 20% of all cases.[1] The physical signs that commonly accompany APAC do not always correlate with the long-term visual prognosis of patients, but they are relevant because of the potential (often reversible) impact on visual function. Symptoms after acute attack are typically attributable to lens opacities or a dilated, unresponsive pupil resulting from iris ischemia. If glaucomatous optic neuropathy is seen in the setting of an APAC presentation, it is likely from pre-existing subacute events and not the result of an acute pressure rise spanning only hours or days. APAC requires timely and proactive management that differs from routine care, which makes the acute crisis an important variant in disease natural history.

Epidemiology

Incidence

Incidence rates of APAC vary in different ethnic and racial groups. The rates are typically expressed as the number of cases occurring per year in 100,000 people and usually address the population aged 30 years and older. The European population has the lowest reported rate (between 2–3/100,00/year),[2,3] followed by the intermediate 6–7/100,000/year among the South and Southeast Asian population,[4] and the highest incidence rate ranges between 12–16/100,000/year among the Chinese population.[4,5] These studies typically use hospital episode data to identify cases and might be subject to sampling bias.

A trial of prophylactic laser iridotomy, the ZAP trial, enrolled people with occluded drainage angles (PACS) in a large urban center in the People's Republic of China and quantified the risk of progression from PACS to PAC in untreated eyes of trial participants. The progression risk was 8 cases/1,000 eye-years (36/889 eyes over 6 years of follow-up). There were 5 APAC events with a cumulative risk of 1 case/1,000 eye-years. The findings suggested a low risk of angle-closure disease progression, especially APAC. Therefore, the risk of significant loss of vision is similarly low over this timescale.[6]

Due to the narrow demographics of ZAP trial participants, other populations may not have the same risk as the population in China. Informing all patients with narrow or occluded angles that their risk of an APAC crisis is around 1/1000 per year may not be accurate. For example, based on PACG prevalence data, the risk may be lower by a factor of 3 or 4 for a white European population.[2-5]

Risk factors: demographic, anatomic, genetic, and environmental

APAC is uncommon in people below 30 years old. It is approximately 3 times more common in women than men.[4,5] There is a known familial tendency, likely related to genetics factors, which are gradually being elucidated.[7,8] People suffering APAC episodes have shorter eyes with more crowded anterior segments than normal eyes.[9]

APAC usually occurs unilaterally. In the case of bilateral APAC, complications of systemic medications or disease should be suspected.[10-12] There are various external factors that appear to trigger the onset of an APAC episode, including pharmacological dilation of the pupil during routine ophthalmic examination.[3] However, the onset of APAC is uncommon after pharmacological mydriasis, even in people with partially occluded drainage angles.[13] The use of antidepressant medication, many of which have anticholinergic properties, may increase the risk of disease onset, although evidence is mixed.[14,15] Pupil-dilating agents are associated with a higher risk of APAC episodes.[16] Idiosyncratic reactions to medications (most notably topiramate, but also sulfonamide drugs, including acetazolamide) may also trigger the onset of APAC.[17] Topiramate causes a supraciliary effusion and anterior rotation of the ciliary body.[18] Systemic disease, such as Vogt-Koyanagi-Harada syndrome, may present as bilateral APAC at onset.[11-12] Heightened emotions are associated with onset of an APAC episode.[19] Adverse weather conditions are associated with a spike in APAC presentations for care. These episodes are believed to be related to greater numbers of people remaining indoors, in lower light conditions, carrying out more sedentary activities.[4] Surges in COVID infections in the community have been linked to a 5-fold increase in APAC presentations.[20,21]

Comments

- APAC more commonly affects older individuals, women, and those of Asian descent.
- Exposure to medications with adrenergic or anticholinergic effects may trigger APAC. Some drugs may induce APAC through idiosyncratic reactions, necessitating careful medication review in at-risk individuals.
- The biometric profile of APAC patients is often more extreme than that of those with asymptomatic angle closure.
- APAC usually occurs unilaterally. Systemic medications (such as anticonvulsants and antidepressants) and systemic disease (such as Vogt-Koyanagi-Harada syndrome) may cause bilateral APAC.

References

1. Yip JL, Foster PJ. Ethnic differences in primary angle-closure glaucoma. Curr Opin Ophthalmol. 2006;17(2):175-80. https://doi.org/10.1097/01.icu.0000193078.47616.aa
2. Teikari J, Raivio I, Nurminen M. Incidence of acute glaucoma in Finland from 1973 to 1982. Graefes Arch Clin Exp Ophthalmol. 1987;225(5):357-60. https://doi.org/10.1007/bf02153405
3. Chua PY, Day AC, Lai KL, et al. The incidence of acute angle closure in Scotland: a prospective surveillance study. Br J Ophthalmol. 2018;102(4):539-43. https://doi.org/10.1136/bjophthalmol-2017-310725
4. Seah SK, Foster PJ, Chew PT, et al. Incidence of acute primary angle-closure glaucoma in Singapore. An island-wide survey. Arch Ophthalmol. 1997;115(11):1436-40. https://doi.org/10.1001/archopht.1997.01100160606014
5. ai JS, Liu DT, Tham CC, et al. Epidemiology of acute primary angle-closure glaucoma in the Hong Kong Chinese population: prospective study. Hong Kong Med J. 2001;7(2):118-23.
6. He M, Jiang Y, Huang S, et al. Laser peripheral iridotomy for the prevention of angle closure: a single-centre, randomised controlled trial. Lancet. 2019;393(10181):1609-18. https://doi.org/10.1016/s0140-6736(18)32607-2
7. Waseem NH, Low S, Shah AZ, et al. Mutations in SPATA13/ASEF2 cause primary angle closure glaucoma. PLoS Genet. 2020;16(4):e1008721. https://doi.org/10.1371/journal.pgen.1008721
8. Khor CC, Do T, Jia H, et al. Genome-wide association study identifies five new susceptibility loci for primary angle closure glaucoma. Nat Genet. 2016;48(5):556-62. https://doi.org/10.1038/ng.3540
9. Friedman DS, Gazzard G, Foster P, et al. Ultrasonographic biomicroscopy, Scheimpflug photography, and novel provocative tests in contralateral eyes of Chinese patients initially seen with acute angle closure. Arch Ophthalmol. 2003;121(5):633-42. https://doi.org/10.1001/

archopht.121.5.633

10. Lai JS, Gangwani RA. Medication-induced acute angle closure attack. Hong Kong Med J. 2012;18(2):139-145.
11. Yuan F, Zhang Y, Yan X. Bilateral acute angle closure glaucoma as an initial presentation of Vogt-Koyanagi-Harada syndrome: A clinical case report. Eur J Ophthalmol. 2022; 32(1):Np230-np234. https://doi.org/10.1177/1120672120951442
12. Yang P, Liu X, Zhou H, et al. Vogt-Koyanagi-Harada disease presenting as acute angle closure glaucoma at onset. Clin Exp Ophthalmol. 2011;39(7):639-647. https://doi.org/10.1111/j.1442-9071.2011.02523.x
13. Friedman DS, Chang DS, Jiang Y, et al. Acute Angle-Closure Attacks Are Uncommon in Primary Angle-Closure Suspects after Pharmacologic Mydriasis: The Zhongshan Angle-Closure Prevention Trial. Ophthalmol Glaucoma. 2022;5(6):581-6. https://doi.org/10.1016/j.ogla.2022.04.003
14. Chen HY, Lin CL, Lai SW, Kao CH. Association of Selective Serotonin Reuptake Inhibitor Use and Acute Angle-Closure Glaucoma. J Clin Psychiatry. 2016;77(6):e692-6. https://doi.org/10.4088/JCP.15m10038
15. Chen HY, Lin CL, Kao CH. Long-Term Use of Selective Serotonin Reuptake Inhibitors and Risk of Glaucoma in Depression Patients. Medicine (Baltimore). 2015;94(45):e2041. https://doi.org/10.1097/md.0000000000002041
16. Subak-Sharpe I, Low S, Nolan W, Foster PJ. Pharmacological and environmental factors in primary angle-closure glaucoma. Br Med Bull. 2010;93:125-43. https://doi.org/10.1093/bmb/ldp042
17. Congdon NG, Friedman DS. Angle-closure glaucoma: impact, etiology, diagnosis, and treatment. Curr Opin Ophthalmol 2003;14(2):70-3. https://doi.org/10.1097/00055735-200304000-00002
18. Medeiros FA, Zhang XY, Bernd AS, Weinreb RN. Angle-closure glaucoma associated with ciliary body detachment in patiients using topiramate. Arch Ophthalmol. 2003 Feb 121(2):282-5, 2003.
19. Talluto D, Feith M, Allee S. Simultaneous angle closure in twins. J Glaucoma. 1998;7(1):68-9.
20. Ying Y, Zhai R, Sun Y, et al. The occurrence of acute primary angle closure triggered, aggravated, and accelerated by COVID-19 infection: retrospective observational study. Front Public Health. 2023;11:1196202. https://doi.org/10.3389/fpubh.2023.1196202
21. Zhu M, Yan Y. The surge of acute angle-closure glaucoma during the outbreak of Omicron in a tertiary hospital in Shanghai. Graefes Arch Clin Exp Ophthalmol. 2023;261(9):2709-11. https://doi.org/10.1007/s00417-023-06077-2

Management

The acute management of APAC is based only on a few RCTs; robust data on management is relatively sparse. However, the principles of managing the ophthalmic emergency are widely accepted.

Most patients are in moderate to severe pain with acutely reduced vision. Nausea and vomiting are relatively common. Therefore, the immediate priorities are analgesia, antiemetics, and rapid confirmation of diagnosis, with subsequent topical and systemic medication to reduce the IOP. First, there should be confirmation that angle closure is present and IOP is elevated. Once this has been established, secondary causes of angle closure should be excluded. If lens-induced or retro-lenticular mechanisms of angle closure are not recognized and treated appropriately, the use of topical pilocarpine may aggravate the condition and result in prolonged pain and a delay in IOP control.

A marked asymmetry of the central anterior chamber depth should raise the suspicion of a secondary lenticular or retro-lenticular mechanisms. One reported scenario of angle closure was attributed to the posterior segment mechanisms associated with topiramate, causing supraciliary effusions and anterior rotation of the ciliary body.[1,2] Therefore, the use of topiramate should be assessed on direct questioning in atypical cases of suspected angle closure.

Regardless of the primary mechanism (*i.e.*, pupillary block versus non-pupillary block) the first-line intervention of APAC is typically LPI with or without combined LPIP or LPP, which should be performed as promptly as possible. Initial treatment with medication may be necessary to control IOP and pain as well as to help achieve corneal clarity. The use of highly concentrated pilocarpine drops administered at frequent intervals is not recommended. After an initial instillation of pilocarpine, an appropriate dosage frequency is every 6 hours. Pilocarpine is ineffective when the IOP exceeds 40 mmHg due to iris sphincter ischemia. Other topical glaucoma medications should be used as clinically indicated. Topical steroids should also be used to control inflammation.

References

1. Medeiros FA, Zhang XY, Bernd AS, Weinreb RN. Angle-closure glaucoma associated with ciliary body detachment in patients using topiramate. Arch Ophthalmol. 2003,Feb 121(2):282-5, 2003.
2. Huang W, Li X, Gao K, et al. Combined subconjunctival injection of dexamethasone for the management of acute primary angle closure: a randomized controlled trial. Br J Ophthalmol. 2020;104(1):87-91. https://doi.org/10.1136/bjophthalmol-2018-313473

IOP-lowering strategies

Sasan Moghimi, Xiulan Zhang

Medical management

Sasan Moghimi

Ensuring patient comfort and reducing IOP to prevent significant optic nerve or retinal nerve fibers damage are the highest priorities in managing APAC. This is typically first achieved with medical therapy. Most classes of glaucoma medications can be utilized in treating APAC. Fast-acting medications, such as carbonic anhydrase inhibitors (*e.g.*, oral or parenteral acetazolamide), topical beta-blockers, and alpha-2 adrenergic agents (*e.g.*, apraclonidine or brimonidine), can be used as first-line therapies, either alone or more commonly in combination. Systemic hyperosmotic agents, such as oral glycerin, oral isosorbide, or intravenous mannitol 20%, may also be used when IOP is exceedingly high or not responsive to initial treatment.

Beta-blockers reduce aqueous humor formation and lower IOP within 10–20 minutes, with peak effect occurring after 2 hours.[1] Alpha-2 agonists, which also reduce aqueous humor formation, have a rapid onset of action, with peak IOP-lowering effects at approximately 2 hours.[2]

Carbonic anhydrase inhibitors are particularly suitable for treating APAC due to their rapid onset of action. In these cases, regular acetazolamide should be used instead of slow-release formulations. Topical carbonic anhydrase inhibitors (*e.g.*, dorzolamide and brinzolamide) also reach peak IOP-lowering efficacy within 2 hours.[3]

While prostaglandin analogs, which primarily increase uveoscleral outflow,[4] are potent IOP-lowering medications and are used in chronic angle-closure glaucoma,[5,6] there is a lack of evidence for their use for acute management of APAC.[4]

Systemic hyperosmotic agents, such as oral glycerin (50%), isosorbide (45%), or intravenous mannitol (20%), dehydrate the vitreous and allow the lens-iris diaphragm to move posteriorly. They are often the most effective means of lowering IOP during acute episodes of APAC. However, these agents have systemic adverse effects and should be used cautiously in diabetic patients (glycerin) or elderly patients with cardiovascular disease (mannitol).

The use of miotics (such as pilocarpine) for the treatment and prevention of APAC is controversial due to potential counterproductive effects. While miotics can potentially reduce iridotrabecular contact and open the angle by constricting the pupil, they can also aggravate pupillary block through ciliary muscle contraction, increased zonular laxity, and increased anterior-posterior lens diameter.[7,8] Numerous cases of paradoxical reactions to miotics resulting in triggering or worsening of angle closure have been reported in the literature, often associated with secondary causes.[9,10] These considerations should be take into account when prescribing pilocarpine for treating APAC.

Comments

Initial treatment for APAC focuses on local and systemic medications to lower the IOP, decrease pain, improve corneal clarity and reduce inflammation.

References

1. Dailey RA, Brubaker RF, Bourne WM. The effects of timolol maleate and acetazolamide on the rate of aqueous formation in normal human subjects. Am J Ophthalmol. 1982;93(2):232-37. https://doi.org/10.1016/0002-9394(82)90419-6
2. Robinson JC, Hubbard WC, Peterson CM, Debink N, Wadhwa A, Kaufman PL. Apraclonidine and brimonidine effects on anterior ocular and cardiovascular physiology in normal and sympathectomized monkeys. Exp Eye Res. 1994;59(6):633-44. https://doi.org/10.1006/exer.1994.1149
3. Ingram CJ, Brubaker RF. Effect of brinzolamide and dorzolamide on aqueous humor flow in human eyes. Am J Ophthalmol. 1999;128(3):292-6. https://doi.org/10.1016/S0002-9394(99)00179-8
4. Toris CB, Zhan G, Camras CB. Increase in Outflow Facility With Unoprostone Treatment in Ocular HypertensivePatients. Arch Ophthalmol. 2004;122(12):1782-87. https://doi.org/10.1001/archopht.122.12.1782
5. Chew PT, Aung T, Aquino M, Rojanapongpun P, Group ES. Intraocular pressure-reducing effects and safety of latanoprost versus timolol in patients with chronic angle-closure glaucoma. Ophthalmology. 2004;111(3):427-34. https://doi.org/10.1016/j.ophtha 2003.06.007
6. Chen M-J, Chen Y-C, Chou C-K, Hsu W-M. Comparison of the effects of latanoprost and bimatoprost on intraocular pressure in chronic angle-closure glaucoma. Ocul Pharmacol Ther. 2007;23(6):559-66. https://doi.org/10.1089/jop.2007.0037
7. Francois J, Goes F. Ultrasonographic study of the effect of different miotics on the eye components. Ophthalmologica. 1977;175(6):328-38. https://doi.org/10.1159/000308677
8. Wilkie J, Drance SM, Schulzer M. The effects of miotics on anterior-chamber depth. Am J Ophthalmol. 1969;68(1):78-83. https://doi.org/10.1016/0002-9394(69)94936-8
9. Gorin G. Angle-closure glaucoma induced by miotics. Am J Ophthalmol. 1966;62(6):1063-67. https://doi.org/10.1016/0002-9394(66)92554-2

10. Rieser JC, Schwartz B. Miotic-induced malignant glaucoma. Arch Ophthalmol. 1972;87(6):706-12. https://doi.org/10.1001/archopht.1972.01000020708018

Anti-inflammatory treatment

Fengbin Lin, Xiulan Zhang

APAC is characterized by a sudden and severe increase of IOP.[1] This elevation is closely associated with inflammatory reactions in the anterior chamber.[2-4] Huang *et al.* found a significant elevation of multiple inflammatory and pro-inflammatory cytokines in the aqueous humor of APAC patients, including IL-6, IL-8, G-CSF, MCP-1, and MCP-3.[2] Moreover, studies have shown that the concentration of VEGF in the aqueous humor of APAC patients is significantly increased 5.7 times higher than in chronic PACG and 13.5 times higher than in cataract patients.[5] The elevated concentration of VEGF in the aqueous humor may be associated with ischemia and hypoxia resulting from the sudden increase in IOP. These findings suggest that high IOP in APAC may contribute to vision loss through an inflammatory mechanism, underscoring the importance of early anti-inflammatory treatment. Based on the evidence, Huang *et al.* conducted an RCT, revealing that patients with APAC who received subconjunctival injections of dexamethasone in addition to conventional treatment experienced a greater reduction in IOP. This increased the overall treatment success rate from 54.9% to 79.7%, while significantly reducing anterior chamber inflammation and ocular pain.[6] These results highlight the potential of incorporating targeted anti-inflammatory therapies, including topical steroidal or non-steroidal anti-inflammatory agents, into the management of APAC to improve clinical outcomes and preserve vision.

Comments

- Early administration of anti-inflammatory agents may facilitate a rapid reduction in inflammation and IOP.

References

1. Pokhrel PK, Loftus SA. Ocular emergencies. Am Fam Physician. 2007;76(6):829-836.
2. Huang W, Chen S, Gao X, et al. Inflammation-related cytokines of aqueous humor in acute primary angle-closure eyes. Invest Ophthalmol Vis Sci. 2014;55(2):1088-1094. https://doi.org/10.1167/iovs.13-13591
3. Liu YM, Chen SD, Li XY, Huang WB, Li F, Wang JW, et al. Aqueous proinflammatory cytokines in acute primary angle-closure eyes. Int J Ophthalmol. 2017;10(5):733-737. https://doi.

org/10.18240/ijo.2017.05.12

4. Wang Y, Chen S, Liu Y, Huang W, Li X, Zhang X. Inflammatory cytokine profiles in eyes with primary angle-closure glaucoma. Biosci Rep. 2018;38(6). https://doi.org/10.1042/BSR20181411
5. Huang W, Gao X, Chen S, Li X, Zhang X, Zhang X. Vascular Endothelial Growth Factor is Increased in Aqueous Humor of Acute Primary Angle-Closure Eyes. J Glaucoma. 2016;25(7):e647-e651. https://doi.org/10.1097/IJG.0000000000000242
6. Huang W, Li X, Gao K, Zhang X. Combined subconjunctival injection of dexamethasone for the management of acute primary angle closure: a randomized controlled trial. Br J Ophthalmol. 2020;104(1):87-91. https://doi.org/10.1136/bjophthalmol-2018-313473

Paracentesis of the anterior chamber

Sasan Moghimi

The primary goal of initial treatment for APAC is to quickly lower IOP to alleviate symptoms and prevent further damage to ocular tissues. While IOP is typically lowered by combination of topical and systemic medications, additional treatments may be needed when medications are insufficient or contraindicated. Immediate paracentesis is an alternative method to reduce IOP in APAC. It involves a controlled drainage of aqueous humor from the anterior chamber using a needle or a paracentesis incision. This can be done by using a slit lamp under topical anesthesia and aseptic conditions. Paracentesis has been shown to be safe and effective in reducing IOP rapidly and eliminating the symptoms of APAC.[1-4]

The unique benefit of anterior chamber paracentesis is its ability to rapidly lower IOP and provide almost instantaneous relief of the severe symptoms of APAC. Once IOP is reduced to an acceptable level and corneal edema resolved, LPI can be performed promptly and permits definitive resolution of APAC.[3-5] Paracentesis may be considered if the patients with contraindications to mannitol or acetazolamide, such as congestive heart failure, chronic renal insufficiency, or other systemic illnesses.[1,2,6] It is also useful when LPI cannot be immediately performed or is unsafe due to corneal edema.[1,2]

In a case series involving 10 eyes with APAC and an IOP of ≥ 50 mmHg, each patient received topical hypotensive medications, immediate anterior chamber paracentesis, and systemic acetazolamide and mannitol as the primary treatment.[2] All patients experienced a rapid reduction in IOP and immediate symptomatic relief. The mean IOP dropped to below 21 mmHg within 2 hours and remained at that level.

In a separate comparative study, patients were evaluated who suffered from their first attack of APAC when receiving anterior chamber paracentesis ($n = 31$) or mannitol infusion ($n = 30$). Compared to mannitol infusion, paracentesis more effectively improved visual acuity in APAC patients with an initial IOP below 60 mmHg. This was achieved by rapidly stabilizing the anterior segment through immediate IOP reduction, quickly decreasing corneal edema, and permitting earlier performance of LPI. No complications, such as endophthalmitis, intraocular trauma, choroidal effusion, or choroidal hemorrhage occurred following paracentesis.[7]

It is noteworthy that the IOP after paracentesis may rise again leading to pain and ischemia due to unresolved pupillary block and definitive treatment (*i.e.*, LPI or cataract extraction) is required for APAC patients. Moreover, there are potential risks associated with performing paracentesis in the setting of APAC. An eye with APAC has a shallow anterior chamber, and thus the risk of damaging the corneal endothelium, iris, or lens from the paracentesis blade/needle is present.[2] Malignant glaucoma may result from the rapid anterior movement of the iris and lens. Other complications include hyphema, choroidal hemorrhage, decompression retinopathy, and even endophthalmitis.[8-10] Prospective RCTs are needed to determine whether paracentesis has a role and offers long-term benefits in the management of APAC.

Comments

- Although anterior chamber paracentesis does not relieve pupillary block, it is safe and effective means of rapidly reducing IOP and eliminating the symptoms of acute angle attack. It should be considered if the patient is at high risk for an adverse reaction to mannitol or acetazolamide, or when LPI cannot be immediately performed or is unsafe due to corneal edema. However, the procedure carries risks and should be performed with caution. It should be eschewed when the IOP can be effectively reduced through medication.

References

1. Cheng C-F, Tsai C-L, Lee OK-S, Feng J-J, Ho JH-C. Anterior Chamber Paracentesis Facilitates Laser Peripheral Iridotomy and Restores Vision in Mild-to-moderate Acute Primary Angle-closure Glaucoma. J Exp Clin Med. 2012;4(1):52-57. https://doi.org/10.1016/j.jecm.2011.11.009
2. Lam DS, Chua JK, Tham CC, Lai JS. Efficacy and safety of immediate anterior chamber paracentesis in the treatment of acute primary angle-closure glaucoma: a pilot study. Ophthalmology. 2002;109(1):64-70. https://doi.org/10.1016/S0161-6420(01)00857-0
3. Arnavielle S, Creuzot-Garcher C, Bron AM. Anterior chamber paracentesis in patients with

acute elevation of intraocular pressure. Graefes Arch Clin Exp Ophthalmol. 2007;245:345-50. https://doi.org/10.1007/s00417-006-0465-5

4. Cioboata M, Anghelie A, Chiotan C, Liora R, Serban R, Cornăcel C. Benefits of anterior chamber paracentesis in the management of glaucomatous emergencies. J Med Life. 2014;7(Spec Iss 2):5.
5. Aung T, Friedman DS, Chew PT, et al. Long-term outcomes in Asians after acute primary angle closure. Ophthalmology. 2004;111(8):1464-69. https://doi.org/10.1016/j.ophtha.2003.12.061
6. Pérez-Pérez AJ, Pazos B, Sobrado J, Gonzalez L, Gándara A. Acute renal failure following massive mannitol infusion. Am J Nephrol. 2002;22(5-6):573-75. https://doi.org/10.1159/000065279
7. Yang X, Su W, Wang M, et al. Effect of anterior chamber paracentesis on initial treatment of acute angle closure. Can J Ophthalmol. 2013;48(6):553-8. https://doi.org/10.1016/j.jcjo.2013.04.012
8. Carnahan MC, Platt LW. Serial paracenteses in the management of acute elevations of intraocular pressure. Ophthalmology. 2002;109(9):1604-06 https://doi.org/10.1016/S0161-6420(02)01126-0
9. Helbig H, Noske W, Kleineidam M, Kellner U, Foerster M. Bacterial endophthalmitis after anterior chamber paracentesis. Br J Ophthalmol. 1995;79(9):866. https://doi.org/10.1136/bjo.79.9.866
10. Alwitry A, Khan K, Rotchford A, Zaman A, Vernon S. Severe decompression retinopathy after medical treatment of acute primary angle closure. Br J Ophthalmol. 2007;91(1):121-21. https://doi.org/10.1136/bjo.2006.100479

Approaches and definitive treatment for medically unresponsive APAC

Vijaya Lingam, Xiulan Zhang

LPI

Vijaya Lingam

LPI creates an alternate pathway in the peripheral iris for the aqueous humor to flow from the posterior to the anterior chamber. APAC is primarily the result of pupillary block, which occurs due to the pressure differential created by aqueous flow obstruction between the iris and lens and anterior bowing of the iris root, leading to iridotrabecular contact. LPI helps relieve pupillary block, equalizing the pressure differential and widening the angle. Since non-pupillary block mechanisms may also contribute to APAC, further management of other coexisting causes of angle closure, such as plateau iris, pseudo-plateau iris, increased lens vault, and thick peripheral iris, may be required.

The lasers used for LPI are photodisruptive Nd:YAG and photocoagulative argon or diode. A sequential argon and Nd:YAG laser can be applied in eyes with thick or brown irides and in eyes with an absence of iris crypts.[1,2] Additionally, the treatment area can be positioned beneath the upper eyelid. A diameter size of approximately 200 μm is considered sufficient for IOP reduction.

Success and risk factors for failure

In APAC, LPI controls IOP effectively 65% to 76% of the time in Caucasians eyes and 58.2% in Asian eyes.[3-5] LPI performed within 1 week of developing APAC and an IOP reduction greater than 30% after maximal tolerated medical therapy conferred greater odds of successful IOP control.[6]

Lim *et al.* reported that 41.3% eyes developed elevated IOP within 1 year of LPI (78.9% within 4 months) necessitating treatment.[7] An RCT by Lam *et al.* showed that IOP was controlled in 3.3% of the participants who had undergone LPI following APAC at 18 months.[8] A follow-up study of this RCT showed that APAC eyes that underwent early phacoemulsification required less medication, had less extensive PAS, and a lower incidence of IOP elevation than eyes that underwent initial LPI.[9] Husain *et al.* reported a 38.9% failure at 2 years with cumulative survival of 61.1% at 2 years following LPI, with all failures occurring within 6 months of the procedure.[10] In a 50-month retrospective study, Aung *et al.* reported that 58.2% post-LPI APAC eyes subsequently experienced a rise in IOP, with 44.5% of cases occurring within the first 6 months.[4] Tan *et al.* reported subsequent rise in IOP in 21.4% of post-LPI eyes.[11]

LPI appears to control IOP in the short- to mid-term period. The failure rate of LPI ranges from 3.3% to 58.2% in various studies, depending upon the criteria for failure and follow-up duration.[4-8,10,11] Failure is often seen within the first 6 months in 40%–80% patients.[5,7] Although failure occurs more commonly in Asians, progressive failure of LPI in Caucasians has also been reported. Increased IOP following LPI in eyes with APAC has been reported to occur in the first 6 months. The cause can be trabecular meshwork damage due to iridotrabecular apposition during APAC, progressive angle closure due to PAS formation, and coexisting non-pupillary block mechanisms of angle closure. Other potential causes include angle characteristics at baseline, such as the presence of PAS prior to LPI,[7] increased iridotrabecular contact length in the light, reduced maximum iris bow height in the light, and greater basal iris thickness in the light.[12]

Complications of LPI

LPI is minimally invasive and can be performed as an outpatient procedure. Complications following LPI include transient IOP spikes (≥ 8 mmHg increase from baseline; IOP > 21 mmHg), transient hyphema, dysphotopsia, corneal burns, non-patency, and cataract progression.[12-15] No significant change in corneal endothelial cell count was reported following sequential LPI in an RCT.[10] However, another retrospective study reported a significant decrease in corneal endothelial cell count.[16] LPI may not prevent long-term increase in IOP in eyes post-APAC.

Fellow eye of APAC patients

Owing to the high risk of developing APAC in the fellow eye, a prophylactic LPI is standard in the fellow unaffected eye.[5] LPI results in progressive widening of the angle. Increase in angle width was reported to occur until 12 months post-LPI, with the maximum widening occurring at 4 months post-LPI.[7] A study reported that fellow eyes with prophylactic LPI did not develop APAC over a 4 year follow-up, with nearly 90% free of hypotensive medication.[17] However, according to the ZAP study, the incidence of angle-closure disease is very low over 6 years, suggesting that the benefit of prophylactic LPI through community-based screening is limited.[18] Given that the benefits and risks of LPI in the ZAP study were evaluated in a Chinese population, these results should not be extrapolated to other populations and further research is required.[19]

Comments

- Correcting the pupillary block mechanism is the definitive treatment of APAC, while medical and other interventions are usually temporizing or adjunctive measures.
- LPI is the first-line management of APAC, independently of responsiveness to medical treatment.
- In eyes with a thick iris and lack of iris crypts, sequential argon laser thinning of the peripheral iris followed by YAG:Nd LPI can be effective.
- Close follow-up is essential after LPI, as additional medications or IOP-lowering surgical interventions may be required for long-term IOP control, particularly in Asian populations.

References

1. de Silva DJ, Day AC, Bunce C, Gazzard G, Foster PJ. Randomised trial of sequential pretreatment for Nd:YAG laser iridotomy in dark irides. Br J Ophthalmol. 2012 Feb;96(2):263-6 https://doi.org/10.1136/bjo.2010.200030

2. de Silva DJ, Gazzard G, Foster P. Laser iridotomy in dark irides. Br J Ophthalmol. 2007 Feb;91(2):222-5. https://doi.org/10.1136/bjo.2006.104315
3. Chan PP, Pang JC, Tham CC. Acute primary angle closure-treatment strategies, evidences and economical considerations. Eye (Lond). 2019 Jan;33(1):110-119. https://doi.org/10.1038/s41433-018-0278-x
4. Aung T, Ang LP, Chan SP, Chew PT. Acute primary angle-closure: long-term intraocular pressure outcome in Asian eyes. Am J Ophthalmol. 2001;131:7-12. https://doi.org/10.1016/S0002-9394(00)00621-8
5. Ong AY, McCann P, Perera SA, Lim F, Ng SM, Friedman DS, Chang D. Lens extraction versus laser peripheral iridotomy for acute primary angle closure. Cochrane Database Syst Rev. 2023 Mar 8;3(3):CD015116. https://doi.org/10.1002/14651858.CD015116.pub2
6. Lee JW, Lee JH, Lee KW. Prognostic factors for the success of laser iridotomy for acute primary angle closure glaucoma. Korean J Ophthalmol. 2009;23:286-90. https://doi.org/10.3341/kjo.2009.23.4.286
7. Lim LS, Aung T, Husain R, Wu YJ, Gazzard G, Seah SK. Acute primary angle closure: configuration of the drainage angle in the first year after laser peripheral iridotomy. Ophthalmology. 2004;111:1470-4. https://doi.org/10.1016/j.ophtha.2004.01.036
8. Lam DS, Leung DY, Tham CC, Li FC, Kwong YY, Chiu TY, Fan DS. Randomized trial of early phacoemulsification versus peripheral iridotomy to prevent intraocular pressure rise after acute primary angle closure. Ophthalmology 2008; 115:1134-1140. https://doi.org/10.1016/j.ophtha.2007.10.033
9. Chan PP, Tang FY, Leung DY, Lam TC, Baig N, Tham CC. Ten-Year Clinical Outcomes of Acute Primary Angle Closure Randomized to Receive Early Phacoemulsification Versus Laser Peripheral Iridotomy. J Glaucoma. 2021; 30:332-9. https://doi.org/10.1097/IJG.0000000000001799
10. Husain R, Gazzard G, Aung T, Chen Y, Padmanabhan V, Oen FT, Seah SK, Hoh ST. Initial management of acute primary angle closure: a randomized trial comparing phacoemulsification with laser peripheral iridotomy. Ophthalmology. 2012;119:2274-81. https://doi.org/10.1016/j.ophtha.2012.06.015
11. Tan AM, Loon SC, Chew PTK. Outcomes following acute primary angle closure in an Asian population. Clin Experiment Ophthalmol. 2009;37: 467-472. https://doi.org/10.1111/j.1442-9071.2009.02060.x
12. Ang G, Wells AP. Factors associated with failure of laser peripheral iridotomy- An anterior segment OCT study. Invest Ophthalmol Vis Sci. 2010;51:5538.
13. Radhakrishnan S, Chen PP, Junk AK, Nouri-Mahdavi K, Chen TC. Laser peripheral iridotomy in primary angle closure. Ophthalmology. 2018;125:1110-1120. https://doi.org/10.1016/j.ophtha.2018.01.015
14. Chang DS, Jiang Y, Kim JA, et al. Cataract progression after Nd:YAG laser iridotomy in

primary angle-closure suspect eyes. Br J Ophthalmol. 2023 Sep;107(9):1264-1268. https://doi.org/10.1136/bjophthalmol-2021-320929

15. Azuara-Blanco A, Burr J, Ramsay C, et al. Effectiveness of early lens extraction for the treatment of primary angle-closure glaucoma (EAGLE): a randomised controlled trial. Lancet. 2016 Oct 1;388(10052):1389-1397. https://doi.org/10.1016/S0140-6736(16)30956-4
16. Park H-YL, Lee NY, Park CK, Kim MS. Long-term changes in endothelial cell counts after early phacoemulsification versus laser peripheral iridotomy using sequential argon: YAG laser technique in acute primary angle closure. Graefes Arch Clin Exp Ophthalmol. 2012;250:1673-80. https://doi.org/10.1007/s00417-012-1998-4
17. Ang LP, Aung T, Chew PT. Acute primary angle closure in an Asian population: long-term outcome of the fellow eye after prophylactic laser peripheral iridotomy. Ophthalmology. 2000 Nov;107(11):2092-6. https://doi.org/10.1016/S0161-6420(00)00360-2
18. He M, Jiang Y, Huang S, et al. Laser peripheral iridotomy for the prevention of angle closure: a single-centre, randomised controlled trial. Lancet. 2019;393(10181):1609-18. https://doi.org/10.1016/S0140-6736(18)32607-2
19. Weinreb RN, Moghimi S. Prophylactic laser iridotomy in primary angle-closure suspects (Comment) Lancet. 2019;393(10181):1572-1574. https://doi.org/10.1016/S0140-6736(18)33059-9

LPIP

Vijaya Lingam

LPIP, also referred to as ALPI, involves the application of contraction burns to the peripheral iris circumferentially using an argon laser. Laser application with a larger laser spot size, lower energy, and longer duration burn leads to contraction of the peripheral iris stroma. This flattens the peripheral iris and creates a space between the anterior surface of the iris and the trabecular meshwork, resulting in rapid lowering of IOP and widening of the angle. ALPI alleviates appositional angle closure and prevents PAS formation. Some studies that performed 360° ALPI reported a success rate of up to 100% in achieving rapid IOP reduction.[1-5] ALPI also opens appositional angle closure in eyes with non-pupillary block mechanisms. However, ALPI may not relieve pupillary block. Performing an LPI may be challenging in APAC eyes with severe corneal edema, anterior chamber inflammation, and a dilated pupil with sphincter ischemia. LPI can be performed once corneal clarity is achieved after ALPI.

ALPI has been reported to be effective in breaking an attack of APAC within 2 hours in eyes unresponsive to medical therapy.[1] Lim *et al.* reported a reduction of IOP from 41.8 mmHg to 16.7 mmHg and increased corneal clarity in 20 APAC eyes with a pre-laser IOP of 24-72 mmHg.[2] ALPI was performed within 12 hours of initiating medical therapy and IOP reduction of < 21 mmHg was achieved in 15 of the 20 eyes. Visual acuity improved or remained unchanged in all patients except one who had concurrent central retinal vein occlusion.

In the presence of high IOP and iris sphincter ischemia, pilocarpine may not be effective in inducing miosis and breaking the attack of APAC.[1] On the contrary, pilocarpine may increase pupillary block by causing a forward movement of the lens and increasing lens thickness.[1] ALPI can be performed in cases where LPI is not possible due to corneal edema. ALPI can also be performed in patients with contraindications to systemic or topical IOP-lowering medications.

Fu *et al.* performed ALPI followed by Nd:YAG LPI (within 1 day of ALPI) in medically unresponsive APAC eyes (n = 36) within an average period of 3.2 ± 1.1 days post-APAC.[6] They excluded patients with post-medication IOP greater than 40 mmHg. They found a significant IOP reduction 2 hours after ALPI in all patients (31.6 ± 7.7 mmHg to 18.4 ± 8.7 mmHg; $p < 0.001$) with a complete success rate of 75%. However, 25% patients required additional IOP-lowering medications at 2 hours post-ALPI. IOP was controlled for up to 3 years in all eyes except 1.[6]

Vu *et al.* performed ALPI in 26 eyes of 24 patients with APAC unresponsive to pilocarpine and found a 38.5% reduction in IOP at 15 minutes and 71% at 2 hours.[7] The mean duration of APAC was 7.9 ± 12.3 days (range 1 to 45 days). The mean IOP decreased from 44.8 ± 9.0 mmHg to 21.3 ± 8.7 mmHg after 30 minutes, to 16.5 ± 8.9 mmHg after 1 hour, and 13.1 ± 9.1 mmHg after 2 hours, with a complete success rate of 80.8% and qualified success rate of 11.8%. Corneal edema resolved in 96.1% (n = 25) of the eyes after 2 hours. A significant increase in the mean angle opening distance and trabecular iris angle was noted on UBM and 8.6% (9 quadrants) of the angles still remained fully closed. Failure was observed in 2 eyes (7.7%) with a long duration of APAC (10 and 45 days), presence of a fixed widely dilated pupil, and PAS formation. Interestingly, the researchers also found that the angle did not open in areas where ALPI could not be performed due to the presence of pterygia. Lai *et al.* found 180° ALPI (n = 10) to be as effective as 360° ALPI in treating APAC with a duration of attack ≤ 48 hours (mean 20.3 hours, range 2 to 48 hours).[8]

Ritch reported successful IOP reduction following ALPI in Caucasian patients with light-colored irides (blue and light brown).[1] A reduction in IOP was observed by Ritch in 1 patient after 180° inferior ALPI and sequential LPI.[1]

In a meta-analysis of 4 RCTs comparing ALPI with medical treatment, initial treatment with ALPI resulted in a rapid reduction of IOP in eyes with APAC within 2 hours as compared with systemic medical treatment.[5] ALPI was performed after instilling timolol 0.5% and pilocarpine. There was no significant difference of IOP reduction at 24 hours as compared to eyes which underwent systemic medical management.[5] No significant difference was observed in the percentage of patients requiring topical IOP-lowering medication nor in the mean endothelial count among the 2 groups.

Lam *et al.* performed ALPI within 30 minutes of presentation in 10 APAC patients with corneal edema.[3] They suggested that topical glycerin or hypertonic saline can be used prior to ALPI in eyes with severe corneal edema. They found that 30 minutes post-ALPI the mean IOP was 21.7 ± 13.1 mmHg (63.5% IOP reduction). One patient with PAS showed a delayed response to ALPI. At 2 hours, the cornea cleared and IOP was <18 mmHg for all 10 patients.

Since ALPI does not relieve pupillary block, it must be combined with either a sequential LPI or SPI. In an RCT by Ngyugen *et al.*, there was no significant difference between ALPI followed by SPI and trabeculectomy in terms of absolute surgical success (97.3% versus 93.3%, respectively) at 1 year.[9] However, a significant increase in anterior chamber depth and angle width on UBM was noted in the ALPI-SPI group at 1 year. Although the complication rate was higher in terms of hyphema and corneal edema in the ALPI-SPI arm, it was not statistically significant.

ALPI can also be combined with argon LPP in APAC with a success rate of 74.1% in normalizing IOP within 48 hours.[10] However, subsequent LPI was performed in all eyes once corneal edema subsided. Unresponsive eyes (n = 5) required surgical management in the form of SPI or phacoemulsification with intraocular lens implantation and GSL.[10]

Advantages of ALPI

Medically unresponsive APAC may be encountered when patients are referred to a tertiary center in the setting of poor or limited access to health care and non-availability of LPI laser at the primary point of eye care. These eyes are likely to present with high IOP, corneal edema, and a mid-dilated pupil, making LPI challenging. ALPI can be easily performed in the outpatient clinic in these eyes with corneal edema and a shallow anterior chamber. Given that the burns do not require penetration of the iris and the spot size is larger, ALPI is easier to perform on the peripheral iris in the presence of corneal edema. The IOP-lowering effect starts within 15 minutes. ALPI also relieves non-pupillary block mechanisms. However, it must be followed up sequentially with an additional procedure (LPI or lens extraction) to relieve pupillary block once corneal edema decreases.

Complications

Complications resulting from ALPI include pigment dispersion, iris atrophy, corneal endothelial burns, sluggishly reactive mid-dilated pupil, inflammation, and rarely, decompression retinopathy. Interestingly, patients have been found to develop extensive angle synechiae years after ALPI, though this observation lacks substantial support in the literature.

Contraindications

ALPI is contraindicated in eyes with a flat anterior chamber, very severe corneal edema, PAS, and known corneal endothelial cell dysfunction.

Comments

- ALPI or LPIP helps achieve rapid IOP reduction and corneal clarity (within 2 hours) in eyes with APAC unresponsive to medical therapy. It is helpful in eyes with corneal edema, shallow anterior chamber, thick, mid-dilated, darkly pigmented irides, and appositional angle closure where LPI is challenging. It is also useful in eyes with additional non-pupillary block mechanisms.
- It is more effective in eyes with appositional angle closure and when performed shortly after the onset of APAC. Its efficacy is less in eyes with prolonged APAC with formation of PAS and a widely dilated pupil.
- ALPI is not a substitute for LPI. Subsequent iridotomy is required once adequate corneal clarity is achieved in order to relieve pupillary block as ALPI alone does not address this mechanism and does not prevent APAC recurrence.
- ALPI may be performed in eyes with persistent appositional angle closure despite LPI, such as eyes with plateau iris.

References

1. Ritch R. Argon laser treatment for medically unresponsive attacks of angle-closure glaucoma. Am J Ophthalmol. 1982;94:197-204. https://doi.org/10.1016/0002-9394(82)90075-7
2. Lim AS, Tan A, Chew P, et al. Laser iridoplasty in the treatment of severe acute angle closure glaucoma. Int Ophthalmol. 1993;17:33-36. https://doi.org/10.1007/BF00918865
3. Lam DSC, Lai JSM, Tham CCY. Immediate argon laser peripheral iridoplasty as treatment for acute attack of primary angle-closure glaucoma. A preliminary study. Ophthalmology. 1998;105:2231-2236. https://doi.org/10.1016/S0161-6420(98)92237-0
4. Lam DSC, Lai JSM, Tham CCY, et al. Argon laser peripheral iridoplasty versus conventional systemic medical therapy as the first line treatment of acute angle closure: a prospective randomized controlled trial. Ophthalmology. 2002;109:1591-1596. https://doi.org/10.1016/

S0161-6420(02)01158-2
5. Cai W, Lou Q, Fan J, et al. Efficacy and safety of argon laser peripheral iridoplasty and systemic medical therapy in Asian patients with acute primary angle closure: a meta-analysis of randomized controlled trials. J Ophthalmol. 2019;2019:7697416. https://doi.org/10.1155/2019/7697416
6. Fu J, Qing G, Wang N, Wang H. Efficacy of laser peripheral iridoplasty and iridotomy on medically refractory patients with acute primary angle closure: a three-year outcome. Chinese Med J. 2013;126:41-45. https://doi.org/10.3760/cma.j.issn.0366-6999.20122279
7. Vu AT, Bui TVA., Mai LA, et al. Effectiveness of laser peripheral iridoplasty in the treatment of acute primary angle closure. Spektrum Augenheilkd. 2023;37:101-105. https://doi.org/10.1007/s00717-022-00522-z
8. Lai JS, Tham CC, Lam DS. Limited argon laser peripheral iridoplasty as immediate treatment for an acute attack of primary angle closure glaucoma: a preliminary study. Eye (Lond). 1999;13:26-30. https://doi.org/10.1038/eye.1999.5
9. Nguyen HX, Nguyen ND, Nguyen HT, et al. Comparing combined laser iridoplasty and surgical iridectomy with trabeculectomy in treatment of refractory acute primary angle closure without significant cataract: a randomized controlled trial. Eye (Lond). 2023;37:2139-2144. https://doi.org/10.1038/s41433-022-02311-z
10. Zhou W, Zhao F, Shi D, Qadri M, Jiang L, Ma L. Argon Laser Peripheral Iridoplasty and Argon Laser Pupilloplasty: Alternative Management for Medically Unresponsive Acute Primary Angle Closure. J Ophthalmol. 2019 Aug 14;2019:1876912 https://doi.org/10.1155/2019/1876912

LPP

Fengbin Lin, Xiulan Zhang

Despite its benefits, LPIP alone may not completely and effectively relieve pupillary block, as it may fail to establish adequate communication between the anterior and posterior chambers, which is necessary for rapid and effective IOP reduction.

LPP offers a more effective solution.[1-2] LPP uses a frequency-doubled 532 nm laser to cauterize and shrink the pupillary margin of the iris and turn it outward (Fig. 1). The parameter settings are as follows: spot diameter of 300–500 μm, laser energy of 200–400 mW, and exposure time 0.4–0.5 seconds. The laser action sites are located at the iris on the pupil edge at the 3 o'clock and 9 o'clock positions. The number of laser points is approximately 4 to 6, and the power is set to induce an obvious and visible contraction of the iris matrix. It effectively relieves pupillary block and allows the aqueous humor to flow freely from the posterior chamber into the anterior chamber.

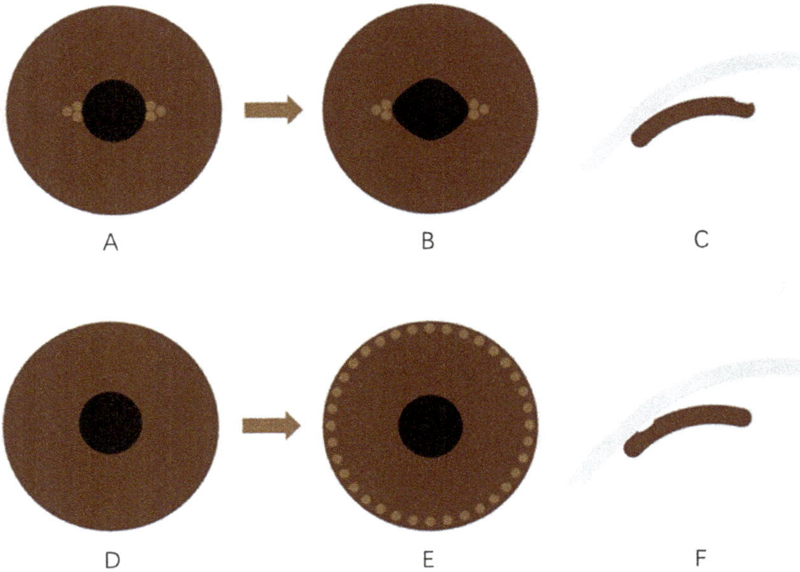

Fig. 1. Schematic diagram of laser pupilloplasty (LPP) and laser peripheral iridoplasty (LPIP). *(A)* Laser site of LPP. *(B)* Changes in the pupil after LPP. *(C)* Changes in the pupil edge and iris after LPP. *(D)* Before treatment. *(E)* Laser site of LPIP. *(F)* Changes of the peripheral iris tissue after LPIP.

Studies have shown that combining LPP with LPIP can significantly relieve pupillary block, widen the peripheral chamber angle, promote aqueous humor outflow, and quickly reduce IOP in patients with APAC. The effective rate of IOP reduction is as high as 71.4% 2 hours after treatment, significantly higher than with LPIP alone (41%).[1]

Advantages of LPP

- Broader indications: LPP requires less corneal transparency, making it suitable for patients with APAC.
- Ease of operation: Many patients with APAC experience symptoms such as ocular pain, headache, and nausea, which can hinder cooperation during treatment. The LPP procedure is performed at the 3 and 9 o'clock positions on the pupillary margin, within the central area of the palpebral fissure, facilitating laser operation.
- Safety and efficacy: LPP avoids the side effects and complications associated with medications, anterior chamber punctures, and surgery while providing a quick reduction in IOP.

Comments

- LPP is an alternative adjunctive treatment that can be combined with ALPI or LPIP to effectively relieve pupillary block in APAC by promoting aqueous humor outflow and rapidly reducing IOP.

References

1. Guo L, Yang Y, Guo L, et al. Comparisons of laser peripheral iridoplasty and laser pupilloplasty in the treatment of acute primary angle closure patients. Chin J Ophthalmol Med. 2022;12(1):12-17.
2. Zhou W, Zhao F, Shi D, Qadri M, Jiang L, Ma L. Argon Laser Peripheral Iridoplasty and Argon Laser Pupilloplasty: Alternative Management for Medically Unresponsive Acute Primary Angle Closure. J Ophthalmol. 2019 Aug 14;2019:1876912. https://doi.org/10.1155/2019/1876912

Primary phacoemulsification

Vijaya Lingam

The principles of APAC management include achieving a reduction in IOP and resolution of angle closure. Although LPI relieves the APAC, IOP can rise again over time despite a patent LPI, at least in Asians and Caucasians.[1-3] This may be due to the presence of non-pupillary block related mechanisms, presence of PAS, or prior functional damage to the trabecular meshwork due to prior episodes of intermittent iridotrabecular contact.[2] On the other hand, medications may help achieve a lower IOP but do not address the underlying angle closure. Although pupillary block is the major mechanism responsible for APAC, non-pupillary block mechanisms, such as increased lens thickness and lens vault, also play a role in angle closure pathophysiology. Eyes with APAC have been reported to have an increased lens vault and a thicker lens than other PACD subcategories.[3-5] Phacoemulsification with intraocular lens implantation addresses both mechanisms in eyes with APAC and visually significant cataract.

Phacoemulsification in eyes with APAC helps increase anterior chamber depth and lower IOP.[6-9] The iris position changes after cataract surgery, leading to an increase in the anterior chamber depth and widening of the angle. Additionally, phacoemulsification can be combined with angle-based procedures such as GSL.[10,11] During phacoemulsification, the use of viscoelastic to deepen the anterior chamber leads to visco-GSL (also known as viscogonioplasty), thereby relieving PAS.[12]

Phacoemulsification reduces IOP in eyes with controlled APAC and APAC unresponsive to medications. In a non-comparative case series of phacoemulsification in APAC eyes ($n = 17$) by Zhang *et al.*, IOP decreased significantly from a median preoperative IOP of 45 mmHg (range 35–70 mmHg) after phacoemulsification.[10] The median IOP just before phacoemulsification was 26 mmHg (range 15-42 mmHg) following topical and systemic medications.[10] Two of these eyes had IOP > 40 mmHg. Intraoperative corneal edema during phacoemulsification was noted in some eyes with high IOP. Significant IOP reduction was noted on the first and seventh postoperative day. Su *et al.* performed phacoemulsification in eyes with medically uncontrolled APAC within 12.94 ± 9.12 days. The IOP decreased from a preoperative value of 48.81 ± 16.83 mmHg to 16.4 ± 10.67 mmHg on day 1, 9.43 ± 3.03 mmHg at 1 week, and 10.70 ± 2.80 mmHg at 3 months.[11]

Husain *et al.* included patients with IOPs of ≤ 30 mmHg within 24 hours of medical management of APAC with visually significant cataract in their study.[13] Phacoemulsification was performed between 5 to 7 days of APAC to achieve better corneal clarity. Success at 2 years was higher in the phacoemulsification than the LPI group (38.2% vs 10.6%, respectively), with a cumulative survival of 89.5% vs 61.1%, respectively. However, the baseline preoperative IOP was 14.6 ± 6.9 mmHg post-systemic medications. At 6 months, no significant change was observed in the corneal endothelium in either group. However, the RCT did not reach the required sample size. Moreover, patients with LPI who underwent phacoemulsification or phacotrabeculectomy were excluded from the analysis. One patient developed an APAC recurrence after LPI.

Jacobi *et al.* compared phacoemulsification with SPI in eyes with uncontrolled APAC. They achieved IOP control in a significantly larger proportion of APAC eyes in the phacoemulsification group (72% vs 35%, respectively).[9] A lower proportion of eyes in the phacoemulsification group required additional surgery (11.5% vs 63%, respectively). The reported rates of conversion to PAC and recurrence of APAC following phacoemulsification are lower compared to LPI. Phacoemulsification also prevents further IOP rise, reduces medication requirement, and reduces the need of subsequent IOP-lowering procedures compared to LPI or SPI.[9]

Anbar *et al.* reported a reduction in IOP from 40.23 ± 10.4 mmHg preoperatively to 11.4 ± 3.3 mmHg 3 months following phacoemulsification within 1 week of APAC attack.[14] They also found a significant increase in anterior chamber volume and depth postoperatively.

Harasymowycz *et al.* combined phacoemulsification with intraocular lens implantation with GSL in eyes with APAC and subacute angle closure and found a mean IOP reduction of 25 mmHg and a 55% reduction in medications over a mean follow-up period of 11 months (range 2–36 months).[15] However, lens removal and GSL does not address all non-pupillary block mechanisms, such as plateau iris and pseudo-plateau iris.[15-17] Although 4 patients with APAC in the study by Harasymowycz *et al.* had plateau iris, they could not compare the outcomes between the pupillary block group and the plateau iris group due to a small sample size.[15]

Tran *et al.* performed UBM pre- and post-cataract surgery in 6 eyes with plateau iris syndrome and found persistence of iridociliary apposition despite cataract extraction.[16] Nonaka *et al.* found that cataract surgery resulted in a significant increase in the angle opening distance at 500 μm after cataract surgery in eyes with PACD (including plateau iris) and residual appositional closure after LPI. However, they noted a persistence of iridociliary contact on UBM. They did not include eyes with APAC in their series. Moreover, IOP changes in the subgroup with plateau iris and follow-up duration were not reported.[18] In a subsequent report in eyes with PAC, the authors reported an attenuation of the anterior positioning of the ciliary processes 3 months following phacoemulsification.[19] Gong *et al.* reported a significant decrease in IOP, number of IOP-lowering medications, PAS, and a significant increase in angle opening distance and trabecular ciliary process angle on UBM following phacoemulsification with visco-GSL in eyes with APAC.[20] No significant change in the trabecular ciliary process distance, which is influenced by the position of the ciliary process, was noted. The rate of PAS recurrence was also not reported. Thus, there is no clear evidence regarding long-term role of phacoemulsification and GSL in eyes with APAC and plateau iris.

It is important to note that the aforementioned studies only included patients with visually significant cataract. Preoperatively, patients received intravenous or oral acetazolamide, intravenous 20% mannitol injection, and topical aqueous suppressants. Clear corneal phacoemulsification was performed. In the study by Jacobi *et al.* in Caucasian participants with APAC, all patients in the phacoemulsification arm received preoperative medications such that IOP was < 35 mmHg prior to surgery.[9] Zhang *et al.* also achieved an IOP reduction from a median baseline IOP of 45 mmHg to 26 mmHg prior to surgery.[11] Lam *et al.* compared phacoemulsification with LPI in an RCT in medically controlled Chinese participants with APAC.[21] They found lower IOP rise in the phacoemulsification group (3.3%) compared to the LPI group (46.7%) at 18 months.

Phacoemulsification also controls IOP in eyes unresponsive to LPI. Although phacoemulsification is effective even when performed early after APAC, it may be preferable to perform the surgery after controlling IOP and inflammation to avoid intra- and postoperative complications.[9,22]

Lin *et al.* compared the clinical outcomes in patients with APAC who underwent primary phacoemulsification, primary LPI, or postponed phacoemulsification following LPI.[22] They found that patients who underwent phacoemulsification had better IOP control, improved vision, deeper anterior chamber depth, and wider angle, and required less antiglaucoma medications than those who underwent LPI alone. Waiting several months to perform phacoemulsification after initial LPI did not appear to adversely affect outcomes when compared with those of early (within days to weeks) phacoemulsification treatment.

Surgical challenges in eyes with APAC

Surgery in APAC eyes can be challenging due to the presence of corneal edema, shallow anterior chamber, posterior synechiae, atonic iris, intraoperative iris prolapse, and poor mydriasis. In addition, there may be associated zonular weakness. Intraoperative use of iris retractors and initial debulking of the nucleus may be useful.[12] Rarely, iridodialysis and cyclodialysis have been reported when phacoemulsification was combined with angle-based procedures. Jacobi *et al.* used iris hooks and performed sphincterotomies in some of their patients.[9] Intra-operative complications include capsular tears, vitreous loss requiring anterior vitrectomy, hyphema, and intermittent iris prolapse.

Moghimi *et al.* suggested that phacoemulsification has lower intra- and post-operative complications when performed after breaking the acute attack and performing LPI.[8] However, their study excluded eyes with APAC with an IOP > 25 mmHg. Postoperative complications following phacoemulsification in APAC eyes include corneal edema, inflammation, and transient IOP spikes. There is also higher risk of corneal decompensation postoperatively. Zhang *et al.* reported a significant decrease in corneal endothelial cell count (median change 166 cells/ mm^2).[11] Biometry may be challenging due to the presence of corneal edema. Central corneal thickness and axial length have been reported to decrease post-phacoemulsification in eyes with APAC.[23] This may lead to prediction errors and refractive errors post-phacoemulsification. A mean surgically induced astigmatism of 0.31 diopters has been reported.[11] A postoperative spherical equivalent of -0.25 ± 1.16 D with no significant change from the preoperative spherical equivalent of 2.07 ± 2.85 D ($p = 0.068$) has been reported by Su *et al.*[12] Phacoemulsification can be combined with additional procedures to address PAS. These include visco-GSL and GSL.[12,14,24] In an RCT, Nguyen *et al.* found that phacoemulsification combined with GSL yielded better postoperative visual outcomes, wider anterior chamber drainage angles, and fewer complications compared to phacotrabeculectomy.[24] Moreover, phacoemulsification can be combined with GSL and goniotomy for

APAC eyes with an underlying chronic PACG component. Zhang *et al.* found that the combination of phacoemulsification, GSL, and goniotomy achieves statistically and clinically significant reductions in IOP in eyes with advanced PACG and cataract.[25-28] For more details, please refer to the surgical management outlined in Section 5.

Comments

- Phacoemulsification in eyes with APAC unresponsive to conventional medical and laser management and visually significant cataract helps to reduce IOP, relieve pupillary block, and widen the anterior chamber angle in APAC.
- Phacoemulsification reduces the long-term need for IOP-lowering medication, recurrence of APAC, and subsequent surgical procedures for IOP control.
- Phacoemulsification in eyes with APAC can be challenging due to the presence of corneal edema, shallow anterior chamber, zonular weakness, and inflammation.
- There is limited evidence regarding the outcomes of phacoemulsification in APAC eyes with a clear crystalline lens, and further research is needed to determine its efficacy in such cases.

References

1. Aung T, Ang LP, Chan SP, Chew PT. Acute primary angle-closure: long-term intraocular pressure outcome in Asian eyes. Am J Ophthalmol. 2001;131:7-12. https://doi.org/10.1016/S0002-9394(00)00621-8
2. Jeong Y, Park KH, Jeoung JW. Long-term prognosis of acute primary angle closure in an east asian cohort. Jpn J Ophthalmol. 2024Jul;68(4):302-310. https://doi.org/10.1007/s10384-024-01065-3
3. Ong AY, McCann P, Perera SA, et al. Lens extraction versus laser peripheral iridotomy for acute primary angle closure. Cochrane Database Syst Rev. 2023 Mar 8;3(3):CD015116. https://doi.org/10.1002/14651858.CD015116.pub2
4. Buckley SA, Reeves B, Burdon M, et al. Acute angle closure glaucoma: Relative failure of YAG iridotomy in affected eyes and factors influencing outcome. Br J Ophthalmol. 1994;78:529-33. https://doi.org/10.1136/bjo.78.7.529
5. Kurimoto Y, Park M, Sakaue H, Kondo T. Changes in the anterior chamber configuration after small-incision cataract surgery with posterior chamber intraocular lens implantation. Am J Ophthalmol. 1997;124:775-80. https://doi.org/10.1016/S0002-9394(14)71694-0
6. Kim M, Park KH, Kim TW, Kim DM. Anterior chamber configuration changes after cataract surgery in eyes with glaucoma. Korean J Ophthalmol. 2012;26:97-103. https://doi.org/10.3341/kjo.2012.26.2.97

7. Boey PY, Singhal S, Perera SA, Aung T. Conventional and emerging treatments in the management of acute primary angle closure. Clin Ophthalmol. 2012;6:417-24. https://doi.org/10.2147/OPTH.S16400
8. Moghimi S, Hashemian H, Chen R, Johari M, Mohammadi M, Lin SC. Early phacoemulsification in patients with acute primary angle closure. J Curr Ophthalmol. 2016 12;27:70-5. https://doi.org/10.1016/j.joco.2015.12.001
9. Jacobi PC, Dietlein TS, Lüke C, et al. Primary phacoemulsification and intraocular lens implantation for acute angle- closure glaucoma. Ophthalmology. 2002;109:1597-1603. https://doi.org/10.1016/S0161-6420(02)01123-5
10. Zhang Z, Chen M, Yin J, Yao K. Microcoaxial phacoemulsification combined with viscogoniosynechialysis for patients with refractory acute angle-closure glaucoma. J Glaucoma. 2014 ;23:119-24. https://doi.org/10.1097/IJG.0b013e318268518d
11. Su W-W, Chen PY-F, Hsiao C-H, Chen HS-L. Primary Phacoemulsification and Intraocular Lens Implantation for Acute Primary Angle-Closure. PLoS One. 2011;6(5):e20056. https://doi.org/10.1371/journal.pone.0020056
12. Ming Zhi Z, Lim ASM, Yin Wong T. A pilot study of lens extraction in the management of acute primary angle-closure glaucoma. Am J Ophthalmol. 2003;135:534-536. https://doi.org/10.1016/S0002-9394(02)02108-6
13. Husain R, Do T, Lai J, et al. Efficacy of phacoemulsification alone vs phacoemulsification with goniosynechialysis in patients with primary angle-closure disease: a randomized clinical trial. JAMA Ophthalmol. 2019;137:1107-1113. https://doi.org/10.1001/jamaophthalmol.2019.2493
14. Anbar MA, Mahmoud HA, Abdellah MM. Angle, anterior chamber parameters, and intraocular pressure changes after early phacoemulsification in acute angle-closure glaucoma. J Cataract Refract Surg. 2023;49:1147-1152. https://doi.org/10.1097/j.jcrs.0000000000001287
15. Harasymowycz PJ, Papamatheakis DG, Ahmed I, et al. Phacoemulsification and goniosynechialysis in the management of unresponsive primary angle closure. J Glaucoma. 2005;14:186-9. https://doi.org/10.1097/01.ijg.0000159131.38828.85
16. Tran HV, Liebmann JM, Ritch R. Iridociliary apposition in plateau iris syndrome persists after cataract extraction. Am J Ophthalmol. 2003;135:40-3. https://doi.org/10.1016/S0002-9394(02)01842-1
17. Tarongoy P, Ho CL, Walton DS. Angle-closure glaucoma: the role of the lens in the pathogenesis, prevention, and treatment. Surv Ophthalmol. 2009;54:211-25. https://doi.org/10.1016/j.survophthal.2008.12.002
18. Nonaka A, Kondo T, Kikuchi M, et al. Angle widening and alteration of ciliary process configuration after cataract surgery for primary angle closure. Ophthalmology. 2006;113:437-41. https://doi.org/10.1016/j.ophtha.2005.11.018
19. Nonaka A, Kondo T, Kikuchi M, et al. Cataract surgery for residual angle closure after peripheral laser iridotomy. Ophthalmology. 2005 Jun;112(6):974-9. https://doi.org/10.1016/j.

ophtha.2004.12.042

20. Gong H, Dong X, Zheng B, et al. Ultrasound Biomicroscopy Might Predict the Outcome of Phacoemulsification-Visco Dissection in Medically Controlled Primary Angle-Closure Glaucoma Eye With Extensive Peripheral Anterior Synechia. Front Med. 2021 Jul 19;8:705864. https://doi.org/10.3389/fmed.2021.705864
21. Lam DS, Leung DY, Tham CC, et al. Randomized trial of early phacoemulsification versus peripheral iridotomy to prevent intraocular pressure rise after acute primary angle closure. Ophthalmology. 2008;115:1134-40. https://doi.org/10.1016/j.ophtha.2007.10.033
22. Lin YH, Wu CH, Huang SM, et al. Early versus Delayed Phacoemulsification and Intraocular Lens Implantation for Acute Primary Angle-Closure. J Ophthalmol. 2020 Mar 24;2020:8319570. https://doi.org/10.1155/2020/8319570
23. Suzuki T, Ueta Y, Tachi N, et al. Refractive outcomes after immediate primary phacoemulsification for acute primary angle closure. Sci Rep. 2023;13:13283. https://doi.org/10.1038/s41598-023-40585-9
24. Nguyen XH, Nguyen DN, Nguyen TH, et al. Comparing the Safety and Efficacy of Phacogoniosynechialysis With Phacotrabeculectomy in the Management of Refractory Acute Primary Closure Angle Glaucoma With Cataract: A Multicenter Randomized Trial. J Glaucoma. 2021;30:552-558. https://doi.org/10.1097/IJG.0000000000001868
25. Song Y, Xie L, Zhu X, et al. Two-year outcome of phacogoniotomy for advanced primary angle-closure glaucoma with cataracts: a multicentre study. Br J Ophthalmol. 2025 Jun 23;109(7):770-774. https://doi.org/10.1136/bjo-2024-325375
26. Song Y, Zhang Y, Li F, et al. One-Year Results of a Multicenter Study: Intraocular Pressure-Lowering Effect of Combined Phacoemulsification, Goniosynechialysis, and Goniotomy for Cases of Advanced Primary Angle-Closure Glaucoma With Cataract. Asia Pac J Ophthalmol. 2022;11(6):529-35. https://doi.org/10.1097/APO.0000000000000579
27. Song Y, Fan S, Tang L, et al. Two-Year Outcomes of Phacogoniotomy vs Phacotrabeculectomy for Advanced Primary Angle-Closure Glaucoma With Cataract: A Noninferiority Randomized Clinical Trial. JAMA Ophthalmol. 2025 Jun 1;143(6):462-469. https://doi.org/10.1001/jamaophthalmol.2025.0685
28. Song Y, Lin F, Lv A, et al. Phacogoniotomy versus phacotrabeculectomy for advanced primary angle-closure glaucoma with cataract: A randomized non-inferiority trial. Asia Pac J Ophthalmol. 2024;13(1):100033. https://doi.org/10.1016/j.apjo.2023.100033

SPI

Vijaya Lingam

SPI relieves pupillary block in eyes with APAC by creating an alternative route for the passage of aqueous humor from the posterior to the anterior chamber.

SPI as an initial procedure for APAC was first proposed by von Graefe in 1856.[1] Patients with APAC present with high IOP and significant corneal edema, and LPI may not be possible in these eyes. Significant improvements in visual acuity and IOP have been reported after SPI in APAC eyes following the termination of the acute attack.[1] A success rate between 70.4% and 75% at 6–12 months (IOP < 21 mmHg without medication) following SPI has been reported.[1-4]

Fleck *et al.* randomized eyes with APAC to SPI and Nd:YAG iridotomy.[3] However, they did not include patients with IOP > 21 mmHg after initial medical treatment. Three patients in the SPI group required Nd:YAG iridotomy to the remaining pigmented layer in eyes with SPI.[3]

Jacobi *et al.* performed SPI in APAC eyes in Caucasians with a clear crystalline and compared it with phacoemulsification in APAC eyes with visually significant cataract and without an obvious plateau iris configuration.[5] SPI was performed after a mean 2.0 ± 0.8 days (ranges 0.5–3 days) following the attack. They reported a success rate of 35% in the SPI arm, which was lower than that observed in the phacoemulsification arm. Additionally, a higher number of subsequent surgeries such as trabeculectomy, cyclophotocoagulation, and lens extraction were required following SPI. Corneal edema and transient IOP spikes were seen in 21.8% eyes and a fibrinous anterior chamber reaction was present in 9.3% eyes.[5] The SPI group required significantly more subsequent surgical interventions (65% vs 16.2%, $p = 0.01$) compared to the phacoemulsification group. However, the most common procedure performed was lens extraction in the iridectomy arm.

Nguyen *et al.* conducted an RCT comparing the complication rates of combined ALPI and SPI with unaugmented trabeculectomy in eyes with medically unresponsive APAC and clear crystalline lenses.[6] Although the complication rate was higher in the ALPI-SPI group, they found it was not statistically significant (45.9% vs 33.3%; $p = 0.23$). There was no difference in complete success rate (97.1% vs 92.6%, respectively) or improvement in visual acuity at 1 year after treatment. No significant difference in the corneal endothelial cell count was noted among the 2 groups. Significant improvement in anterior chamber depth and UBM angle parameters were noted in the ALPI-SPI group compared to the trabeculectomy group, indicating greater widening of the anterior chamber angle.

The initial approach to APAC management also depends on lens status. While phacoemulsification with intraocular lens implantation is an option in eyes with visually significant cataracts, there is a paucity if evidence supporting its efficacy in APAC eyes with clear crystalline lenses. The recommended procedures in eyes with a clear crystalline lens include LPI, ALPI, or LPIP, trabeculectomy, and SPI. SPI theoretically causes less pigment release compared to LPI, which may be problematic when the trabecular meshwork is already compromised. Anterior chamber reformation during SPI may also break newly formed PAS.[6] LPI can be challenging when the anterior chamber is extremely shallow or when the iris is very thick, as is often the case in Asian eyes, as observed under UBM. In these situations, SPI offers advantages over LPI. SPI can be performed in eyes with a clear crystalline lens and/or severe corneal edema. Additionally, it does not need special instrumentation, such as an Nd:YAG or argon laser. The conjunctiva is preserved for future filtering surgery if required.

Limitations
SPI does not prevent PAS formation. Moreover, IOP may rise over time in some eyes. It does not address non-pupillary block mechanisms such as an anteriorly located lens-iris diaphragm or thick crystalline lens.

Trabeculectomy
Vijaya Lingam

Trabeculectomy in eyes with APAC has been described in eyes with APAC unresponsive to medical management (with or without LPI), especially in the presence of severe corneal edema, PAS, or delayed presentation. Trabeculectomy has been performed in cases with prolonged symptoms and delayed treatment for more than 48 hours,[7] ranging from 1–57 days in various studies.[4,7-9] The percentage of eyes with APAC undergoing trabeculectomy has been reported from 1% to 51% in various studies.[4,7-9] Krishnamurthy *et al.* reported that 1% of APAC eyes required trabeculectomy,[8] whereas 15.3% of APAC eyes in a case series by Buckley required trabeculectomy.[4] Aung *et al.* reported that 32.5% patients with APAC underwent trabeculectomy (without antimetabolites) with a complete success rate of 56.2% and a qualified success rate of 9.4%.[7] The mean duration of symptoms was 4.5 days (range 1–14) in the medical failure group ($n = 32$) with a mean of 4.1 ± 2.5 (range 1–10) days between presentation and surgery. The success rate was lower than in eyes with medically controlled APAC (87.5%). The most common cause of failure was scarring of the bleb, possibly due to surgery in an inflamed eye. Eyes with medically uncontrolled APAC had more complications than medically controlled eyes. These included shallow anterior chamber, hyphema, and transiently elevated IOP. Alternatives to trabeculectomy should be considered in eyes with these features due to higher risk of failure. If required, trabeculectomy should be performed when preoperative inflammation is optimized and with intraoperative use of antimetabolites. In a retrospective series by Sihota *et al.*, 51.6% of 136 eyes with APAC unresponsive to LPI and medications underwent trabeculectomy with a 3-month success rate of 64.1%.[9]

Sawada *et al.* reported a success rate of 40.0% ± 29.7% in 10 eyes of Japanese patients with medically unresponsive APAC.[10] In a retrospective case series (*n* = 35) of refractory APAC unresponsive to medical and laser treatment, Krishnamurthy *et al.* reported a complete success rate of 81% (95% CI: 56% to 92%) and a complete plus qualified success rate of 97% (95% CI: 81%–99%) at 7 years which was maintained until 10 years.[8] Among the 35 eyes that underwent trabeculectomy, mitomycin C was used in 15 eyes intraoperatively. The median time to surgery was 13 days (range 1–57), and the median interval from the time of symptom onset to the date of surgery was 22.5 days (range 14–34). Only 31% eyes underwent trabeculectomy within the first week of presentation.

Aung *et al.* had a qualified success rate of 56.2% (*n* = 32) and a complete success rate of 9.4% after trabeculectomy without mitomycin C at 4.1 ± 2.5 days following APAC.[7] Krishnamurthy *et al.* performed trabeculectomy in APAC eyes without visually significant cataracts and with uncontrolled IOP despite LPI and medical management.[8] Median time to surgery was 13 days (range 1–57) post presentation with a median duration of symptoms of 10 days (interquartile range 4,16). Complete success was seen in 88% (95% CI: 72%–95%) at 1 year. The authors hypothesized that their better outcomes were due to preoperative control of inflammation with topical corticosteroids and shorter duration of APAC.

Despite the variability in outcomes, short follow-up durations, and lack of control group, these studies suggest trabeculectomy is a viable option in eyes with uncontrolled APAC despite medication and LPI or ALPI, or where laser is not possible due to corneal edema and shallow anterior chamber. Use of preoperative topical steroids and intraoperative antimetabolites is recommended. The risk of failure is higher than trabeculectomy in chronic PACG eyes.

Complications

The potential complications of trabeculectomy include inflammation, hyphema, hypotony, shallow anterior chamber, choroidal detachment, aqueous misdirection, scarring of the bleb, corneal edema, cataract formation, bleb leaks, and retinal hemorrhages, among others.

Comments

- SPI is an option for the short-term management of APAC, especially in eyes with severe corneal edema that precludes other interventions. This is particularly relevant when resources such as argon and Nd:YAG lasers are unavailable, or in cases where LPI cannot be performed, such as when the anterior chamber is very shallow and the iris is very thick. SPI can be performed in eyes with either clear crystalline lenses or visually significant cataracts.

- SPI may not prevent long-term increases in IOP and development of PAS in all eyes. Additional IOP-lowering medications and subsequent surgeries, including lens extraction, may be required.
- Trabeculectomy has a low to moderate success rate in eyes with medically uncontrolled APAC. It can be considered in eyes with extensive PAS or advanced glaucomatous optic nerve head damage, such as in APAC eyes with an underlying chronic PACG component. The most common cause of failure is bleb fibrosis, likely due to performing the procedure in an inflamed eye. Careful perioperative inflammation control is essential to optimize surgical outcomes.

References

1. Playfair TJ, Watson PG. Management of acute primary angle closure glaucoma: a long-term follow-up of the results of peripheral iridectomy used as an initial procedure. Br J Ophthalmol. 1979;63:17-22. https://doi.org/10.1136/bjo.63.1.17
2. Krupin T, Mitchell KB, Johnson MF, Bernard B. The long-term effects of iridectomy for primary acute angle closure glaucoma. Am J Ophthalmol. 1978;86:506-9. https://doi.org/10.1016/0002-9394(78)90297-0
3. Fleck BW, Wright E, Fairley EA. A randomised prospective comparison of operative peripheral iridectomy and Nd: YAG laser iridotomy treatment of acute angle closure glaucoma: 3 year visual acuity and intraocular pressure control outcome. Br J Ophthalmol. 1997;81:884-8. https://doi.org/10.1136/bjo.81.10.884
4. SA, Reeves B, Burdon M, et al. Acute angle closure glaucoma: relative failure of YAG iridotomy in affected eyes and factors influencing outcome. Br J Ophthalmol. 1994;78: 529-33. https://doi.org/10.1136/bjo.78.7.529
5. Jacobi PC, Dietlein TS, Lüke C, Engels B, Krieglstein GK. Primary phacoemulsification and intraocular lens implantation for acute angle-closure glaucoma. Ophthalmology. 2002;109:1597-603. https://doi.org/10.1016/S0161-6420(02)01123-5
6. Nguyen HX, Nguyen ND, Nguyen HT, et al. Comparing combined laser iridoplasty and surgical iridectomy with trabeculectomy in treatment of refractory acute primary angle closure without significant cataract: a randomized controlled trial. Eye. 2023;37:2139-2144. https://doi.org/10.1038/s41433-022-02311-z

7. Aung T, Tow SL, Yap EY, Chan SP, Seah SK. Trabeculectomy for acute primary angle closure. Ophthalmology. 2000;107:1298-302. https://doi.org/10.1016/S0161-6420(00)00137-8
8. Krishnamurthy R, Senthil S, Rao HL, Mandal AK, Garudadri C. Outcomes of trabeculectomy in eyes with refractory acute primary angle closure in Indian eyes. Indian J Ophthalmol, 2022;70:580-584. https://doi.org/10.4103/ijo.IJO_1065_21
9. Sihota R, Agarwal HC. Profile of the subtypes of angle closure glaucoma in a tertiary hospital in North India. Indian J Ophthalmol. 1998;46:25-29.
10. Sawada A, Aoyama A, Yamamoto T, Takatsuka N. Long-term therapeutic outcome of acute primary angle closure in Japanese. Jpn J Ophthalmol. 2007;51:353-359. https://doi.org/10.1007/s10384-007-0464-z

Predicting incident APAC and its outcomes

Fei Li, Xiulan Zhang

Predicting incident APAC

Identifying individuals at risk of developing APAC is crucial for implementing preventive strategies and reducing potential complications associated with this urgent ocular condition. Risk factors for APAC can be identified by anterior segment OCT, including shallower anterior chamber, narrower anterior chamber angle, and higher lens vault. These anatomical features are also associated with angle closure overall.[1-7] While it is possible to stratify people according to their risk of APAC, it remains impossible to accurately predict who will suffer from APAC.

UBM offers insights into the morphology of the iris and ciliary body. APAC is typically associated with pupillary block, characterized by iris bombe. In contrast, non-pupillary block conditions, including plateau iris, ciliary body hypertrophy, anteriorly positioned ciliary body, or mixed mechanisms, are linked to chronic PACG. Tension in the suspensory ligament can influence lens positioning and has also been linked to APAC.[8,9] Additionally, patients with PACG who have a thicker choroid may also have a higher risk of APAC, as choroidal thickening correlates with a shallower anterior chamber depth and narrower angles.[10]

Predicting the outcome of APAC

APAC can lead to significant visual impairment if not diagnosed and treated promptly. Predicting outcomes in patients with APAC could enhance management strategies and improve patient prognoses.

Several factors are associated with APAC outcomes, with the duration of symptoms before treatment being particularly critical.[11-13] Specifically, a delay of 24 to 72 hours is associated with an increased risk of developing chronic glaucoma compared to a delay of less than 24 hours,[12] as prolonged attacks may result in irreversible damage to the optic nerve and other ocular structures.[14]

Age is another important factor influencing the prognosis of APAC.[15] Older patients often experience poorer visual outcomes due to age-related changes in the eye and a higher likelihood of pre-existing ocular conditions.[16,17] This demographic may also have a more complex clinical picture, complicating treatment and recovery.

The initial response to medical management is useful in predicting long-term outcomes.[13,18] Patients who can achieve effective IOP control with initial treatment are more likely to have favorable results. Conversely, those requiring additional procedures, such as laser or surgical treatment, after initial medical management experience a higher risk of developing chronic glaucoma.[19] The type of subsequent treatment also matters. For instance, patients undergoing early phacoemulsification after an acute attack tend to have better long-term visual outcomes than those who do not receive such interventions.[20]

Retinal microvasculature damage revealed by OCT angiography correlated with visual acuity and visual field deficits even after APAC remission.[21] Early reductions in vessel density and a long-term decrease in circumpapillary retinal nerve fiber layer thickness were observed during the first 8 months after APAC attack.[22] Glaucomatous progression should be suspected in eyes with reduced vessel density even after the remission of an APAC episode.[22] Monitoring these indices may predict visual recovery or deterioration, thereby influencing ongoing management strategies, such as opting for a more aggressive IOP-lowering approach or considering surgical interventions.

Additionally, the state of the pupil during the acute attack can provide important prognostic information. A non-reactive pupil may indicate more severe damage, leading to a poorer prognosis.[12,23] Overall, timely intervention is critical in managing APAC, as it significantly enhances the chances of preserving vision and preventing irreversible damage.

Comments

- Identifying the risk factors for forecasting APAC incidence and outcomes is important. However, translating this knowledge into effective preventive and intervention strategies remains a significant challenge.

References

1. Huang W, Li X, Gao X, Zhang X. The anterior and posterior biometric characteristics in primary angle-closure disease: Data based on anterior segment optical coherence tomography and swept-source optical coherence tomography. Indian J Ophthalmol. 2021;69(4):865-70. https://doi.org/10.4103/ijo.IJO_936_20
2. Wang Y, Dong XX, Hou XW, Pan CW. Risk Factors for Primary Angle-closure Glaucoma: A Systematic Review and Meta-analysis of 45 Studies. Optom Vis Sci. 2023;100(9):606-13. https://doi.org/10.1097/opx.0000000000002050
3. Liu T, Li M, Chen X, et al. Anterior Lens Curvature Matters in the Course of Primary Angle Closure: An Analysis Based on Ultrasound Biomicroscopic Imaging. J Ophthalmol. 2022;2022:5570633. https://doi.org/10.1155/2022/5570633
4. Senthilkumar VA, Pradhan C, Rajendrababu S, et al. Comparison of uveal parameters between acute primary angle-closure eyes and fellow eyes in South Indian population. Indian J Ophthalmol. 2022;70(4):1232-8. https://doi.org/10.4103/ijo.IJO_1561_21
5. Moghimi S, Fathollahzadeh N, Chen R, et al. Comparison of Fellow Eyes of Acute Primary Angle Closure and Phacomorphic Angle Closure. J Glaucoma 2019;28(3):194-200. https://doi.org/10.1097/ijg.0000000000001167
6. Lee JR, Sung KR, Han S. Comparison of anterior segment parameters between the acute primary angle closure eye and the fellow eye. Invest Ophthalmol Vis Sci. 2014;55(6):3646-50. https://doi.org/10.1167/iovs.13-13009
7. Atalay E, Nongpiur ME, Baskaran M, et al. Biometric Factors Associated With Acute Primary Angle Closure: Comparison of the Affected and Fellow Eye. Invest Ophthalmol Vis Sci. 2016;57(13):5320-5. https://doi.org/10.1167/iovs.16-20006
8. Pei XT, Wang SH, Qing GP, et al. Zonular instability-associated morphologic features in eyes with primary angle closure disease using the swept-source anterior segment - optical coherence tomography system. BMC Ophthalmol. 2024;24(1):203. https://doi.org/10.1186/s12886-024-03462-1
9. Huang H, Zhang X. The efficacy of capsular tension ring in the treatment of acute angle-closure glaucoma caused by lens suspensory ligament relaxation. Chinese Journal of Ocular Trauma and Occupational Eye Disease. 2020;42(01):26-30. https://doi.org/10.3760/cma.j.issn.2095-1477.2020.01.006
10. Li F, Li H, Yang J, et al. Upside-down position leads to choroidal expansion and anterior chamber shallowing: OCT study. Br J Ophthalmol. 2020;104(6):790-4. https://doi.org/10.1136/bjophthalmol-2019-314418
11. Buckley SA, Reeves B, Burdon M, et al. Acute angle closure glaucoma: relative failure of YAG iridotomy in affected eyes and factors influencing outcome. Br J Ophthalmol. 1994;78(7):529-33. https://doi.org/10.1136/bjo.78.7.529
12. Wong JS, Chew PT, Alsagoff Z, Poh K. Clinical course and outcome of primary acute an-

gle-closure glaucoma in Singapore. Singapore Med J. 1997;38(1):16-8.

13. Hamid S, Matarazzo F, Sun Z, et al. Long-term outcomes after acute primary angle closure: case series from Moorfields Eye Hospital, UK. Br J Ophthalmol. 2024;108(12):1659-64. https://doi.org/10.1136/bjo-2023-324748
14. Chan PP, Pang JC, Tham CC. Acute primary angle closure-treatment strategies, evidences and economical considerations. Eye. 2019;33(1):110-9. https://doi.org/10.1038/s41433-018-0278-x
15. Jeong Y, Park KH, Jeoung JW. Long-term prognosis of acute primary angle closure in an east asian cohort. Jpn J Ophthalmol. 2024;68(4):302-10. https://doi.org/10.1007/s10384-024-01065-3
16. Tañá-Rivero P, Ruiz-Mesa R, Aguilar-Córcoles S, et al. Lens-vault analysis and its correlation with other biometric parameters using swept-source OCT. J Optom. 2022;15(1):88-99. https://doi.org/10.1016/j.optom.2021.04.001
17. Kolenko OV, Sorokin EL, Pashentsev E, et al. Age-related increase in lens thickness and changes in the profile of anterior chamber angle in patients with moderate and high axial hyperopia. National Journal Glaucoma. 2024;1:36-43. https://doi.org/10.53432/2078-4104-2024-23-1-36-43
18. Suzuki T, Fujishiro T, Tachi N, et al. Three-Year Outcomes of Immediate Primary Phacoemulsification on Acute Primary Angle Closure Eyes and the Fellow Eyes. Clin Ophthalmol. 2023;17:1035-45. https://doi.org/10.2147/opth.S406067
19. Qu J, Tian Z, Li X, Zhang Y. Anterior segment pars plana vitrectomy combined with posterior capsulorhexis, phacoemulsification and trabeculectomy in treatment of medically uncontrolled acute primary angle-closure glaucoma: A retrospective study. Medicine. 2022;101(40):e30946. https://doi.org/10.1097/md.0000000000030946
20. Xie J, Li P, Han B. Meta-Analysis of Phacoemulsification and Laser Peripheral Iridotomy in the Treatment of Primary Angle-Closure Glaucoma. J Ophthalmol. 2023;2023:6732424. https://doi.org/10.1155/2023/6732424
21. Nie L, Xu J, Fu L, et al. Changes in circumpapillary retinal vessel density after acute primary angle closure episode via OCT angiography. Int Ophthalmol. 2021;41(7):2389-97. https://doi.org/10.1007/s10792-021-01793-2
22. Moghimi S, SafiZadeh M, Xu BY, et al. Vessel density and retinal nerve fibre layer thickness following acute primary angle closure. Br J Ophthalmol. 2020;104(8):1103-8. https://doi.org/10.1136/bjophthalmol-2019-314789
23. Nongpiur ME, Aung T. Mechanisms underlying acute angle closure. Clin Exp Ophthalmol. 2017;45(4):331-2. https://doi.org/10.1111/ceo.12967

Future directions

Fei Li, Paul Foster, Xiulan Zhang

The management of APAC is evolving, propelled by technological advancements, refined surgical techniques, and an enhanced understanding of its pathophysiology (Fig. 1). The incidence of APAC should decrease as cataract surgery rises globally. However, this trend may be offset by a rebalancing of preventive strategies, such as more selective treatment of PACS with prophylactic LPI. Timely IOP-lowering and anti-inflammatory treatments promote more rapid control of the disease. However, future optimization in managing APAC may focus on the following areas.

Precise patient-centered care

The advancement anterior segment OCT imaging, with enhanced semi or fully automated biometric tools, allows rapid, highly sophisticated assessment of structural risk factors, such as shallower anterior chamber depth and higher lens vault. Although the role of this technology in clinical management is yet to be

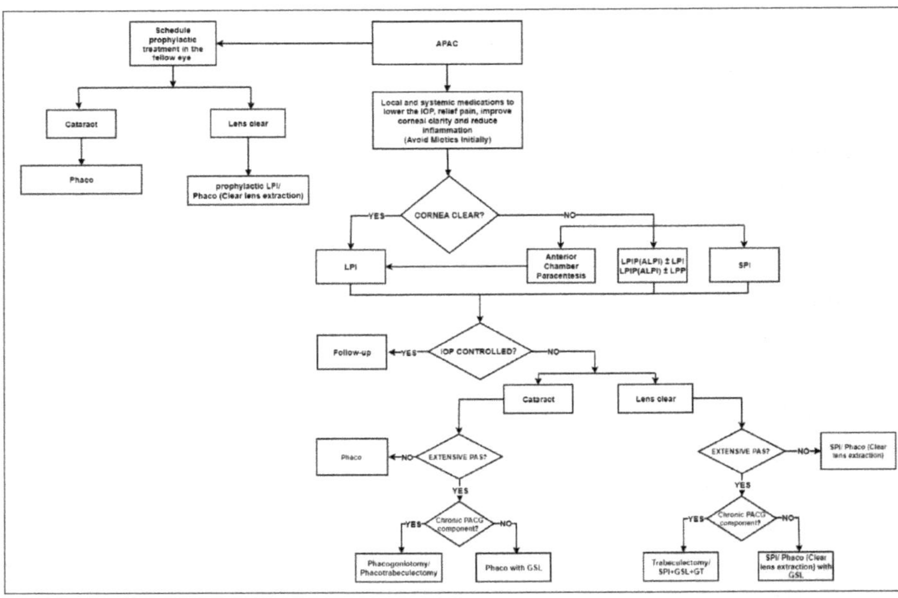

Fig. 1. Management strategies of acute primary angle closure. APAC: acute primary angle closure; LPI: laser peripheral iridotomy; LPIP: laser peripheral iridoplasty; ALPI: argon laser peripheral iridoplasty; LPP: laser pupilloplasty; GSL: goniosynechialysis; PAS: peripheral anterior synechiae; PACG: primary angle-closure glaucoma; SPI: surgical peripheral iridectomy; Phaco: phacoemulsification or phacoemulsification with intraocular lens implantation; GT: goniotomy, ab interno trabeculotomy; IOP: intraocular pressure.

established, the data from anterior segment OCT and large-scale genome-wide association studies may offer greater insights into the biological mechanisms underpinning the development of this disease in individual patients. The development of tools such as polygenic risk score may further advance personalized risk-stratification and care.[1,2]

With the increasing importance of patient-centered care, customizing the APAC treatment approach to fit each patient's unique needs and preferences can ensure effective care that aligns with their values. By including patient perspectives in decision-making, clinicians can improve treatment adherence and overall satisfaction. Future advancements in personalized medicine will allow more tailored interventions, taking into account genetic predispositions, lifestyle factors, and patient-specific risk profiles. Additionally, employing shared decision-making tools and patient education initiatives can empower patients to actively manage their condition. This holistic approach will improve clinical outcomes and foster a stronger doctor-patient relationship, leading to better long-term management of APAC.

Neuroprotective agents

Adjuvant therapies with neuroprotective and anti-inflammatory properties may better protect vision. Future research should focus on identifying effective neuroprotective compounds, optimizing their delivery, and understanding their long-term impact on visual outcomes.

In conclusion, while there is optimism about advancements in APAC management, especially in precise patient-centered care and neuroprotection strategies, much of this still is aspirational. Continued research is essential to translate these hopes into viable clinical practices that improve patient outcomes.

Comments

- Personalized care provides the promise for optimizing APAC management and improving patient outcomes. However, there is a need for more robust clinical trials to validate these approaches and ensure their effectiveness in practice.

References

1. Hao L, Kraft P, Berriz GF, et al. Development of a clinical polygenic risk score assay and reporting workflow. Nat Med. 2022;28(5):1006-13. https://doi.org/10.1038/s41591-022-01767-6
2. Li F, Zhang X. The Role of Polygenic Risk Scores in Glaucoma Management. JAMA Ophthalmology. 2024;142(4):364. https://doi.org/10.1001/jamaophthalmol.2024.0220

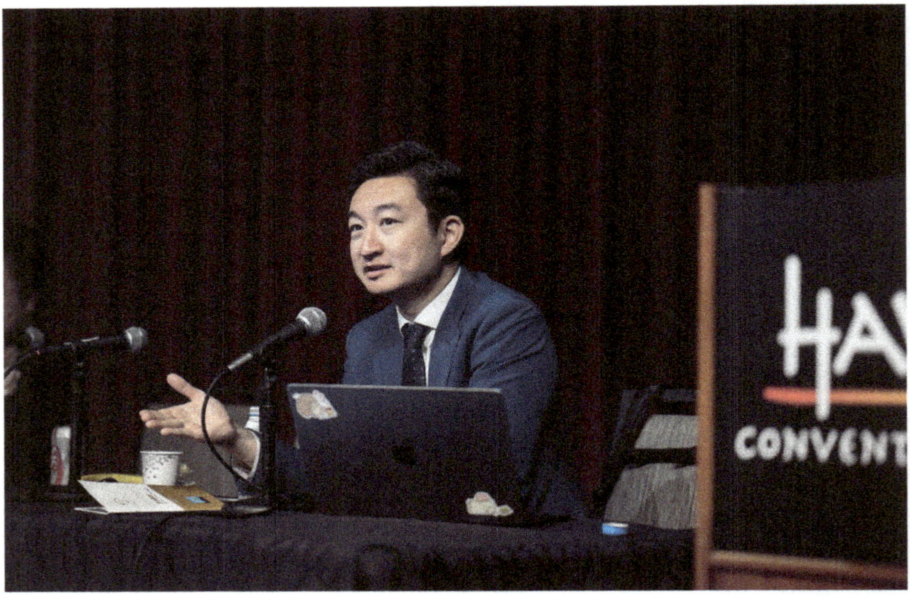

Benjamin Xu

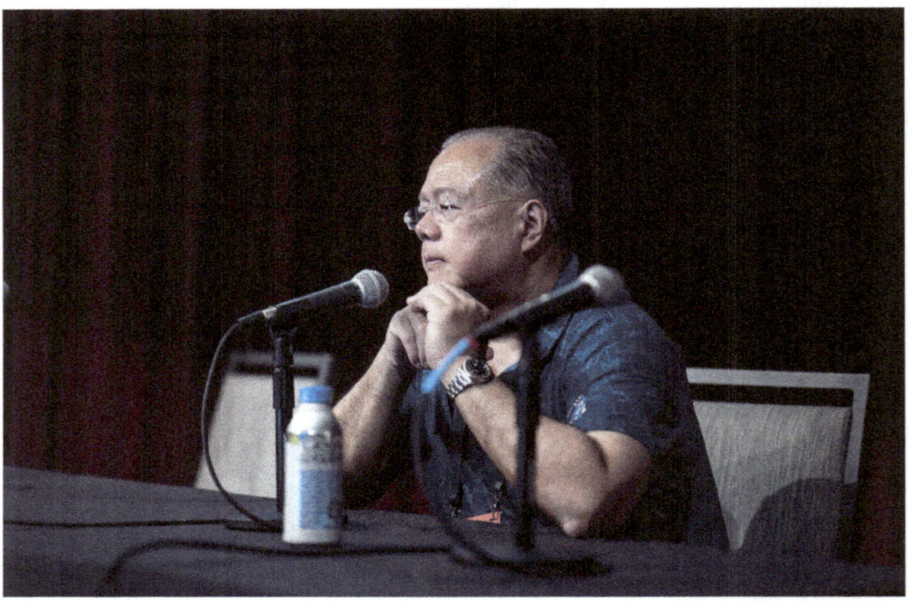

Tin Aung

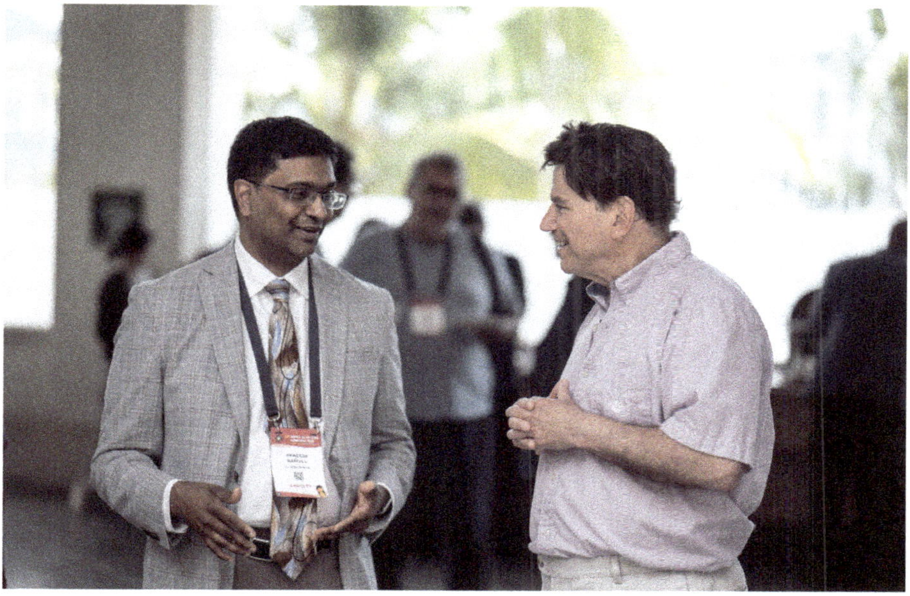

Pradeep Ramulu and Robert N. Weinreb

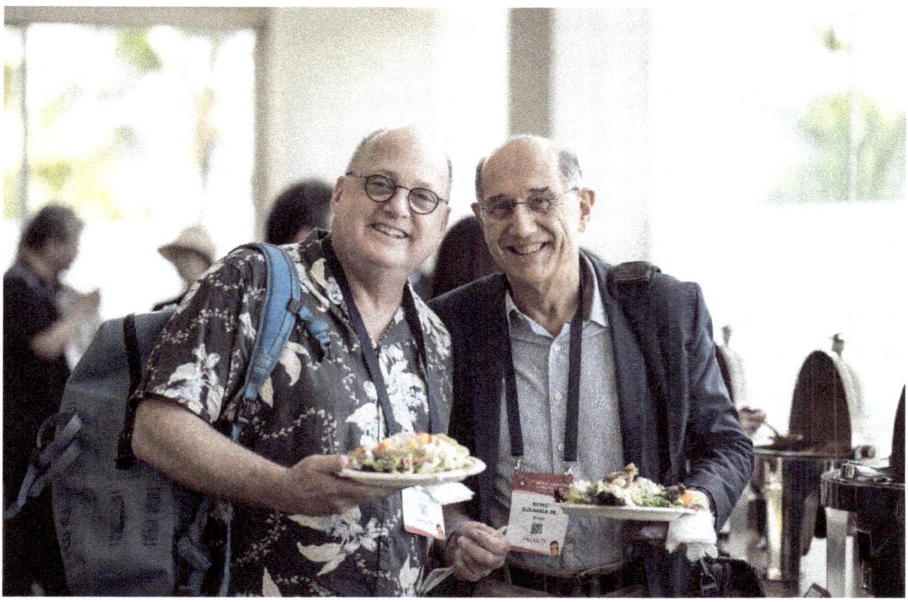

Robert Feldman and Remo Susanna Jr.

SUMMARY OF CONSENSUS POINTS

SECTION 1 - EPIDEMIOLOGY

Angle closure

1. Angle closure prevalence appears to be increasing due to population aging.
2. Angle closure appears to be more common in many Asian populations than in European-derived or African-derived populations.
    - More epidemiologic data are needed, particularly in African-derived populations.
3. Women and the elderly are at higher risk of angle closure.
4. The risk of progression from primary angle-closure suspect to primary angle closure is low for most primary angle closure suspect eyes.
    - There is a higher risk of progression from primary-angle closure suspect to primary angle closure with older age.
    - The low rate of progression in clinical trials is not consistent with the prevalence of primary angle-closure glaucoma in epidemiological studies.
5. Primary angle closure is a higher risk state for primary angle-closure glaucoma.
    - Data on the clinical significance of peripheral anterior synechiae are limited.

Primary angle-closure glaucoma

6. The number of individuals with primary angle-closure glaucoma is projected to rise.
    - Projections do not account for the increasing rates of cataract surgery and myopia prevalence, which are strongly protective against primary angle-closure glaucoma.
7. Primary angle-closure glaucoma is most common among individuals of Asian ancestry.
    - Data in non-Asians are limited.
8. As blindness is associated with over 25% of primary angle-closure glaucoma cases worldwide, a focus on detecting primary angle-closure disease (defined as primary angle closure or primary angle-closure glaucoma) at a treatable stage is needed to prevent vision loss from primary angle-closure glaucoma.

9. Primary angle-closure glaucoma can occur in myopic eyes, although the proportion varies by race and ethnicity.
   - Primary angle-closure glaucoma is uncommon in high myopes.
   - The relationship between myopia and angle closure depends on the effects on anterior segment biometrics more than overall axial length.

Future directions

- Data are sparse from individuals aged 70 years and older, which is a growing demographic group. Cross-sectional biometry in populations shows mean anterior chamber depth declines with age, peaking between 30 to 50 years of age. This decline slows and potentially reverses at age 70 years, but more research is needed.
- Further research is required to investigate individuals who may be at higher risk of progression from primary angle-closure suspect to primary angle closure, such as those with connective tissue abnormalities.

SECTION 2 - GENETICS AND PATHOPHYSIOLOGY

1. First-degree relatives of individuals with spectrum of primary angle closure, defined as primary angle-closure suspect, primary angle closure, or primary angle-closure glaucoma, are at significantly higher risk of angle closure supporting its genetic basis.
   - Large-scale genome-wide association studies have identified genetic loci associated with primary angle-closure glaucoma.
   - Known genetic variants associated with primary angle-closure glaucoma have small effect sizes.
2. Evidence to recommend genetic testing for primary angle-closure disease, defined as primary angle closure or primary angle-closure glaucoma, is limited.
3. Risk conferred by hyperopic refractive error is secondary to its association with ocular biometrics, specifically shorter AL and shallower anterior chamber depth.
   - Anterior chamber depth alone does not explain racial and ethnic differences in angle-closure prevalence.
4. Pupillary block is the major mechanism, accounting for 75% of all primary angle closure.

5. Association studies suggest that dynamic changes in iris and choroidal volume are involved in the pathogenesis of primary angle-closure disease.
    - Choroidal effusion can be found in primary angle closure and primary angle-closure glaucoma eyes.
    - Primary angle-closure suspect, primary angle closure, and primary angle-closure glaucoma are associated with greater choroidal thickness.
    - Supraciliary effusion can result in anterior rotation of the ciliary body and angle closure.
    - Accumulation of aqueous in the vitreous cavity and greater resistance to fluid exchange across the anterior hyaloid can precipitate angle closure from aqueous misdirection (also sometimes termed vitreous block).
    - Malignant glaucoma is an ambiguous term that is not adequately descriptive of the disease process.
6. Vitreous block, collagen abnormalities, autonomic dysfunction, and zonulopathy likely contribute to angle-closure pathogenesis but are not directly measurable using available tools.

Future directions

More research is needed on iris thickness, which has emerged as an important anatomical risk factor for primary angle-closure disease.

- Serial studies, including follow-up on the ZAP study cohort, are needed to establish the precise nature of the relationship between primary angle-closure glaucoma with dynamic changes in iris volume and choroidal volume.

SECTION 3 - DIAGNOSIS AND EVALUATION

1. The definitions of spectrum of primary angle closure are based on gonioscopy and clinical findings:
    - Angle closure on gonioscopy is defined as when the posterior, usually pigmented, trabecular meshwork is not visible, possibly indicating the presence of iridotrabecular contact.
    - Primary angle-closure suspect: 2 or more quadrants of angle closure on gonioscopy.
    - Primary angle closure: primary angle-closure suspect plus peripheral anterior synechiae and/or elevated intraocular pressure, or an acute primary angle closure attack.

- Primary angle-closure glaucoma: primary angle-closure suspect or primary angle closure plus glaucomatous optic neuropathy.

2. One way of characterizing the spectrum of primary angle closure is:
   - The term primary angle closure disease includes primary angle-closure and primary angle-closure glaucoma.
   - The term spectrum of primary angle closure includes primary angle-closure suspect and primary angle-closure disease.
3. Gonioscopy is the clinical standard for evaluating the anterior chamber angle. However, it is subjective and variable.
   - Gonioscopy is a vital but underutilized part of the eye exam.
   - The patient should be examined in a dark room and with the use of a short, narrow slit-beam to avoid constricting the pupil and artifactually opening the angle.
   - Indentation gonioscopy remains the gold standard for identifying peripheral anterior synechiae.
   - Tilting of the goniolens can be performed to visualize the angle recess in eyes with a high lens vault.
4. The Van Herick test of limbal anterior chamber depth only has moderate sensitivity or specificity in detecting eyes with gonioscopic angle closure and is not a replacement for gonioscopy.
   - Limbal anterior chamber depth can be used for opportunistic case detection when followed by gonioscopy but is less useful for population-based screening as it could generate an unacceptably high number of false positives.
5. Anterior segment optical coherence tomography and ultrasound biomicroscopy are adjunctive tools to gonioscopy for evaluating the anterior chamber angle.
   - Angle closure on anterior segment optical coherence tomography and ultrasound biomicroscopy is defined as presence of contact between the anterior iris surface and inner corneal curvature or angle wall anterior to the scleral spur, which indicates the presence of iridotrabecular contact.
   - Iridotrabecular contact can be described in terms of circumferential extent and anterior-posterior length (also referred to as height or width). There is no consensus about clinically significant thresholds in extent or length.
6. There may be disagreement between gonioscopy and anterior segment optical coherence tomography in detecting angle closure due to differences in definitions.
   - A wide range of factors, including anatomical configurations, examination

techniques, refraction correction, level of ambient lighting, and pupillary constriction due to light or accommodation, contribute to the disagreement.
  - The extent of iridotrabecular contact on anterior segment optical coherence tomography is more strongly associated with primary angle-closure disease severity than cumulative gonioscopy grading.
7. Gonioscopy is poorly able to identify which primary angle-closure suspect eyes are at high risk for primary angle-closure disease.
  - Anterior segment optical coherence tomography measurements have been found to be associated with progression from primary angle-closure suspect to primary angle closure.
  - No precise iridotrabecular contact or measurement cutoffs have been demonstrated to be clinically significant or widely adopted for routine care.
  - Longitudinal studies assessing the clinical significance of anterior segment optical coherence tomography findings alone for risk stratifying primary angle-closure suspect eyes are needed.
8. Ultrasound biomicroscopy remains the gold standard for evaluating the ciliary body.
  - Newer anterior segment optical coherence tomography devices utilizing longer-wavelength swept-source lasers and image averaging provide reproducible visualization and analysis of the ciliary body in some eyes.
9. Plateau iris configuration is characterized by anteriorly positioned ciliary processes causing posterior angulation in the peripheral iris and the absence of the iridociliary sulcus.
  - Plateau iris syndrome is persistence of angle closure despite a patent iridotomy in the presence of plateau iris configuration
10. Goniophotographs are useful to capture anatomical findings (*e.g.*, iris nevus) but are not commonly used to evaluate the angle recess.
11. There is no consensus about which biometric parameters describing the anterior segment are the most clinically relevant for detecting individuals at high risk for primary angle-closure glaucoma.
  - Anterior chamber depth cutoffs have been tested but are not effective for identifying individuals at high risk for primary angle-closure glaucoma in the community.
  - Anterior chamber volume has better diagnostic performance in detecting angle closure compared to anterior chamber angle width parameters, such as angle opening distance.
12. There are no widely accepted provocative tests to identify individuals at high

risk for primary angle-closure glaucoma.

- The dark room prone provocative test is unable to risk-stratify primary angle-closure suspect for progression to primary angle-closure disease.

SECTION 4 - MANAGEMENT: MEDICAL AND LASER

General approach

1. Gonioscopy is an indispensable part of the ophthalmic examination.
   - Gonioscopy should be performed with indentation to differentiate appositional from synechial closure.
   - The Van Herick test is not a substitute for gonioscopy.
   - Anterior segment imaging modalities can be used to augment the clinical examination but are not a substitute for gonioscopy, as features such as trabecular pigmentation, angle recession, and neovascularization cannot be reliably identified using anterior segment optical coherence tomography or ultrasound biomicroscopy.
2. Long-term follow-up with gonioscopy in phakic eyes is needed, as age-related lens thickening can further narrow the angle, increasing the risk of primary angle-closure glaucoma.
3. Evaluation of the optic disc, visual field, and retinal nerve fiber layer is critical for detecting glaucomatous damage and progression.
4. An important goal of treatment in primary angle-closure disease is to alleviate iridotrabecular contact and prevent further impairment of aqueous drainage due to angle closure.
5. Even when the angle-closure process is controlled, further treatment may be necessary to avoid glaucoma progression.
   - Medications, lasers, and surgeries can recover or improve aqueous outflow in angle-closure eyes.

Medical treatment

6. In eyes with primary angle-closure disease, prostaglandin analogues are the most effective medical agent for intraocular pressure lowering regardless of the extent of synechial closure once pupillary block has been controlled.
7. Carbonic anhydrase inhibitors, beta blockers, and alpha-adrenergic agonists can be considered for second-line medical treatments.
   - Evidence on the intraocular pressure-lowering efficacy of Rho kinase

inhibitors in angle closure is limited.

8. The role of miotics in primary angle closure is unclear.
   - Miotics generally should not be used long-term as intraocular pressure-lowering agents in angle-closure eyes.
   - Miotics should be used in cases of acute primary angle closure but may not be effective due to iris ischemia while the intraocular pressure is high.
   - Miotics may be considered for long-term use in plateau iris syndrome.
9. Cycloplegics should be considered in the setting of anterior chamber shallowing from secondary angle closure, such as aqueous misdirection.

Laser treatment

10. Laser peripheral iridotomy is used to relieve relative pupillary block, which is the main mechanism in most patients with angle closure.
    - Angle closure persists in around a quarter of post-laser peripheral iridotomy eyes.
    - Angle assessment (gonioscopy or anterior segment optical coherence tomography) should be performed post-laser peripheral iridotomy to assess the effect of LPI and identify other mechanisms, including plateau iris.
11. LPI is a safe procedure with very low risk of serious adverse events.
    - Sequential argon/Nd:YAG technique (argon first followed by Nd:YAG) requires less overall energy in patients with thick irides, specifically those of Asian and African descent or Hispanic ethnicity.
    - Laser peripheral iridotomy location near the lid margins should be avoided to reduce risk of dysphotopsias.
    - Laser peripheral iridotomy size should be a minimum of 200 μm in diameter.
    - There is an increased risk of intraocular pressure spikes when performing LPI in eyes with elevated intraocular pressure and 2 or more quadrants of peripheral anterior synechiae.
12. Laser peripheral iridotomy is not indicated in most primary angle-closure suspect eyes (ZAP and ANA-LIS trials), although risk assessment for progression is suboptimal.
    - Factors to be considered for performing laser peripheral iridotomy include, for example, history of primary angle-closure disease in the fellow eye, older age, positive family history of primary angle-closure glaucoma, need for frequent dilation (e.g., in diabetics or glaucoma

suspects), limited access to care, and need for hemodialysis.

- Biometric features associated with greater risk for progression include higher intraocular pressure, smaller AOD500, smaller limbal anterior chamber depth, and shallower anterior chamber depth.

13. In acute primary angle closure, laser peripheral iridotomy should be performed as soon as possible in the contralateral eye, which is at very high risk for a similar event.
14. Early lens extraction is an effective method of intraocular pressure lowering that is more cost-effective and results in better quality of life compared to laser peripheral iridotomy at certain stages of primary angle-closure disease (EAGLE trial).
    - Participants of the EAGLE trial were aged 50 years or older and had primary angle closure with intraocular pressure > 30 mmHg or primary angle-closure glaucoma.
    - Patients who do not fulfill the EAGLE criteria may still benefit from early lens extraction, although these data are lacking.
15. In acute primary angle closure, laser peripheral iridoplasty or laser pupilloplasty may help to break the attack prior to definitive treatment.
    - Laser peripheral iridoplasty widens the angle recess by contracting the iris away from the trabecular meshwork.
    - Laser pupilloplasty contracts the iris tissue near the pupil, creating a peaked pupil and relieving pupillary block.
16. Iridoplasty can widen the angle in eyes with plateau iris syndrome that have persistent appositional angle closure after laser peripheral iridotomy.
    - Evidence does not support improved long-term intraocular pressure control.
    - Iridoplasty is not useful for synechial angle closure.
    - Iridoplasty may be associated with adverse effects, such as pupillary dilation, corneal endothelial damage, and progressive peripheral anterior synechiae formation.
17. Selective laser trabeculoplasty can be effective for intraocular pressure reduction in angle-closure eyes that have had laser peripheral iridotomy and/or lens extraction, allowing for visual access to the trabecular meshwork.

Future directions

- Additional data are needed on the efficacy of laser peripheral iridotomy treatment in diverse populations, especially with demographics differing from those of the ZAP and ANA-LIS trials.

- Further studies are needed to identify features of individuals who may be poorly responsive to laser peripheral iridotomy treatment and should be considered for alternative treatments, such as lens extraction, instead.

SECTION 5 - SURGICAL MANAGEMENT

1. Lens extraction can lead to significant reduction in intraocular pressure and medication burden in primary angle-closure disease
   - Lens extraction can effectively lower intraocular pressure regardless of whether the glaucoma is controlled or uncontrolled preoperatively.
   - Lens extraction alone may not achieve target intraocular pressure or medication-free control in those with poorly controlled primary angle-closure glaucoma and advanced disease.
   - Glaucoma surgery (e.g., trabeculectomy, minimally invasive glaucoma surgery) at the time of lens extraction may be indicated to achieve intraocular pressure control, particularly when the glaucoma is moderate to severe.
   - Lens extraction can alter visual field and optical coherence tomography results, necessitating a new baseline for subsequent glaucoma monitoring.
2. Lens extraction is an option as a first-line treatment for primary angle-closure glaucoma and primary angle closure with raised intraocular pressure (EAGLE trial).
   - Lens extraction demonstrated superior effectiveness in lowering intraocular pressure, medication needs, the rate of subsequent glaucoma surgeries, and was associated with better quality of life score compared to standard care with laser peripheral iridotomy and topical medications.
   - Phacoemulsification with intraocular lens placement in the capsular bag is the recommended method of lens extraction.
   - If phacoemulsification is not available, the benefits and risks of the available surgical techniques must be carefully evaluated.
3. There are inconclusive data on the benefit of phacoemulsification + goniosynechiolysis for better intraocular pressure lowering as compared to Phaco alone in patients with primary angle-closure glaucoma, cataract, and peripheral anterior synechiae.
   - Evidence is inconclusive that phacoemulsification + goniosynechiolysis is superior to phacoemulsification alone in terms of intraocular pressure control, reduction of peripheral anterior synechiae, and the need for

medications.

4. Combining phacoemulsification with goniosynechiolysis and minimally invasive glaucoma surgery, including goniotomy, may be more effective than phacoemulsification alone in reducing intraocular pressure in patients with primary angle-closure glaucoma.
    - Data are limited on the types of minimally invasive glaucoma surgery and the specific stages of primary angle-closure disease appropriate for this treatment.
    - Some minimally invasive glaucoma surgery devices are off-label for use in primary angle-closure disease.
    - Goniosynechiolysis may need to be performed to access the trabecular meshwork.
    - Phacoemulsification with goniosynechiolysis and goniotomy (phacogoniotomy) can be a viable option for intraocular pressure reduction in patients with primary angle-closure glaucoma and cataract.
    - One randomized controlled trial reported similar cumulative rates of surgical success between phacogoniotomy and phacotrabeculectomy in advanced primary angle-closure glaucoma eyes.
5. Trabeculectomy alone can provide effective intraocular pressure lowering in primary angle-closure glaucoma eyes, particularly in the pseudophakic eye.
    - In the phakic eye, trabeculectomy promotes cataract progression and there is an increased risk of shallow AC and iris incarceration in the sclerectomy.
    - Subsequent cataract surgery can increase the risk of bleb scarring.
6. Combining phacoemulsification with trabeculectomy (phacotrabeculectomy).
    - Phacotrabeculectomy is a viable option for primary angle-closure glaucoma eyes.
    - Phacotrabeculectomy addresses the underlying issue of a crowded anterior chamber or a bulky lens and reduces the risk of further shallowing of the anterior chamber.
7. Glaucoma drainage device implantation is typically reserved for primary angle-closure glaucoma eyes at higher risk for failure and/or complications than with other interventions or for those patients who have unsuccessful outcomes with other intraocular pressure-lowering surgeries.
    - Combined phacoemulsification and glaucoma drainage device implantation can be considered in eyes with significant cataract or very shallow anterior chamber due to a thick crystalline lens.
8. Cycloablation is an alternative treatment for the management of primary

angle-closure glaucoma.

- Results are variable and treatment often needs to be repeated.
- It may be particularly useful when the patient wishes to avoid the risks of incisional surgery or is not systemically fit for or unable to access the operating room.
- Large prospective randomized controlled trials on the use of cycloablation for primary angle-closure glaucoma are needed.
- Endoscopic cyclophotocoagulation combined with phacoemulsification may provide greater intraocular pressure lowering than phacoemulsification alone.

SECTION 6 – ACUTE PRIMARY ANGLE CLOSURE

1. Acute primary angle closure is an ophthalmic emergency that can cause sudden, pronounced, but typically transient reduction in vision.
   - Acute primary angle closure typically presents with severe ocular pain, headache, nausea, and a fixed mid-dilated pupil.
   - Secondary causes of angle closure should be excluded.
   - Acute primary angle closure more commonly affects older individuals, women, and those of Asian descent.
   - A range of medications may precipitate acute primary angle closure, including those with adrenergic or anticholinergic effects. Careful medication review should be performed in at-risk individuals.
   - Acute primary angle closure usually occurs unilaterally. Systemic medications (such as anticonvulsants and antidepressants) and systemic disease (such as Vogt- Koyanagi-Harada syndrome) may cause bilateral acute primary angle closure.
2. Initial treatment with topical and systemic medications can lower the intraocular pressure, relieve pain, improve corneal clarity, and reduce inflammation.
   - Miotics should be used in cases of acute primary angle closure but may not be effective due to iris ischemia while the intraocular pressure is high.
   - Early administration of anti-inflammatory agents may facilitate a more rapid reduction in intraocular pressure.
3. Laser peripheral iridotomy should be performed as soon as possible.
   - If laser peripheral iridotomy is not possible due to corneal edema, anterior chamber paracentesis, diode laser, or laser peripheral iridoplasty, with or

without laser pupilloplasty, can be performed.
    - If the iris is thick and there are no convenient iris crypts, argon laser pretreatment should be considered, followed by YAG:Nd laser peripheral iridotomy.
4. Anterior chamber paracentesis is an option for immediate intraocular pressure reduction and symptom relief in acute primary angle closure.
    - It is particularly useful when systemic intraocular pressure-lowering agents such as mannitol or acetazolamide are contraindicated or when laser peripheral iridotomy or laser peripheral iridoplasty cannot be performed. However, the procedure carries risks and should be performed with caution.
5. Lens extraction (once intraocular pressure and inflammation have been controlled) is the definitive treatment for acute primary angle closure, as it alleviates pupillary block, deepens the anterior chamber angle, lowers intraocular pressure, and improves vision.
    - Surgical challenges include corneal edema, a shallow anterior chamber, intraocular inflammation, and zonular weakness or dehiscence.
6. Surgical peripheral iridectomy can be performed in eyes with medically uncontrolled acute primary angle closure when an appropriate laser is unavailable, when laser peripheral iridotomy is not possible, or in cases with both severe corneal edema and a clear lens.
7. Trabeculectomy can be considered for uncontrolled intraocular pressure after acute primary angle closure resolution if there are extensive peripheral anterior synechiae after iridectomy or if the iridectomy could not be performed.
    - Phacoemulsification and combined goniosynechiolysis with or without goniotomy is an alternative to trabeculectomy.
8. Patients with spectrum of primary angle closure should be educated about acute primary angle closure symptoms and the need to see an eye care specialist urgently if they present.
9. There is no effective method to identify individuals at high risk for acute primary angle closure. The use of anterior segment imaging or polygenic risk score is unproven.
10. Additional research is needed to identify anatomical features predictive of acute primary angle closure.

INDEX OF AUTHORS

EXTENDED TABLE OF CONTENTS

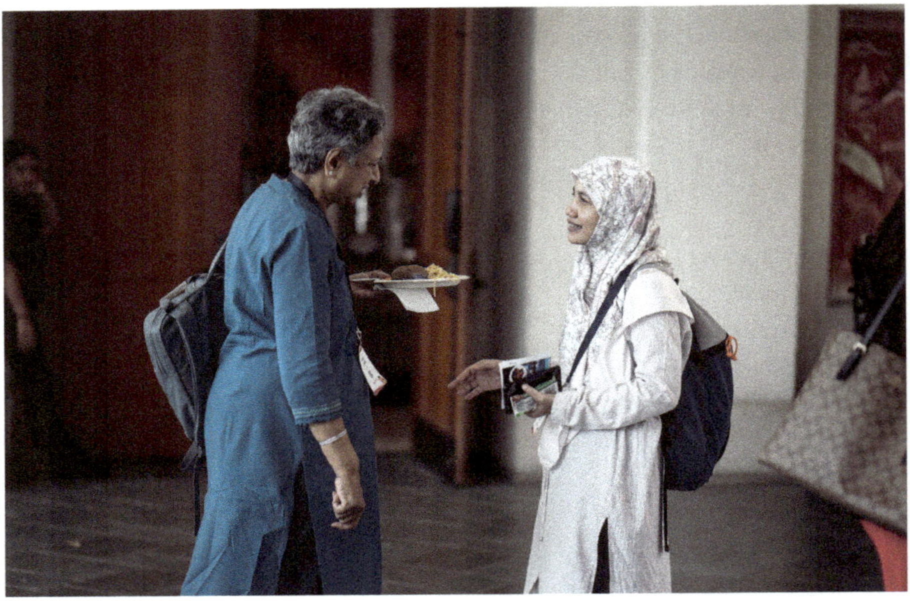

Vijaya Lingam, and Virna Dwi Oktariana Asrory

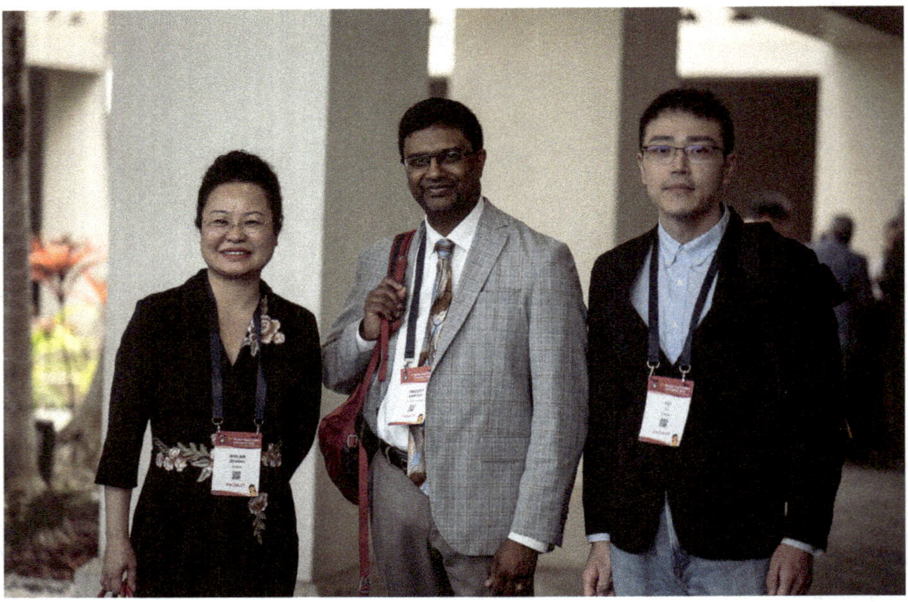

Xiulan Zhang, Pradeep Ramulu, and Fei Li

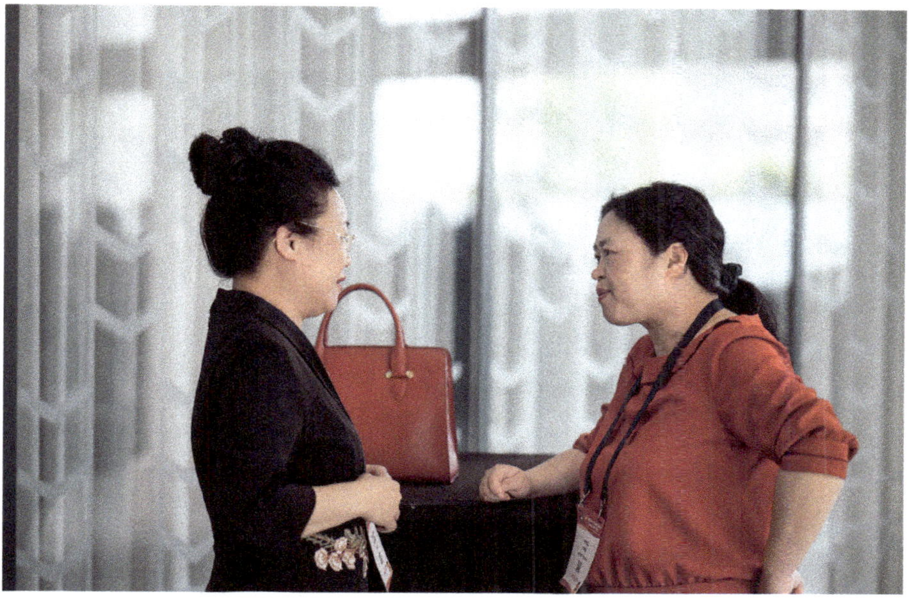

Ying Han and Zhang Xiulan

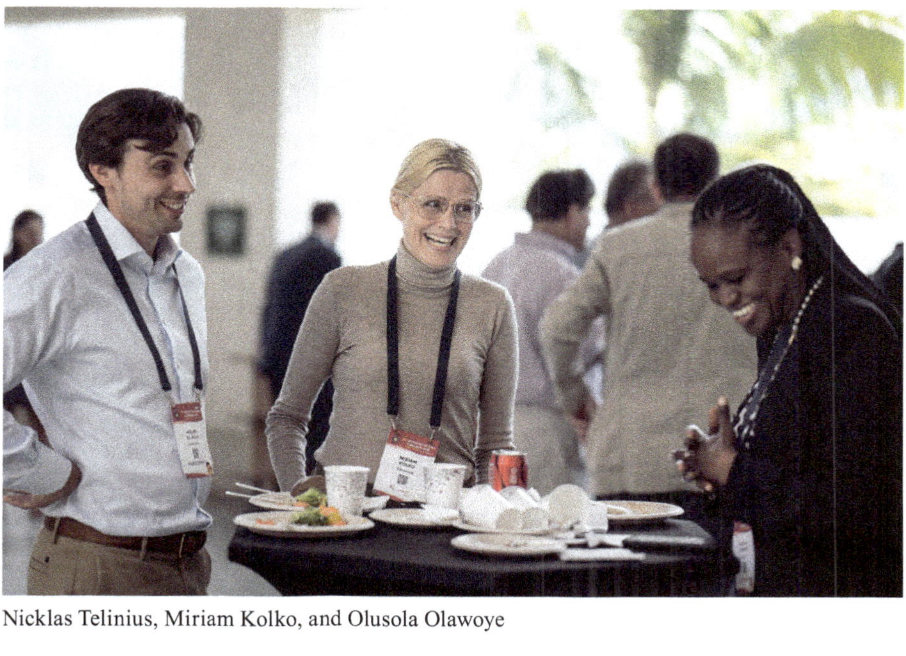

Nicklas Telinius, Miriam Kolko, and Olusola Olawoye

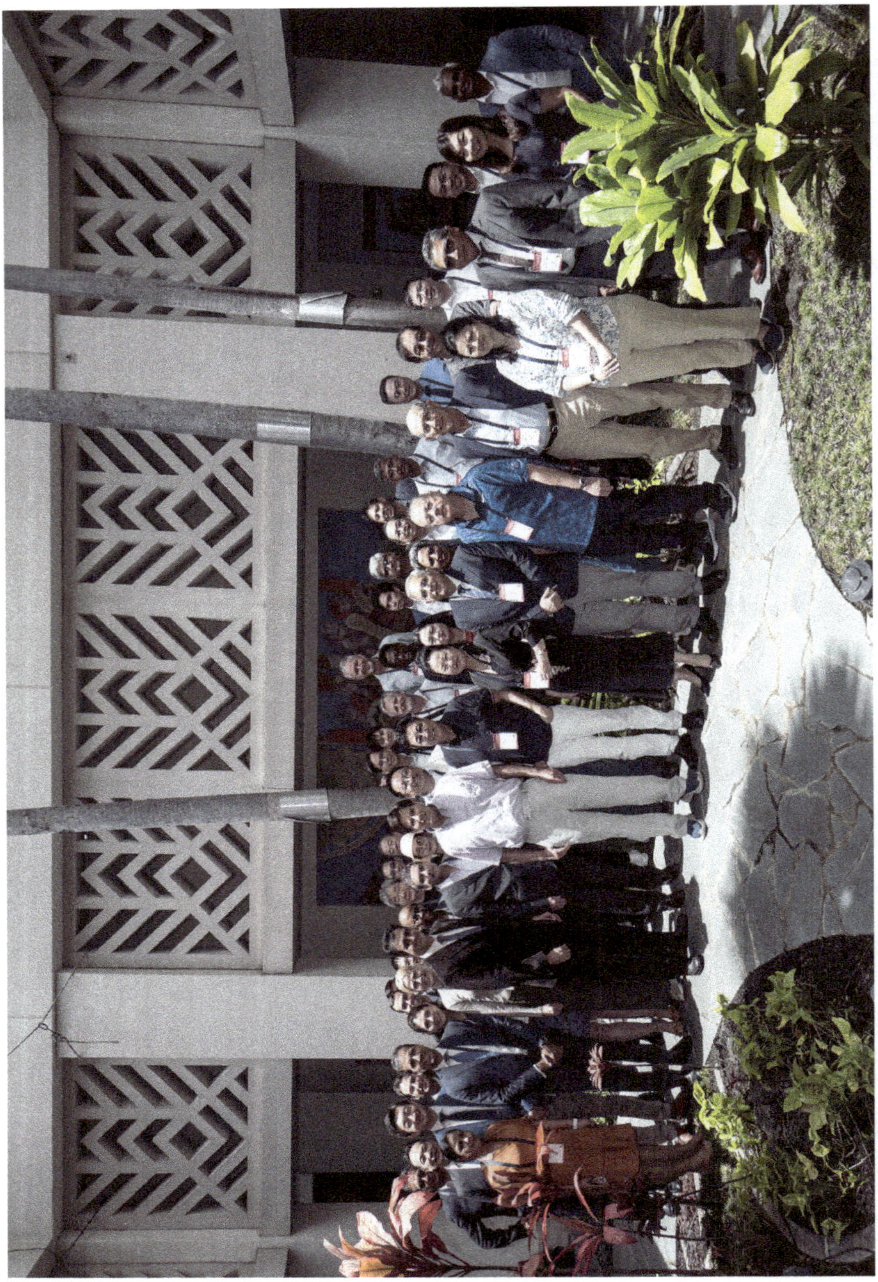

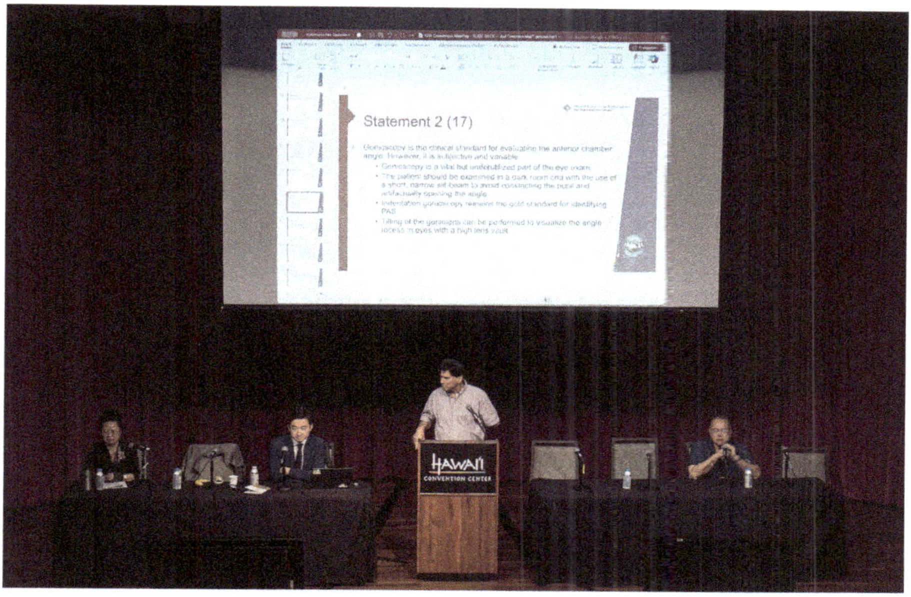

Zhang Xiulan, Benjamin Xu, Robert Weinreb, and Tin Aung

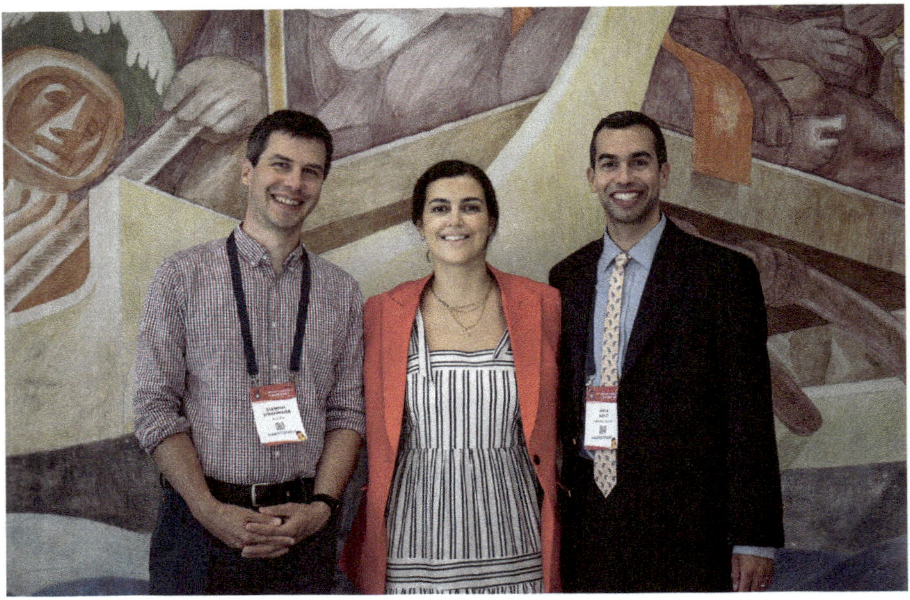

Meeting Scribes: Clemens Strohmaier, Natalia Porporato, and Kyle Bolo

We appreciate the excellent support of the Consensus Scribes (Kyle Bolo, MD; Natalia Porporato, MD, PhD; Clemens Strohmaier, MD, PhD) who diligently and thoughtfully revised the consensus statements throughout the course of
We appreciate the excellent support of the Consensus Scribes (Kyle Bolo, MD; Natalia Porporato, MD, PhD; Clemens Strohmaier, MD, PhD) who diligently and thoughtfully revised the consensus statements throughout the course of the meeting as participants introduced new ideas and proposals for discussion by the entire consensus group. Silvia Sanchez di Martino, sorted through the diversity of presentations within the text and brought greater order and clarity to the Consensus Report.

Simon Bakker, our publisher from Kugler Publications, Amsterdam, once again rose to the occasion to have the Consensus Report available in a timely fashion. We remain grateful for his support with this and other endeavors.

WGA Consensus Series

The Glaucoma Consensus Initiative of the World Glaucoma Association is based on the idea that the collective wisdom of a group is better than the opinion of a single expert. Assembling a sufficiently large and sufficiently diverse group of glaucoma specialists and scientists provides recommendations and insights that are likely to be superior to those of a single clinician. These recommendations and insights form the foundation for the Glaucoma Consensus Reports.

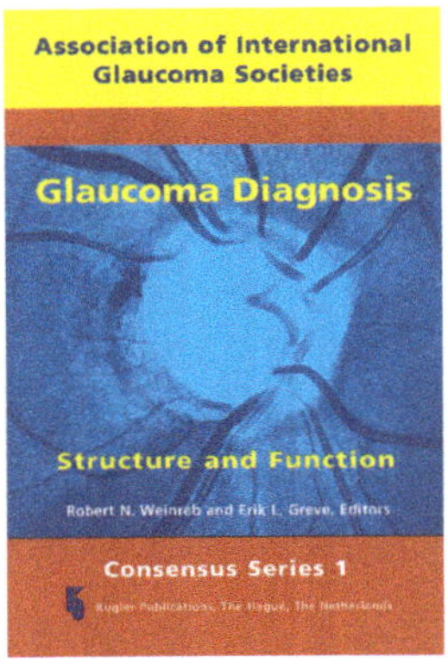

2004

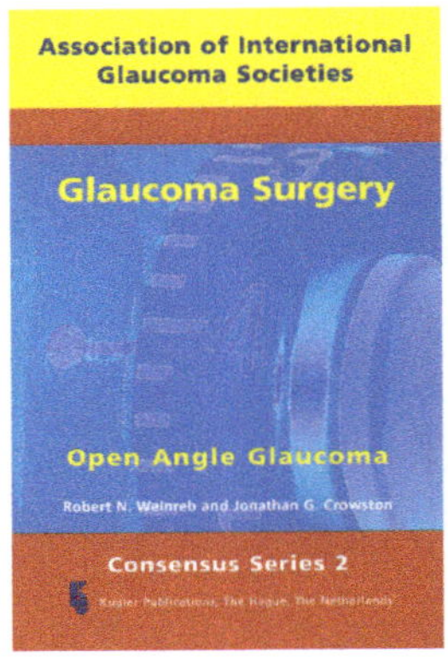

2005

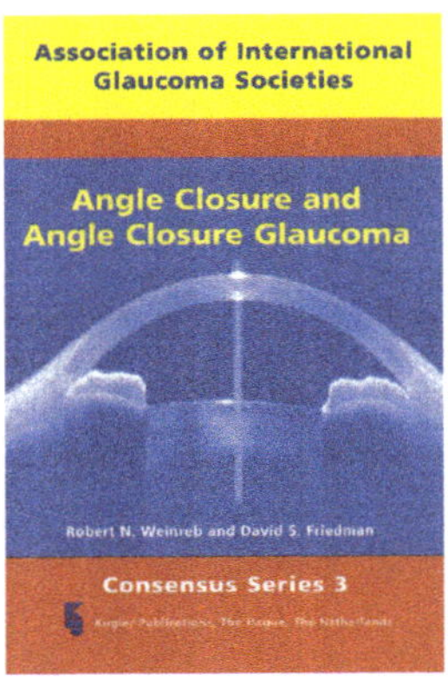

2006

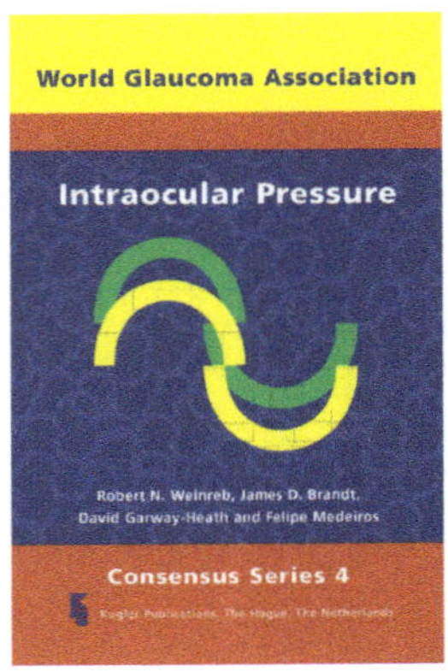

2007

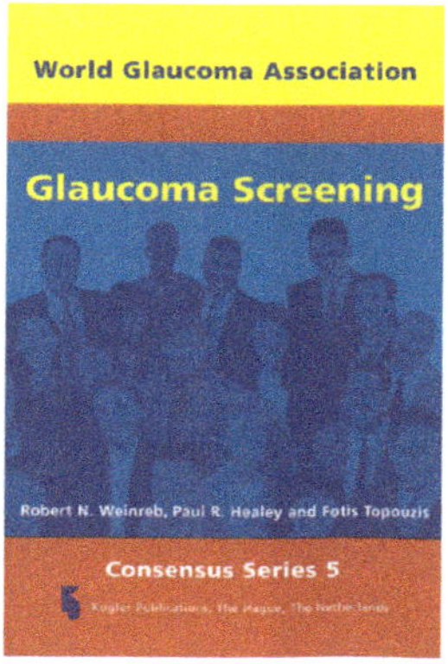

2008

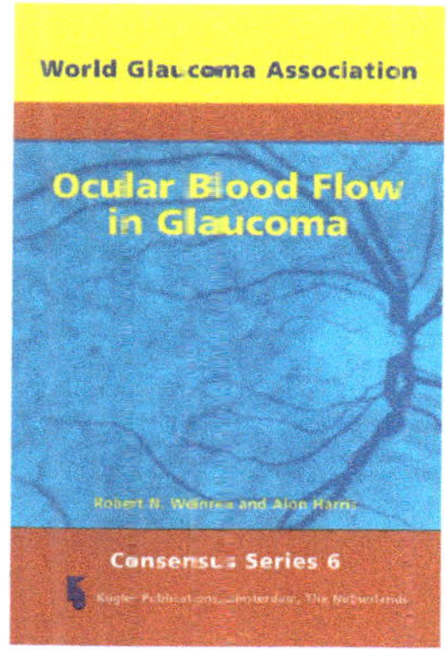

2009

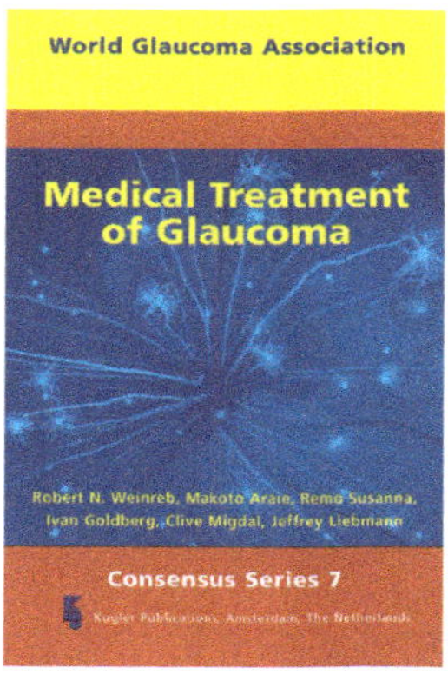

2010

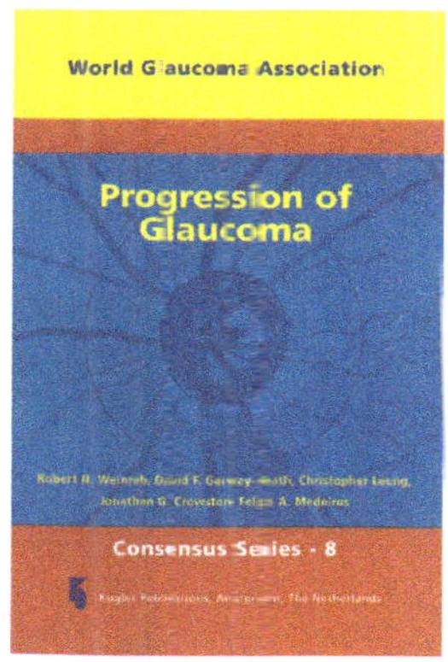

2011

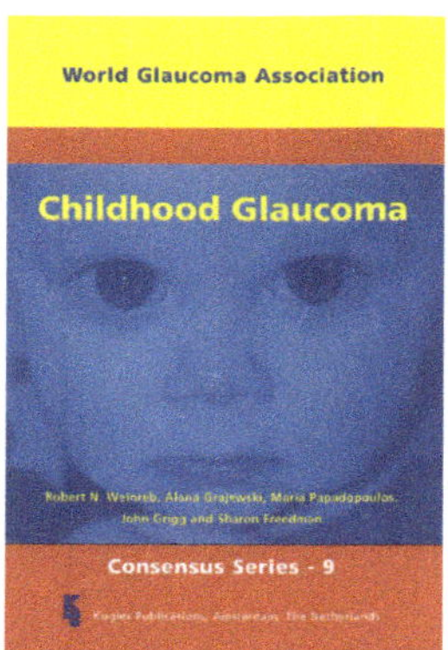

2013

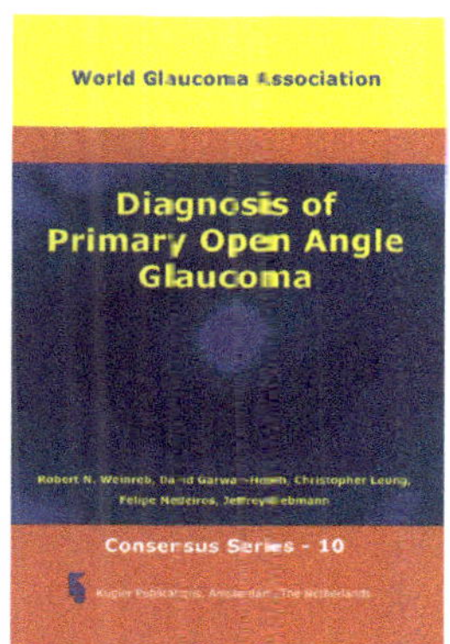

2017

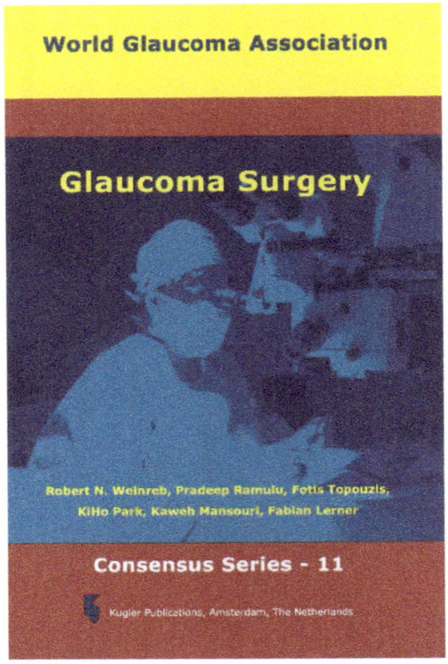
World Glaucoma Association
Glaucoma Surgery
Robert N. Weinreb, Pradeep Ramulu, Fotis Topouzis,
KiHo Park, Kaweh Mansouri, Fabian Lerner
Consensus Series - 11
Kugler Publications, Amsterdam, The Netherlands

2019

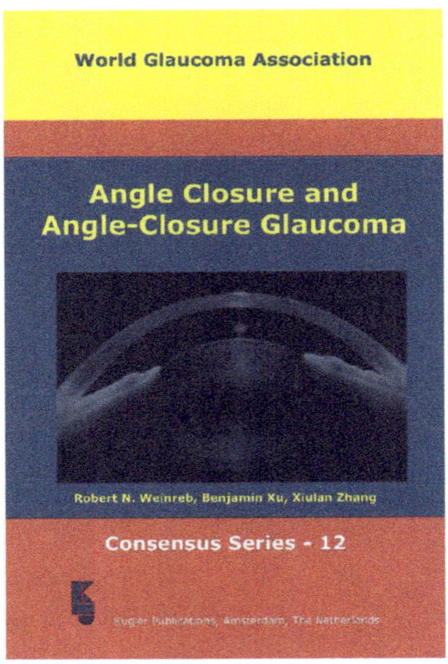
World Glaucoma Association
Angle Closure and
Angle-Closure Glaucoma
Robert N. Weinreb, Benjamin Xu, Xiulan Zhang
Consensus Series - 12
Kugler Publications, Amsterdam, The Netherlands

2026

www.ingramcontent.com/pod-product-compliance
Lightning Source LLC
Chambersburg PA
CBHW050521240926
51846CB00003B/642
* 9 7 8 9 0 6 2 9 9 3 3 9 0 *